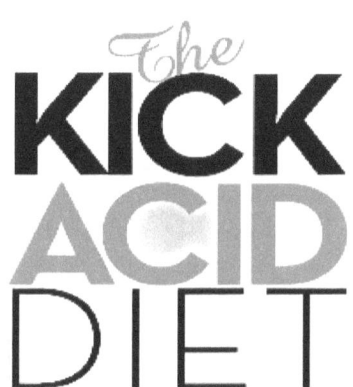

The KICK ACID DIET

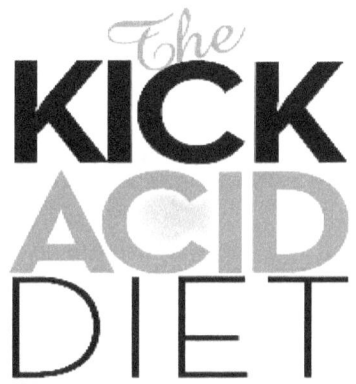

Reduce Acidity. Improve Your Health. Enhance Your Performance. Reduce Your Waistline.

Dr. Alwyn Wong

Copyright © 2010 Alwyn Wong
ISBN 978-0-9811215-0-5

All rights reserved. No part of this publication may be used for any purpose other than personal use. Therefore, reproduction, modification, storage in a retrieval system or retransmission, in any form or by any means, electronic, mechanical or otherwise, for reasons other than personal use, is strictly prohibited without prior written permission.

Printed in United States by Lulu Enterprises Inc.

This publication contains opinions of the author. It is not designed to provide a medical diagnosis, nor is it intended to provide treatment or consultation related to a medical condition or health issue. The reader should consult with a medical or qualified health professional before engaging in any of the practices referred to in this book.

The author specifically disclaims all liability, loss, or risk, personal or otherwise, which is incurred as a consequence, directly or indirectly, of the use or application of any of the contents of this book.

LIBRARY AND ARCHIVES CANADA CATALOGUING IN PUBLICATION

Wong, Alwyn

The Kick Acid Diet: Reduce Acidity. Improve Your Health. Enhance Your Performance. Reduce Your Waistline/ Alwyn Wong

Cover Design by Damian Box

Photos credited to Glen Grant and Wil Nah

Website design by Colin Valnion

First Edition: October 2010

This book is dedicated to my parents - without your support, guidance, and unconditional love, this book would not be possible. Your generosity and kindness forever inspire me.

I only hope this makes you proud.

Table of Contents

Preface   *i*

Part I - Introduction   1

    My Story
    State of the Nation
    Riddle Me This
    Lives Transformed
    How to Use This Book
    Step by Step Plan
    The Challenge

Part II - What are Acids?   13

    Waging the War on Fat Loss
    What Are Acids?
    What Is pH?
    Regulating the Body's pH
    Range of Physiological pH
    Buffers
    Step 1: Are You Acidic?

Part III - Acidity and It's Effects   25

    Metabolic Acidosis and Its Consequences
    Two Few Calories
    Two Few Calories…and Too Much Exercise
    Bones Burn Body Fat
    Muscle Wasting
    Growth Hormone
    Insulin
    Thyroid Hormone
    Summary
    Step 2: Assessing Hormone Function

Table of Contents

Part IV - Nutrition and Acidosis — 45

    Nutrition
    Protein
    Grains
    Fruits and Vegetables
    Nutritional Grading
    Using the PRAL
    Step 3: Determine the Acid-Base Status of Your Diet using the PRAL
    PRAL Density Tables
    Putting It All Together

Part V - The Kick Acid Diet Meal Planner — 71

    Step 4: Using the Kick Acid Diet Meal Planner
    PRAL Density
    Using the Food Tables in Appendix A
    Food Journal
    Phases (Muscle Up, Fat Loss, Maintenance, Performance)
    Food Preparation and Mineral Loss
    Why were these foods chosen?

Part VI - The Kick Acid Diet Recipes — 89

Part VII - The Kick Acid Diet Workout Program — 117

    Step 5: Biomarker Health Assessment
    Step 6: *The Kick Acid Diet – Workout*
    Exercise Descriptions

Conclusion and Acknowledgments — 167

Appendix A: PRAL Tables — 171
Appendix B: Hormone Screens — 345
Appendix C: Biomarker Assessment Tables — 353
Glossary — 359
References — 367

"Our greatest glory is not in never failing, but in rising up every time we fail. "

Ralph Waldo Emerson

Preface

Are you like the girl who always wants to hide in her itsy-bitsy, teeny-weeny bikini at the beach? Does the thought of being in your birthday suit make you want to do anything *but* have a party? Take a look at those around you. Do you know a co-worker, friend, or family member that looks great, is full of energy and is enjoying the quality of life that has always seemed to have eluded you?

If you answered "yes" to any of these questions, you are not alone. Do you know what separates those with the six-packs, shapely shoulders, and muscular legs from the 90 pound weaklings? The answer is simple - knowledge and habits.

The study of nutrition can be complicated, but the understanding and implementation of sound nutritional habits can be made quite simple. While newly-made discoveries may strengthen our knowledge and dispel long-held beliefs, clinicians, scientists, and most importantly, you, the reader, are often left searching for answers. As Thomas Edison has stated, "The doctor of the future will give no medicine, but will interest his patients in the care of the human frame, in diet and in the cause and prevention of disease."

To complicate matters further, there is a gap between knowledge and application; between theory and practice. What good is all this nutrition knowledge if we do not apply it to our own lives? The gap that lies between knowledge and application is habit. Our health and nutritional habits are, in turn, largely dictated by our behaviours.

The relationship between acids and alkaline substances, (also referred to as bases) must be in perfect harmony to ensure that metabolism works. Almost all of life's processes require a particular equilibrium between acids and bases in order to run smoothly. A change in the actual acid concentration may inhibit or stimulate the activity of virtually all biochemical processes in our bodies. A stable metabolism cannot tolerate a change in acid levels. Therefore, a consistent acid-base balance is paramount. I am fascinated and inspired by Lance Armstrong, one of the greatest athletes of our time. I will use him to shed light on the importance of the point I just made. Think of your metabolism as Team Radio Shack and your acid levels as Lance Armstrong. In order for the team to do well, Lance must do well. This goal is so important that other team members will sacrifice their individual success to ensure Lance's success. Other team members can be compared to other body systems, such as your muscular, skeletal and your hormonal systems.

Preface

The goal of *The Kick Acid Diet* is to combine science with art. The science is taken from the research and writing of great minds who are at the forefront of nutritional science today. In fact, parts of this book will be a combination of many of these prevailing theories. The art is blending and incorporating these vast ingredients of nutritional knowledge into bite-size, easy-to-implement and enjoyable recipes. Through an understanding of the science of acidity and alkalinity, you can form new behavioural habits that contribute to the art of living a healthier life.

The Science will offer you the *what*, *where's*, and *why's*. It will be divided into sections in order to facilitate understanding. I strongly urge you to dive into this section to gain the understanding and base (no pun intended) to put these healthy practices into action. I've also added a subsection, with terms italicized and their corresponding meaning found in the glossary providing further clarification of the terms and concepts used in this book. The Art will offer you the *how's* and *when's*.

Part I: Introduction

"The doctor of the future will give no medicine, but will interest his patients in the care of the human frame, in diet, and in the cause and prevention of disease."

Thomas Edison

Introduction

There is nothing more satisfying than seeing all of your hard work pay off. Here's how it should work: go the gym, eat well, and get enough rest, and voila, perfect body! Unfortunately, life doesn't always work out that way. Do you workout regularly, but don't notice a difference in the mirror? Let's be honest, we all want to look good naked. I'm a gym rat, but if I wasn't getting results, I wouldn't stick with a program for too long. Have you read every nutritional book on the shelves at Chapters and spent countless hours in the gym but still get frustrated in your attempts to improve your health, body composition, and athletic performance? If this scenario describes you, then this book is for you.

When it comes to weight loss, we usually follow one plan of action. We reduce the amount of calories we consume in order to put ourselves into a caloric deficit. We then couple with this, copious amounts of strenuous exercise, hoping to burn off any extra calories that may be drifting around our midriff.

Don't get me wrong. I love exercise, especially weight training. Like I mentioned before, I'm a gym rat. I have competed as a bodybuilder, and my clientele has consisted of people who engage in strenuous physical activity – from professional and Olympic athletes, mixed martial artists to fitness enthusiasts. We need exercise to be healthy, to perform well, and to increase our vitality. However, starving oneself is not the answer to your weight loss woes. Let me explain. When your body enters a state of starvation, certain processes occur. First, our body starts breaking down muscle tissue in order to provide fuel for itself. This breakdown not only results in less lean tissue, it causes the release of the stress hormone cortisol. Cortisol, as we'll see later, can wreak havoc on your health. Finally, when our bodies break down the amino acids found in muscle tissue, ketone bodies are released. While vital organs, such as your brain, use these *ketones* as an energy source, they are also very acidic and potentially harmful.

Fortunately, many of us now realize that not only can we lose weight, we can be healthy, and have lots of energy by consuming the foods we enjoy, and not limiting ourselves to restrictive, bland diets. Now, if Michael Phelps can look the way he does (and win 8 gold medals) by consuming a reported 12 000 calories a day, we can safely say that restricting calories is not the answer. I'm not recommending anywhere near this amount of food intake, by the way. It is the aim of this book to show you how and why. Doctors, researchers and many of you recognize that food is

Introduction

more than just an energy source. We're beginning to look at food for its non-nutritive qualities and components. We now know that food can influence our moods, our pain levels, our appearance, and even our libido.

My Story

It seems as if every author has a story – a raison d'etre, an inspiring story that lead to their work. I too have a story, albeit not your typical one.

In fact, it's not as much a story, but more a philosophy and a blueprint for future living. Fortunately, I have never suffered a debilitating illness nor have I struggled with weight gain. Let me clarify, I have never struggled with *fat* gain, but I was a skinny little fellow. That is my story.

I was taught from an early age the benefits of healthy eating and regular physical activity. Growing up, we were rarely allowed to have junk food – whether it was chips, pop or sweets. As any typical child, I wanted what I could not have. Now I thank them (my parents).

With these habits instilled in me, I was allowed to live a healthy life, free of disease, and having the body I've always wanted. (I've never taken a prescription drug, which I not only attribute to diet, but also is a reason why I can always stay in shape).

My story is this. It's important, as a health professional, educator, and author, to not only live the lifestyle, but to look the part. I am surprised by how many people in the field of health and fitness cannot maintain a healthy weight, while giving their patients and clients nutritional advice. You would be surprised at how many doctors, trainers, and nutritionists who smoke. I won't even get started on this.

We have become so politically correct that we have lost sight of the fact that a body free of excess body fat is the norm. Obesity, is mainly due to lifestyle, and as such can be reduced and prevented. Obesity is more than just a cosmetic problem, as you'll read in the introduction. We need to wage the war on fat loss!

Now, I'm not perfect. I do not always eat according to the rules of this book. But incorporating these principles into my life has allowed me to enjoy life's indulgences, with moderation, and with continued success.

There was a period in my life, a tragic and difficult time for me that, as the saying goes – "I fell off the wagon". It was through my faith and with the help of my family and friends that I got through it. I didn't turn to drugs or alcohol or the typical "self-destructive" behaviour, but what I did, I consider just as bad. I ate poorly. *Very* poorly. All of my meals consisted of take-out and fast-food. I had protein and meal-replacement shakes, and

Introduction

supplemented with a multi, but these cannot form the foundation of one's diet.

After a month on this "diet", I began to notice changes. I began to lose muscle mass. A chronic neck injury resurfaced so badly that I couldn't move my head for two days. I had less energy. And even though I was still lean by society's standards, I was getting fat. And I could only imagine what was happening inside of me.

This had to change, and fortunately, I committed to once again living a healthy lifestyle, consisting of regular exercise and high quality natural foods. I am reaping the benefits of these changes – I am full of energy, lean, and on the path to longevity and optimal health!

State of the Nation

The obesity rate has been climbing steadily for the last 25 years. The entire adult population has grown heavier, and the heaviest have become much heavier. The Centers for Disease Control and Prevention now estimate that adult obesity rates in the US are holding steady at 34% or 72 million Americans. That's one in three adults! Sadly, in Canada, the situation is similar.

Obesity has been defined by the National Institutes of Health (the NIH) as a body mass index (BMI) of 30 and above. ***BMI*** is calculated by dividing your height in meters by your weight in kilograms squared. We are born with a specific number of fat cells. When we gain fat weight, these cells increase in both size (hypertrophy) and number (hyperplasia). ***Hyperplasia*** has been shown to occur when BMI is 35 or above. Problems arise because we cannot lose fat cells once they form.

Obesity is one of the leading risk factors for heart disease and stroke, type 2 diabetes, cancer, hypertension, arthritis, infertility, gastrointestinal dysfunction, sleep apnea, mental health conditions, and premature death. Obesity is far more than a cosmetic problem. It is estimated that obesity is the cause of 300 000 deaths a year in the US. The stats, unfortunately, are similar north of the border. In fact, Argentinean senators recently approved the passage of a bill that classifies obesity as a disease.

What's even more frightening is the alarming rate of obesity amongst our children. Not only are we getting fat, but our children are getting fat! Over the last 25 years, we have witnessed an alarming rise in the proportion of overweight and obese children. Obesity rates among children and youth have nearly tripled during this period. Childhood obesity is a

Introduction

particular concern because excess weight over time increases the risk of developing chronic health problems. By the time today's teens are middle age, the rate of heart disease could be 16 per cent higher because of the extra pounds they are carrying around today, a U.S. study suggests.

Experts warn that if childhood obesity rates continue to rise, the children of tomorrow could be the first generation in history to have shorter life spans than their parents. Obesity is already causing a wide range of complications in children. Some children as young as seven are developing cardiovascular risk factors.

Not only is the incidence of obesity climbing, the rate of *degenerative disease* is also on the rise. What's most disturbing about this is that these conditions are preventable. Their risk can be modified through lifestyle, namely physical activity and nutrition. The rate of degenerative diseases, much like the obesity epidemic, is a major problem facing the 21st century. In 1900, only one in seven died of cardiovascular disease, and one in thirty died of cancer. According to recent stats from US Surgeon Generals Report, 68% of people die from cardiovascular disease, cancer, and diabetes. The one thing these conditions have in common is the connection between lifestyle and nutrition.

Processed foods, drugs, lack of physical activity, and pollution are all attributable for this dramatic rise. The good news is that many of these degenerative conditions can be reversed by the consumption of nutrient-rich foods, such as fruits and vegetables. Due to our consumption of nutrient void foods, we end up consuming a lot of calories to compensate for the lack of nutrients. As a result, we are in a caloric excess, leading to increased fat, but are lacking many of the essential nutrients needed to prevent disease, and to achieve optimal health. What's more, is that the foods that make up the typical North American diet result in *metabolic acidosis*, a condition characterized by an accumulation too much acid and not enough *buffering*.

Riddle Me This

In my years as a clinician and trainer, I've constantly looked for better ways to improve the health of my patients and clients, to hasten recovery time, to assist in weight loss and muscle gain, and to improve athletic performance. While my goal has always been to help my patients, I was also looking for principles I could apply to my own life.

I often wondered how the same diet plan or nutritional strategy could work for one individual and not another. I was aware of individual

Introduction

differences, such as genetics, overall health, and nutritional history – but I knew there was something more. The deeper I looked, the more I realized that the answer lay in the finer details. As a clinician, it was not enough to simply look at an individual's nutritional plan from a "big picture" perspective. I needed to look beyond just the macronutrients and micronutrients .Why, for example, did I have a different reaction when I ate one source of protein versus when I ate the same amount of another protein source? Now, some may call me picky, but I tried to account for the amount of fats in this food and also tried to keep the other foods constant. I noticed the same thing for carbohydrates. Certain carbohydrates, despite accounting for fibre content and such, caused me to feel different than others. I will answer these questions for you in *The Kick Acid Diet*.

Lives Transformed

Due to the agricultural revolution, our diets have been transformed. Wild animals and uncultivated plants, characteristic of our hunter-gatherer diets, have been largely replaced by saturated fats, simple sugars, and table salt. Similarly, the amounts of fibre, magnesium, and potassium have decreased. Diseases of civilization, a term commonly used to describe the constellation of atherosclerosis, type 2 diabetes, osteoporosis, and some forms of cancer are all attributable to this dietary transformation.

One of the major consequences of this dietary shift is the increase in acid producing foods, along with the decrease in alkaline forming foods. The resulting low-grade acidosis, and subsequent response of the body's regulatory mechanisms has resulted in detrimental effects on the body, including bone destruction, muscle wasting, and kidney stone formation.

Now for those of you who didn't pay attention in high school chemistry, here's a refresher of acid-alkaline balance. All substances are classified as either acidic or alkaline based on pH levels, which range from 0 to 14. Pure water has a neutral pH of 7. Foods can be categorized as either acid forming or alkaline forming. The aim is to maintain an alkaline or, at the very least, neutral environment within our bodies.

An interesting point must be made. Our ancestors consumed more protein, and, therefore, produced more acid than we do today. The shift from an alkaline diet to an acidic diet occurred due to lower bicarbonate production, an important buffer which we'll discuss later. This significant reduction in ***bicarbonate*** production is due to a displacement of alkaline-rich plant foods by cereals and calorie-dense, nutrient-poor foods, such as refined sugars and saturated fats.

Introduction

All foods, based on their *bioavailability*, vitamin and mineral content, protein content, as well as other factors, will lead to fluctuations in acid levels of the body. In other words, foods will directly affect your body's acid-alkaline levels. Now, I didn't discover this, but it has helped me find the questions I was looking for. Read this paragraph over and over and over again, as it forms the basis for the remainder of this book.

Our body's digestive and metabolic machinery is adapted for an alkali rich diet. Our bodies are alkaline by design, but acidic by function. Therefore, modern man not only has to deal with the negative effects of acidosis, which we'll soon discuss, but the absence of the alkaline milieu that our bodies are accustomed to.

This book is about acidosis. The word acid when translated from the Latin word, acidus, means sour. This is just one of the properties of acids. When consumed, acids often cause a stinging feeling inside the walls of the mouth. They can also conduct electricity, depending on the strength of the acid, as in batteries.

Originally, acids were thought to be liquids. In fact, acids exist in many forms, including gases and solids. The strength of the acid will determine its chemical reactivity and corrosiveness, and ultimately its danger risk upon contact. Due to this chemical reactivity, acids have many uses. These include pickling, which is the process that removes rust and other corrosive elements from metals. They can also be used to produce salts and gasoline. Finally, acids are often used as preservatives and flavour enhancers in many cola products.

We can see, even without going into detail, how the reactive nature of these substances can be harmful to our bodies. Keep in mind, however, some acids are naturally occurring substances within our bodies. For example, hydrochloric acid is secreted by the stomach to help break down proteins and carbohydrates. Lactic acid is a by-product of energy metabolism.

This book is also about metabolism. Your body gets the energy it needs from food through metabolism. Metabolism is simply the chemical reactions that take place in the body required to sustain life. That is, to think, move, and reproduce. Metabolism can be further broken down into anabolic and catabolic processes. *Anabolism* is the process by which various building blocks are put together to form other structures, such as protein and fat. *Catabolism* is the process of breaking down substances, usually from food, into smaller, more usable substances with the aim of producing energy. This energy release provides fuel for building the body, heating the body, and

Introduction

enabling muscle contraction and movement. As complex chemical units are broken down into more simple substances, the waste products released are removed from the body through the skin, kidneys, lungs, and intestines. When we undergo severe or constant stress, our muscles catabolize or break down. This happens because our body's priority is to provide fuel for the brain, not to maintain muscle mass.

Metabolism can also be looked at as the sum of all the metabolic pathways involved in the body. Each of the reactions in these pathways requires *enzymes*. These enzymes, or proteins, control the chemical reactions of metabolism, and each chemical reaction is coordinated with other body functions. Enzymes are involved in a reaction, without being consumed. Essentially, enzymes speed up a reaction. A shift in acidity will affect your enzymes and your entire metabolism.

When somebody says they have a fast metabolism, what they're referring to is their ability for these reactions to occur quickly and efficiently. A sluggish metabolism, on the other hand, is one that doesn't result in much energy production or turnover. To maintain lean healthy tissue requires energy. Your muscles are in a dynamic state, alternating between protein synthesis and breakdown. This interplay is important. When we subject ourselves to too much stress or do not feed our bodies the right foods, the balance moves toward protein breakdown.

When people think of metabolism, we think of it as something that influences how our body loses or gains weight. It is common to assess our metabolism by the amount of calories that we burn, especially at rest. A calorie, in nutritional terms, may be easier understood with the following explanation: a gram of protein or carbohydrates has four calories, and one gram of fat has nine calories. To lose a pound of body fat requires one to burn 3500 calories in excess to what one is consuming.

I've had the pleasure and honour to meet many great minds, in the field of nutrition, to whom I am greatly indebted. These people helped to make a lot of the book-based theory come to life in a practical, real way. Each shone in their area of expertise (be it fats, athletic performance, supplementation or anti-aging) and brought a unique perspective to the table. Despite their different backgrounds and experience, each viewed nutrition as a holistic concept, comprised of many equally important facets, ranging from macronutrient and micronutrient intake to meal timing and frequency. I also learned was that while nutrition may be the cornerstone of optimal health, it is incomplete without regular physical activity and adequate rest. Finally, the most important concept shared by these

Introduction

nutritional leaders is that eating is behavioural. We can read all of the books and memorize all of our essential amino acids, but if we do not commit to applying these principles to our lives, this information is useless. As a wise man once said, 'knowledge is not power; applied knowledge is power'.

How to Use This Book

The Kick Acid Diet will provide you with a step-by-step plan to control acidity, lose fat, and improve the quality of your life. The plan is best followed in the order outlined, as establishing baseline levels will provide you with information required to know the extent of your problem, and more importantly, how to correct it.

Step-by-Step Plan

Step 1: Measure pH by testing urine/saliva
Step 2: Complete hormone assessment to assess status
Step 3: 3a) Determine the acid content of your diet using PRAL
3b) Eliminate acidic foods and increase alkalizing foods
3c) Supplement with alkalizing supplements
Step 4: Kick Acid Diet Meal Planner
Step 5: Assess your body composition and other health indices using the Biomarker Health Assessment
Step 6: Kick Acid Diet Workout Program

The Challenge

The reason I decided to write this book was very personal. A commitment that I made to myself and my patients as a clinician and an educator was to practice what I preach. I'm proud to say, that through my lifestyle choices, including my eating habits, I have fulfilled this commitment.

Gone are the days where you, the public, are willing to accept that your leaders are not engaging in the practices they deem critical. We need to be held accountable, and we cannot hide behind our credentials and white coats, when our guts start protruding and we lack the energy and vitality that only comes through regular physical activity and a good diet!

Looking the part has given me credibility with my patients. Whether I'm treating a frozen shoulder or advising on nutrition and diets, my patients are happy and willing to listen to somebody who has committed his life to health and wellness.

Introduction

I challenge all healthcare professionals – doctors, nutritionists, nurses, etc to take our own advice and put our recommendations into action in our own lives as well as our families.

I now offer you, the reader, a challenge. Challenge yourself to see your health as a gift. Your health is truly a gift that keeps giving. Only when you are healthy can you truly enjoy life. Health is a gift that must be cherished.

If you are serious about being healthy, getting fit, and performing at your peak, a well-balanced diet that provides all the vital nutrients and maintains an alkali environment is essential. It's time to kick some acid!

Part II: What Are Acids?

"The superior doctor prevents sickness; The mediocre doctor attends to impending sickness; The inferior doctor treats actual sickness."

Chinese proverb

What Are Acids?

Waging the War on Fat Loss

A well respected coach once said that fat loss is a war. He recommends "assaulting" fat for 28 days, with a single-mindedness that borders on obsessive. All other pursuits should take a back seat. Then you can ensure success. While, I do like this approach, it is not realistic for everyone. Most people cannot commit to this type of plan, whether it's due to family, work, or other obligations. We've been inundated with numerous approaches, mostly dietary, that I'll now touch upon briefly.

The majority of diet books on the market, and there a lot of them, typically follow the same approach. Limit, or nearly eliminate all carbohydrates. The common premise behind these books is that the consumption of excessive carbohydrates leads to insulin production, and eventually insulin sensitivity. Their recommendation, which is founded by both science and experience, is that high levels of insulin lead to increased fat storage.

These approaches vary in that some recommend limiting all carbohydrates, while others recommend only limiting refined carbohydrates and grains. Furthermore, some approaches recommend increasing your fat levels, while others say to avoid fat at all costs. What most of these approaches have in common is their insistence on adequate levels of proteins, thereby blunting the insulin response.

The next set of books to hit the market attribute weight gain and health problems to hormone imbalance. These experts ascertain that conditions, ranging from obesity to infertility, are a result of your body's hormonal dysfunction. With regards to shedding fat, these authors focus again on insulin, but also on the hormones cortisol and thyroid hormones.

Fortunately, these books are backed by sound research and have a lot of clinical validity. In other words, they work…to a certain extent. *The Kick Acid Diet* not only addresses the insulin conundrum and balances your hormones, it also provides the missing link to the war on fat loss – acid-alkaline balance.

What are Acids?

There's a new enemy in the war on fat loss, and its name is acidity. The good news is, there's also an old sheriff in town, and its name is food!

What comes to your mind when you hear the term acid? When I think of the term acid, strangely, I remember growing up playing hockey on outdoor rinks. For many years of my childhood, my dad would build an ice-rink in our backyard. From time to time, there would be a yellow patch of

What Are Acids?

ice that was softer and slushier than the rest. This was due to the acid rain. I also think of vinegar, and the bitter aftertaste that it leaves, or its strong, pungent odor. What we all know is acids are very reactive, and can be dangerous if exposed to.

Technically speaking, an acid is a substance that will release a hydrogen molecule when placed in water. Bases, on the other hand, have the ability to soak up extra hydrogen molecules. It is these hydrogen molecules that are dangerous and must be neutralized by substances known as buffers. It is difficult to discuss acids, without first describing pH.

What is pH?

Potential hydrogen (pH) is a measure of acidity or alkalinity. The pH scale measures the amount of hydrogen molecules in a solution. The pH scale was developed as a way of simplifying the measurement of hydrogen in the body. Hydrogen concentration can vary over an enormous range. The hydrogen molecule is so reactive that it has profound effects on biological systems even at very low concentrations.

The terms acidity level and pH level will be used interchangeably throughout this book. Your body is largely made up of water, which allows nutrients, oxygen and other chemicals to be transported from place to place. Without water, chemical reactions cannot take place. This water-based solution is acidic, alkaline or neutral. A pH from 1.0 to 6.9 is considered acidic, 7.0 is neutral, and 7.1 to 14.0 is alkaline. In other words, the lower the pH number, the greater the acidity, and the higher the pH number, the greater the alkalinity. Normal blood has a pH of 7.3.

Since our bodies are comprised of 50-60% water, the pH level has profound effects on the body's internal chemistry, thus effecting health and metabolism. When the pH level of the body becomes too acidic or too alkaline for a prolonged period of time, the body is said to be imbalanced. The body does not tolerate extended pH imbalances of any kind. In fact, the management of pH is so important that the body will do what it must to maintain a healthy range, even if that means sacrificing other facets of health. This will be discussed later.

Buffers, which we'll discuss in more detail later, limit the change in pH. They are like a sponge soaking up extra hydrogen ions, and similarly, hydrogen can be squeezed out when more hydrogen is needed.

Most enzymes, which are made of proteins, function within a narrow pH range (7.35 to 7.45). Certain digestive enzymes, such as the enzyme pepsin, work best in an acidic environment, as in the stomach,

What Are Acids?

where pH is between 1.5 to 3.0. Enzyme function is disturbed, even with subtle changes in pH. This can affect systems such as the cardiovascular and respiratory, to name a few.

Let me now illustrate the relationship between pH and one of your body's systems: the cardiovascular system. During times of intense exercise, your body's cell's become acidic (which is normal). The acidity of your cells serves a purpose. When red blood cells, carrying oxygen become acidic due to the exercise performed, their ability to hold on to oxygen molecules decreases. The oxygen is released from the red blood cell and is transported into the muscle cell, where it's now needed. This can be represented by the oxygen dissociation curve.

In cases of metabolic acidosis, an abnormal state, red blood cells also lose their ability to hold on to oxygen. The problem here is that oxygen is not transported as effectively to where it's needed. Furthermore, when oxygen is released, but is not needed by muscle cells, it, being very reactive, causes free-radical damage.

All regulatory mechanisms (breathing, circulation, digestion, hormonal production) essentially serve the purpose of maintaining normal pH levels, usually by removing excess acids (Remember the Lance Armstrong analogy we used?) from body tissues without damaging living cells. Ironically, if the cell becomes too acidic or too alkaline, these same cells will become poisoned by their own toxic waste.

Just as acid rain can destroy plants and other vegetation, a pH outside of the normal range can erode and destroy the body's cells and tissues. More importantly, yet much more subtle, altered pH levels will cause functional havoc, that is, altering your body's normal physiology and metabolism, which often goes undetected on standard laboratory or diagnostic tests. Unregulated pH states will cause muscle dysfunction, bone weakness, and neurological problems.

Diets appear to be the major factor in maintaining appropriate pH levels throughout the body. This is a good thing! Why? We can control what we put into (and don't put into) our bodies. The objective of this book is to show you not only the why's behind nutritional acid-base physiology, but what we can do to live a healthier life, lose fat, and improve our physical performance by making simple, yet effective food choices.

Regulating the Body's pH

The pH level of our internal fluids affects every cell in our bodies. The entire metabolic process depends upon an alkaline environment.

What Are Acids?

Chronic over acidity corrodes body tissue, and if left unchecked will interrupt all the body's functions, from the beating of your heart to the neural firing of your brain. In other words, over-acidity interferes with life itself.

Every cell in the body functions within an optimal pH range between 7.35-7.40. Although the optimal range may differ between various types of cells, the net pH of the body must be tightly regulated. This wouldn't pose a problem if the pH remained constant. Challenges, both internal and external, cause subtle, yet significant changes in the pH, altering the function of enzymes, hormones, neurological function, and muscle contractility, to name a few. Let's now explore some of these influences.

It is critical for the human body to maintain the alkalinity of its blood at a pH range of 7.35-7.40. A blood sample is a convenient method of assessing the entire body's pH status. Any deviation, albeit slight, will activate the body's homeostatic mechanisms. If the body is too acidic, it has to borrow minerals such as calcium, potassium, and magnesium from vital organs and bones, as they act as buffers, safely removing it from the body. With time, the entire system will weaken.

Furthermore, if the body's pH levels are off, and it's either too acidic or too alkaline, nutrients from food and supplements may not be absorbed properly. This is especially true of minerals, which are important for many body functions including enzyme production and cellular metabolism.

Finally, as we'll see, acidity also affects the ability of your hormones to function properly.

Can a person end up too alkaline? Yes, this does happen when people limit their diets to only fruits and vegetables. Over alkalinity is a potentially serious problem which may take longer to correct than over acidity. However, due to the nature of our lifestyle, this is next to impossible for most people.

Balance is the key. If changes in the diet are not sufficient to correct an over-acidic pH, supplements may be needed for a while. These might include the correct forms of calcium, magnesium and trace minerals, as well as enzyme supplements to help the body digest foods, which we will discuss later.

If our body's buffering systems are overloaded, and normal pH range is exceeded, blood loses its normal properties and the transport of oxygen, nutrients, and metabolic waste-products is dramatically impaired. In medical terms, excess acid load in the blood is called "acidosis". Acute acidosis is a life threatening condition requiring immediate steps of

What Are Acids?

emergency treatment for instant reconstitution of physiological blood pH. In practice, acute acidosis is rather uncommon and usually the consequence of diseases of the lung and kidney. These organs are significantly involved in the regulation of acid-alkaline balance. Acute acidosis is not subject to dietary influences and therefore we will not go into detail with it in this book.

Our attention is concentrated on chronic ***metabolic acidosis*** which is also called *latent acidosis*. The term latent means disguised and refers to a chronic condition which is not recognizable at first. Chronic metabolic acidosis is much more commonly observed featuring a slight shift of blood pH in the acid direction within the normal range (7.34 –7.45). At the same time, blood buffering capacity is diminished. This type of acidosis progresses without any specific symptoms, that is, we do not feel any physical changes.

Range of Physiological pH

The ratio of acid and base in our bodies must not be rated as a rigid system but rather as a dynamic equilibrium in permanent motion to keep a stable pH. Although in our bodies the concentration of acids and bases currently changes, the pH in different organs and tissues as well as blood pH remains almost constant within narrow ranges. Each organ or metabolic unit has its own optimum pH.

Sample pH values of common substances.

   pH 0 battery acid
   pH 1 hydrochloric acid
   pH 2 lemon juice, vinegar
   pH 3 grapefruit
   pH 4 tomato juice
   pH 5 black coffee
   pH 6 urine/saliva
   pH 7 fresh water, milk
   pH 8 sea water
   pH 9 baking soda
   pH 10 Milk of Magnesia®
   pH 11 ammonia
   pH 12 soap
   pH 13 bleach
   pH 14 liquid drain cleaner

What Are Acids?
Buffers

Buffers are substances that resist changes in pH when an acid (or base) is added to a solution. Remember from the previous section that acids are compounds that release those pesky hydrogen ions. And it is these hydrogen ions that cause changes in pH.

In other words, buffers act like sponges, soaking up hydrogen ions. If your dish sponge gets saturated with water, water leaks out. The same thing happens in your body. When your body's first line of buffering defense gets saturated or overwhelmed in the presence of hydrogen ions, they leak out, wreaking havoc and slowing your metabolism!

Your body has automatic mechanisms that work around the clock to keep your body in acid-alkaline balance by handling the onslaught of excess acids.

Kidneys

The body eliminates excess acids by way of the urine. A chemical known as *ammonia* comes to the rescue when your body cannot deal with these excess acids. Ammonia neutralizes excess acids. When your urine smells like a combination between bleach and vinegar, it is a sure sign that your body is overly acidic!

Protein

Certain amino acids circulate in the blood, lymph and *inside* the cells to buffer excess acids.

Fat

A fat known as LDL, or the "bad" cholesterol circulating in the blood, lymph, and *outside* the cells also buffers these acids. Some theories suggest that in order to protect your body from these acids, fat storage is impaired, resulting in bigger hips and bellies.

Hormones

The hormones that control water balance at the kidneys aid in buffering by retaining water, and diluting these acids.

Bicarbonate

The buffer, bicarbonate, is produced in red blood cells, and circulates throughout the body.

Lungs

Breathing out causes the release of the acid waste product, carbon dioxide. Aaah, alkalinity.

What Are Acids?

Water Consumption
> Since pH is a function of the concentration of hydrogen ions, drinking water is a simple, yet effective way of neutralizing acids by diluting the solution.

Electrolytes
> Finally, circulating electrolytes help buffer excess acids. We've all heard about electrolyte, but what are they? These substances, commonly found in sports drinks, are required for your body to function as they control water balance and nerve conduction. The relevant electrolytes with respect to acid-base balance are the minerals sodium, magnesium, potassium, and calcium.

> These minerals are stored primarily in bone and muscle. In times of need, they are released into the body to perform their buffering jobs. Fortunately, these minerals can be obtained through diet, sparing precious bone and muscle tissue.

What Are Acids?
STEP 1: ARE YOU ACIDIC?

Measuring pH

Measuring pH with the use of pH strips is easy and convenient. Certain steps must be taken in order to ensure an accurate reading. Furthermore, knowledge of the daily fluctuations in pH will help determine the interpretation of the reading. For example, urine pH is 6-6.5 in the morning and 6.5-7 in the evening. Saliva pH ranges from 6.5 to 7.5, all day.

Essentially, an increased acidity (or reduced pH) of these two bodily fluids, is reflective of the borrowing of minerals (calcium, sodium, potassium, and magnesium) from vital organs to buffer the acids, and subsequently, remove them from the body.

Urine

Urine pH is reflective of un-buffered hydrogen ions. Urine pH is related to the function of the kidneys, adrenal glands, lungs, and gonads to regulate pH. Urine pH is also related to the stomach pH (acidic) and small intestinal pH (alkaline). Finally, urine pH changes with climate, being lower in warmer climates, and higher in colder climates. If the urine pH is less than 6.5, the body's buffering systems are overwhelmed.

Saliva

Salivary pH is said to be reflective of the activity of digestive enzymes, mainly those manufactured in the stomach, liver, and pancreas. If the salivary pH is too high, the body may be producing too many acids or may be overwhelmed by the un-buffered acids produced in various metabolic processes. Others believe that saliva pH is reflective of the level of emotional stress. Saliva is the mirror of blood with respect to pH. The blood is in turn an indicator of the health of the fluid outside of our cells, which is said to reflect the state of our alkaline reserves. Furthermore, blood pH can tell us the condition of the liver, lymphatic and pancreatic enzymes. Saliva pH is very slow to change, so when it does, the problem is chronic.

What Are Acids?

Steps to Measuring pH

Fortunately, measuring pH is simple and can be done by anybody. As mentioned above, taking certain steps will ensure an accurate reading.

1. The best time to measure pH is one hour prior to a meal or two hours post-meal.
2. Test at least twice a week, under the same conditions, to ensure accuracy.

Knowing how to measure your own acidity is just the first step. It's not good enough to know if you're acidic or not, we need to know how to prevent acidity *by measuring the acidity of your diet.* Let's take a look at what happens when we don't neutralize these acids through dietary means.

Part III: Acidity and Its Effects

"Let food be thy medicine, and let thy medicine be food."
Hippocrates

Acidity and Its Effects

Let's just cut to the chase. In addition, to destroying body tissue and impairing transport of nutrients, acidity is going to make you fat.

Acidity makes you fat for two reasons. First, your body has to buffer these acids to prevent damage and to allow your metabolism to function properly. In so doing, your two most metabolically active tissues, bone and muscle, are broken down to release the calcium and other chemicals that perform this buffering.

The other way reason that acidity makes you fat is its negative affect on your hormones. To make matters worse, the hormones most affected by acidity are those responsible for fat loss. Ironic, isn't it?

Metabolic Acidosis and Its Consequences

Metabolic acidosis is a state where the body's pH is below its optimal range. Remember, the lower the pH, the more acidic the solution. Essentially, metabolic acidosis is a pH imbalance in which the body has accumulated too much acid and cannot, for various reasons, neutralize this acid. This may occur, for example, when the body uses fats and protein for energy instead of carbohydrates, as in extreme dieting or diabetes.

Other causes of metabolic acidosis include kidney and liver dysfunction and infection. Furthermore, it may be one of the first signs of drug overdose, including alcoholism. Another common cause of metabolic acidosis is diet. Members of industrialized nations suffer from metabolic acidosis due to their disproportionate intake of acid precursors (protein and grains) compared to alkaline-rich foods (fruits and vegetables). This may partly be attributed to the reduced content of essential alkaline minerals, such as potassium, magnesium, and calcium in our food supply. Acid rain depleted soils may be a contributing factor. Finally, industrial food processing contributes to a further reduction of the original content of vital bases.

Too Few Calories

Let's take a look first how calorie restricted diets will slow your metabolism down. Weight reduction diets and fasting, often characterized by a decrease in caloric intake, as well as full abstinence from solid food, are known to disturb acid-alkaline balance. The goal with these diets is to release fat stores as our bodies rely on their own energy reserves due to lack of adequate fuel intake. This may be hoped for, but as the concentration of acidic ketone bodies increases, (from the breakdown of fat, and protein) metabolism suffers. This may result in a pronounced acidosis, ironically,

Acidity and Its Effects

impairing overall metabolism. *Successful long-term fat loss through dieting can only be achieved if the additional acid production is offset by an adequate intake of fruits and vegetables.*

Two Few Calories...and Too Much Exercise

Sport and exercise are healthy and increase general well-being. However, if one is not consuming enough calories, exercise can lead to increased acidosis and a sluggish metabolism. Here's why - The electrolytes, which are also alkaline minerals, such as potassium, magnesium, sodium, and calcium are quickly lost when sweating, but are urgently needed by the body to neutralize the acids formed via intensive muscular activity. If the loss of alkaline minerals and fluid via sweating is not accounted for from the diet, acidosis will occur. Symptoms of exercise related acidosis include fatigue, muscle cramps and aches. If you're an athlete, what this translates is to reduced performance and increase risk of injury. A detailed workout program is outlined later in the book which will provide you with a guide to use exercise as a method of preventing acidity.

In the body's attempt to buffer this acidic state, several consequences will occur.

Acidity and Its Effects
Bones Burn Body Fat

Your knee bone's connected to your thigh bone. Your thigh bone's connected to your hip bone. Your hip bone's connected to your ability to shed fat! Even though our skeleton only accounts for about 15% of our total body weight, it is very metabolically active. It undergoes constant turnover, continually breaking itself down and rebuilding in response to daily stressors and diet. There is a misconception that bones are not metabolically active because they cannot move themselves. However, there is lots of "movement" going on in bones, even when we're resting. This activity, invisible to the naked eye and most microscopes, is a large part of basal metabolic rate or BMR. BMR is the amount of calories we burn at rest. It is essentially the energy required to move, breathe, and reproduce. Sound familiar?

Your bones not only act as a site for muscle attachment and the protector of your vital organs. It serves another, equally important function. Bone stores the body's minerals. These include calcium, potassium, magnesium and sodium. This isn't a one- sided relationship, however. In return for safe and secure storage, these minerals provide bone with the structural integrity that gives bone its distinct hardness. In other words, our bones house the majority of our alkalizing minerals: calcium, magnesium, potassium, and sodium.

The strength of bone comes mainly from calcium. Although many other systems depend on calcium for proper function, the majority of it is stored within bones and teeth. The amount of calcium in bone represents 99% of the body's calcium stores. Magnesium represents the next largest mineral in bone, accounting for approximately 50-80% of the body's magnesium stores. Finally, normal bone also contains considerable amounts of potassium. In fact, the amount of potassium in bone is more than that found in the entire rest of the body.

Acidosis

When the lungs and kidneys can no longer get rid of excess acids, potassium and sodium are the body's next line of defense in buffering. Once these reserves are depleted, the body calls upon its calcium and magnesium stores.

Calcium, stored as calcium carbonate and calcium apatite, is released from the bone to buffer the excess acids. The mineral loss from the skeleton results in weakened, fragile bone, characteristic of osteoporosis. It must be mentioned that other minerals found in bone, such as magnesium and zinc, are also depleted in response to increased acidity.

Acidity and Its Effects

When the body becomes acidic, bone formation ceases and bone destruction increases. This is so profound that bone destruction increase sixfold with a decrease in pH from 7.25 to 7.15. Once the acidosis becomes chronic, other factors perpetuate the process. At a pH of 6.9, bone formation comes to a complete halt. It must be noted that these changes in occur at the *DNA* level, which may explain why there is a lag in the normalization of function after alkalizing measures have been taken. A chemical known as prostaglandin E (pgE) is also stimulated in response to a drop in pH, causing further breakdown of bone. Once pH returns to 7.4, bone destruction stops.

The Protein Paradox

The calcium and other mineral content of skeleton appear to be markedly influenced by nutrients other than calcium itself; namely dietary protein and other alkalizing minerals. We also know that consuming protein results in increased acidity. However, a strange situation occurs when it comes to bones. Long-term protein intake increases the strength of bones as long as two conditions are met. This bone forming property of protein has been shown to occur only in animal proteins, and in the presence of alkalizing minerals.

Starvation in the Midst of Aplenty

Osteoporosis is a condition that features loss of the normal density of bone and fragile bone. Individuals with osteoporosis often have a distinct look. The disease most often affects older women of Caucasian or Asian descent. Many of these people are smaller, have little muscle mass, and present with a hunched over posture. On the other hand, this disease may go unnoticed for years, and can affect men, younger individuals, and people of all races.

In North America, a strange irony exists. Calcium intake is one of the highest in the world, but it also has one of the highest rates of osteoporosis. We are literally starving in the midst of aplenty! Bone mineral content is dependent not just upon calcium intake but upon total calcium balance. When the body is acidic, calcium is leeched from bone, weakening it. Supplementation with both calcium and vitamin D has been shown to be effective in preventing osteoporosis, as long as there doesn't exist an underlying acidosis.

Acidity and Its Effects

Summary

When we look after our bones, we create an environment conducive to fat loss. What's more is this bone activity takes place while you're not exercising, and is even taking place while you're sleeping! The take point is that if you want to increase your body's ability to lose fat, even while you're resting and sleeping, take care of those bones!

If buffering at the lungs and kidneys fail, and the calcium (and magnesium, sodium, and potassium) from the bones is no longer an adequate supply, the body will then turn to its next largest supply of calcium, skeletal muscle.

Acidity and Its Effects
Muscle Wasting

In order for the calcium stored in muscle to be released, muscle tissue must be broken down. When muscle is being destroyed, the body is said to enter a negative *nitrogen balance*. Protein, unlike carbohydrates or fat, contains nitrogen. Nitrogen elimination, or the amount of protein being eliminated from the body, can be measured to determine the amount of protein present in the body. Since 70% of protein is found in muscle tissue, this gives an excellent indication of the body's muscle building potential.

The scientist who first linked nitrogen wasting to metabolic acidosis noted that the nitrogen wasting was directly related to the acidosis, not some underlying cause. This was evident in all acidic conditions and was reversed by the administration of bases, thereby correcting the acidosis, and not the actual cause of the acidosis.

The benefits of muscle as related to physical performance and sport cannot be refuted. What is not as well known, nor as extensively researched, is muscle's positive effect on health and the prevention of disease, which is beyond the scope of this book.

Muscle is the principal reservoir of amino acids to be used by our vital organs in the absence of adequate dietary protein. Our vital organs rely on a steady supply of amino acids to serve as building blocks for new proteins to balance a persistent rate of protein breakdown. Furthermore, between meals, amino acids are also used for the production of glucose, a process which occurs in the liver and is known as gluconeogenesis. The brain and nervous system require glucose to function. In disease states, muscle is so important that there exists a direct effect between lean muscle mass and the length of survival in terminally ill AIDS patients.

Stress and Disease

During periods of stress, there is increased production of proteins involved in immune function and wound healing. The production of these proteins places a significant demand on the body's amino acid pools. For example, the amount of dietary protein required to recover from burns has been shown to be 3g/kg of body weight. For the average size male at 175lbs, that is 240g of protein a day! As such, individuals with limited reserves of lean body mass do not respond well to stress, as is evident in survival rates of burn/cancer victims and individuals with HIV.

Heart disease and cancer are the main chronic diseases in the US and are both associated with the rapid and extensive loss of muscle mass, strength, and metabolic function. Keep in mind, that there is an indirect effect of the loss of muscle that occurs with chronic disease. That is, the loss

Acidity and Its Effects

of muscle strength required for recovery.

Obesity

Another benefit of muscle is its contribution to basal metabolic rate (BMR). This can be explained as the minimum calorific requirement needed to sustain life in a resting individual. To further simplify, it is the amount of calories you would burn staying in bed all day. Our basal metabolic rate accounts for the largest portion of energy expenditure, and muscle is the only part of BMR that is variable. For example, every 10 kg of muscle results in 100 extra calories burned. Put another way, 3lbs of muscle results in a seven percent increase of BMR and daily caloric requirement by 15%; or one pound of muscle burns approximately 35 calories/day.

Muscle also affects your body's ability to metabolize sugars. As we just learned, the body is continually using energy, even while at rest. Though this energy use is constant, the rate in which food metabolizes energy is irregular and intermittent. In one study, after four months of strength training, there was a 236% increase in glucose uptake. This increase was attributed to changes in the muscles' metabolic function. In other words, the muscle became more responsive to insulin, improving insulin sensitivity.

Acidosis

Increased acidity directly contributes to muscle loss by increasing the metabolism and breakdown of specific amino acids: glutamine and the branched-chain amino acids or BCAA's.

Glutamine has increased in popularity amongst athletes, bodybuilders, and fitness enthusiasts in the recent years. Even though most people take it for its direct effect on muscle building, supplementing with this product has the additional benefits. These include the provision of fuel for the small intestine and brain, and stimulating immune function. It also helps regulate acid-base balance.

Glutamine is produced primarily in the muscles, fat, and lungs. Under normal conditions, most glutamine is used in the liver and the small intestine. However, in metabolic acidosis, the kidney is the major site of glutamine utilization and metabolism. In fact, during periods of increased acidity, one third of the glutamine is extracted from the kidney in one pass. Glutamine is required to generate ammonium, which helps the body to eliminate acids in the urine.

In order to meet the need for glutamine at the kidneys, glutamine is released from muscle. Production is increased at the liver (at the expense of other amino acids), and is made less available for the small intestine.

Acidity and Its Effects

Glutamine is so important that the body sacrifices other amino acids to maintain an adequate supply. As the body's amino acid pool dwindles, there are fewer and fewer building blocks to build and repair tissue; to serve as the substrate for enzyme production; and to act as immune system messengers. What results is a weakened system that is not able to perform its necessary functions optimally. It also results in less muscle mass and ultimately, a slower metabolic rate. In summary, chronic metabolic acidosis, results in an increased production of proteins and enzymes involved in glutamine metabolism, and less protein for other functions.

The Branched-Chain Amino Acids or BCAA's are *leucine, isoleucine,* and *valine*. The combination of these three essential amino acids make up approximately one third of the protein found skeletal muscle in the human body, and play an important role in protein synthesis. **Essential amino acids** are those amino acids that are required for survival, but cannot be manufactured by the body. BCAA's have numerous functions, that mainly involve anabolic processes and protein synthesis. Other functions include reducing nervous system fatigue, improving immune function and increasing the use of glucose by muscle tissue. As such, BCAA's are used by many athletes and bodybuilders.

The breakdown of branched-chain amino acids (BCAA's) in the presence of excess acids is indirect, and is under control of a group of chemicals known as glucocorticoids, the main one being cortisol.

Cortisol

Cortisol, or the stress hormone as it is commonly known, is produced by the adrenal glands. Each adrenal gland sits atop their respective kidney. Stress, whether it's mental, physical or emotional, results in the release of cortisol from the adrenal glands.

Cortisol is known as a **glucocorticoid**, because of its involvement in glucose or sugar metabolism. When blood sugar levels fall to critical levels, cortisol maintains blood sugar concentration, via many different processes. In the liver and muscle tissue, it causes the production of glucose from non-carbohydrate sources, such as protein and fat, leading to muscle wasting. Cortisol also blocks the uptake of glucose in muscle and fat tissue, conserving blood glucose construction. Finally, cortisol causes the breakdown of fat in fat cells, releasing energy, and the substrates for gluconeogenesis.

In response to excess acidity, the adrenal glands release extra cortisol. This not only leads to muscle wasting, but can lead to the inhibition of bone formation, suppression of calcium absorption and delayed wound

Acidity and Its Effects

healing. Other symptoms of cortisol excess include weight gain; an abnormal accumulation of fatty pads throughout the body; stretch marks; high blood pressure; weakness; lethargy; thin, fragile skin; insulin resistance; kidney stones; increased risk of infection; irregular menstruation; decreased libido; emotional disturbances; and abnormal hair growth in women.

Since cortisol promotes the development of abdominal obesity, and has a direct negative impact on insulin function throughout the body, even a modest, but sustained increase in cortisol production can increase the risk of insulin resistance and type II diabetes. Furthermore, increased cortisol levels will make you fat.

Summary

Muscle is so important to not only our health, but to our metabolic rate. As we'll see in the *Kick Acid Diet* Workout Program, muscle keeps your engine revving and fat loss at an all time high!

Normal hormone function and secretion is disrupted during metabolic acidosis. Changes in hormone status include increased cortisol secretion described above, as well as decreased thyroid hormone production and function, and reduced insulin sensitivity, and growth hormone resistance, all of which will have negative effects on your body composition, and all of which, we'll discuss in detail.

Acidity and Its Effects

Growth Hormone

It seems as if the new drug of choice in professional sports is growth hormone. It's touted to enhance muscle mass, increase energy levels, and reduce fat and such, numerous athletes have turned to it to improve their performance. The debate rages on as to whether growth hormone actually does improve performance, by scientists and researchers. However, athletes are not waiting for double-blind, placebo controlled studies to wait for the answers!

It's not only millionaire athletes and celebrities that are turning to growth hormone, but elderly people and those determined to fight the effects of aging.

Growth hormone (GH) is a hormone that is synthesized and secreted by the ***anterior pituitary gland***. GH is a major participant in the control of several processes including growth and metabolism. Despite receiving none of the glory, it is the lesser known hormone, insulin-like growth factor (IGF-1) that is responsible the direct of effects of growth hormone. IGF-1 is produced by the liver and is considered a hormone, but may act directly on neighboring tissues, bypassing the blood. Together, these two hormones operate as the GH-IGF-1 axis.

The amount and pattern of GH secretion change throughout life. Resting levels are highest in early childhood. The amplitudes and peaks are greatest during the pubertal growth spurt. Both resting levels and the amplitude of the peaks decline throughout life.

Production of GH and IGF-1 is controlled by many factors, including stress, exercise, nutrition, sleep, and GH itself. The most intense period of GH release is shortly after the onset of deep sleep. On the other hand, IGF-1 levels are highest during the day.

The direct and indirect functions of GH of mainly anabolic, and include the following: tissue repair and recovery; muscle and bone growth; fat breakdown, increased appetite; better exercise capacity; increased lung capacity; and faster wound healing. Wow – it's no wonder why so many people are turning to this wonder hormone!

Specifically, GH exerts its effects on the following macronutrients as follows: protein synthesis is increased (increased amino acid uptake, increased rate of protein synthesis, and reduced protein breakdown), normal blood sugar levels are maintained (controls insulin and increases glucose production at liver), and fat is broken down.

Although growth functions are the best known attributes of GH, it serves many other metabolic functions as well. It increases calcium retention in the bone; it increases muscle mass via the production of new muscle cells,

Acidity and Its Effects

which is known as hyperplasia, which is different than hypertrophy; it stimulates the immune system; and preserves the health of the pancreas.

There is considerable interest in the use of GH as a pharmaceutical and biotechnical agent. Although describing these in detail is beyond the scope of this book, some of these applications include the following; anti-aging; reversing conditions resulting in short stature, such as dwarfism; increasing the size of livestock; and stimulating increased milk production in cows.

With age, there are changes in the GH-IGF-1 axis. GH secretion from the anterior pituitary is highest around puberty, with a progressive decline thereafter. What results is lower levels of GH and IGF-1.

Acidosis

I'm going to include the symptoms of GH deficiency to further illustrate the effects that excess acidity may have on this hormone and health. In children, GH deficiency results in growth failure. In adults, these age-related changes in GH and IGF-1 levels are mainly catabolic: reduction in lean body mass; increased fat mass; and a reduction in bone density. Despite accounting for many age-related changes, it has been shown, on the other hand, that excess GH may reduce one's lifespan.

There are certain diseases which may cause GH deficiency, which are beyond the scope of this book. If you suspect a GH deficiency, consult with your doctor for proper treatment and to rule out non-diet and lifestyle related causes. These include mutations, congenital conditions involving the endocrine system and damage to the pituitary itself from surgery, trauma, and disease. As we'll now see, metabolic acidosis can cause a functional GH deficiency.

Metabolic acidosis has been shown to reduce the effects of GH and IGF-1, by lowering the body's responsiveness to the hormone and altering the secretion patterns of GH itself. Whether this is a direct or indirect effect has not been established, but metabolic acidosis has also resulted in reduced concentrations of blood IGF-1 in humans.

This reduced GH secretion resulted in reduced body mass and food efficiency. Reducing the effects of chronic metabolic acidosis by the ingestion of alkali salts improved the function of the GH-IGF-1 axis. Interestingly, the administration of GH also reduced the acidity, by increasing bicarbonate production and increasing ammonium excretion at the kidney.

Acidity and Its Effects

Summary

Instead of turning to the potentially dangerous practice of taking growth hormone, we can simply make our own growth hormone function more efficiently. When this system is working optimally, the result will be increased muscle mass and a reduction of body fat.

Acidity and Its Effects

Insulin

In order to function properly, the body must maintain its blood glucose levels within normal limits. It does so through various mechanisms, most notably the pancreas. In response to elevated blood sugar (and amino acid and fat) levels, the pancreas secretes insulin into the blood stream. The release of insulin causes an increased uptake of nutrients into the cells, and as the blood concentrations of these substances drop, insulin secretion is suppressed.

Glucagon, insulin's partner, is also secreted by the pancreas in response to lowered blood sugar levels. The main target of glucagon is the liver, where it stimulates the breakdown of glycogen to glucose and the production of glucose from non-carbohydrate sources, and causes the release of glucose into the blood stream. Glucagon secretion also results in a drop in amino acid concentration as these substances are required for the formation of glucose in the liver.

In addition to increasing the cellular uptake of all nutrients, insulin increases protein, fat and glycogen synthesis, decreases fat and protein breakdown, and modifies the activity of numerous enzymes.

To summarize, insulin is your body's main storage hormone. Not only does it directly increase the storage of fat into cells, it acts to make you fat through other mechanisms. First, the body only has a limited capacity to store protein and carbohydrates, but its ability to store fat is unlimited. As such, excess protein and carbohydrates get converted and stored as fat. Next, insulin shuts down your fat burning hormone, lipase. Lipase is responsible for the breakdown of your body's fats.

Theoretically, one could starve despite consuming many calories if insulin did not function or did not exist. When we speak of or read about insulin, we are often referring to diabetes.

Syndrome X, Insulin Resistance and Diabetes

Insulin resistance occurs when the normal amount of insulin secreted by the pancreas is not able to perform its functions, most notably, glucose uptake by the cell. In other words, there is a defect in the body's ability to uptake glucose in response to insulin. In response, the pancreas secretes more insulin, leading to a condition known as hyperinsulinemia.

The medical community recently coined a term syndrome X, or metabolic syndrome, to describe the cluster of symptoms related to, and potentially caused by insulin resistance. These include the following: elevated triglyceride levels, reduced HDL (good cholesterol), hypertension, glucose intolerance and elevated insulin levels. Unfortunately, insulin

Acidity and Its Effects

resistance can go unnoticed for years. When symptoms do arise, they include lethargy, inability to focus, and accelerated aging.

Insulin resistance and syndrome X is usually caused by poor dietary habits, including a diet high in refined carbohydrates, such as breads, pastas, cookies, and doughnuts. As we'll see later, metabolic acidosis can also lead to this condition. If caught early enough, not all syndrome X sufferers will progress to diabetes.

There are two types of diabetes: diabetes insipidus and diabetes mellitus. Simply, diabetes insipidus involves damage to the pituitary gland and results in the production of large amounts of urine regardless of the amount of liquid consumed.

Diabetes mellitus is characterized by insufficient production of insulin by the pancreas, resulting in abnormally high levels of blood sugar. Since sugar cannot enter the cells, the body breaks down muscle and fat, the final by-product being acidic ketone bodies. This process results in a drop in pH of the blood, a condition known as ketoacidosis. Ketoacidosis, if severe enough, can result in death.

Acidosis

Insulin resistance not only causes increased acidity, but insulin itself is also affected by metabolic acidosis. In numerous studies, there is a reduced sensitivity to insulin with chronic metabolic acidosis. In other words, the cells do not respond to insulin as well, and as a result, glucose metabolism is altered. Furthermore, metabolic acidosis also reduces the secretion of insulin by the pancreas.

Finally, since chronic metabolic acidosis has been shown to increase cortisol levels, and cortisol has been shown to reduce insulin sensitivity, there is a third mechanism explaining the effects of metabolic acidosis on insulin function.

Summary

I'm consulting with patients or if I'm teaching a class on nutrition, I always stress the importance of insulin control. My lecture normally starts by drawing a chart, indicating what happens when you eat a food that causes a rapid rise in insulin levels, such as a donut or candy bar. I then show people why it's important to keep your insulin levels low, because it is during these insulin spikes that we get fat.

Acidity and Its Effects

Thyroid Hormone

Your thyroid gland is a small gland located in the front of the neck, just below one's Adam's apple or larynx. It is made up of two halves, called lobes that lie along the windpipe (trachea) and are joined together by a narrow band of thyroid tissue, known as the isthmus.

In response to thyroid stimulating hormone (TSH) from the pituitary gland, the thyroid gland takes iodine, found in many foods, and converts it into thyroid hormones: thyroxine (T4) and triiodothyronine (T3). Collectively, the thyroid hormones are so important that every cell in the body depends upon thyroid hormones for regulation of their metabolism. Thyroid hormones increase metabolic rate, control the body's response to the stress hormone adrenaline, and regulates the overall metabolism of protein, fats, and carbohydrates. Generally speaking, lower levels of the thyroid hormones entering cells will slow their metabolism.

Individuals with hypothyroidism will have symptoms associated with a slow metabolism. This condition is so common that many people are unaware they have it. Based on blood tests, which are not very sensitive at detecting mild hypothyroidism, it is estimated that between one percent and four percent of adults have moderate to severe hypothyroidism, and 10 percent to 12 percent have mild or sub-clinical hypothyroidism.

Symptoms of hypothyroidism include the following: fatigue; weakness; weight gain or increased difficulty losing weight; coarse, dry hair; dry, rough pale skin; hair loss; cold intolerance; muscle cramps and aches; constipation; depression; irritability; memory loss; abnormal menstruation; decreased libido

Because the body is expecting a certain amount of thyroid hormone, the pituitary gland will make additional thyroid-stimulating-hormone (TSH) in an attempt to entice the thyroid to produce more hormones. This constant bombardment with high levels of TSH may cause the thyroid gland to become enlarged, forming what is known as a goiter.

Acidosis

Even the thyroid gland is not safe from the effects of chronic metabolic acidosis. In normal adults, acidosis causes reduced levels of T3 and T4 in the blood and a rise in TSH, suggesting a problem with thyroid gland function. As a result, a functional state of hypothyroidism occurs. It has also been shown that this dysfunction can be fully corrected by eliminating the acidosis.

Acidity and Its Effects

Summary

Unlike the other substances, such as growth hormone and amino acids, the practice of supplementing with thyroid hormones is not common. Rather, when somebody cannot lose weight despite dieting and exercising, thyroid dysfunction is often suspected.

Dysfunction of all of the systems described above – bone, muscle, growth hormone, cortisol, thyroid hormones, and insulin – all lead to a reduction of metabolism, and a subsequent increase in fat.

Due to the constant turnover of fat cells, bone is a metabolically active tissue. With increased bone mass, one can not only burn more calories at rest, but they also have the strength to perform the necessary exercise required for permanent fat loss.

Similarly, muscle is a fat burning machine. It is said that we start losing muscle tissue at age 30, and this loss of muscle accounts for not only many of our degenerative diseases, but also the expansion of our waistlines as we age.

Growth hormone, and its partner, insulin-like growth factor, are directly responsible for growth and metabolism. So much so, many athletes and individuals looking to fight the effects of aging, turn to the use of these drugs.

Anybody with a sluggish thyroid can attest to the difficulty in keeping the pounds off. What makes this situation worse, is that these individuals lack the energy to give their metabolism a kick start!

Insulin sensitivity, characteristics of type II diabetes and syndrome X, prevents fat loss due to the abnormally high amounts of circulating insulin required to maintain normal blood sugars. The problem with all of this is that insulin is the body's main anabolic hormone, causing the storage of fat.

The stressors we face on a daily basis, if left unchecked, result in the production of cortisol, results in weight gain and muscle loss as discussed above.

Finally, one of the most common consequences of metabolic acidosis is the production of kidney stones. The formation of kidney stones does not have an effect on metabolism, but I included it out of a sense of completeness. The exact details are beyond the scope of this book, however.

Acidity and Its Effects
STEP 2: ASSESSING HORMONE FUNCTION

The great thing about the *Kick Acid Diet* is that if pH imbalance is the underlying cause, all hormone dysfunction, ranging from insulin resistance to low growth hormone levels, can be corrected with one approach!

Once you've determined your level of acidity, you should assess your level of hormone function. Refer to the Appendix for the following hormonal questionnaires: growth hormone; insulin; thyroid hormone;, and cortisol. If you suspect an underlying hormonal dysfunction unrelated to acidity, consult with your healthcare professional for further testing.

Part IV: Nutrition and Acidosis

God, in His infinite wisdom, neglected nothing and if we would eat our food without trying to improve, change or refine it, thereby destroying its life-giving elements, it would meet all requirements of the body."

Jethro Kloss

Nutrition and Acidosis

Food as fuel? Yeah, right. Food is not only a fuel, but it is so much more. Food is the window by which we can peak into one's culture, revealing one's history, traditions, and comforts. Think back at the last time you gathered with family and friends. Maybe it was a wedding or a celebration of some kind. I'll bet that your choice of foods had less to due with calorie count, than it did with taste and culture.

In the 20th century, thanks to many great researchers, we were witness to an expanding knowledge of the biological effects of non-nutritive substances. It was during this time that we began to recognize nutritional deficiency disorders were often caused by vitamin deficiencies and minerals, and that the biological value of proteins was based partly on their amino acid content.

All foods, based on their *bioavailability*, vitamin and mineral content, as well as their protein content, and certain other factors, will lead to fluctuations in the pH levels of the body. In other words, your food choices can and will effect your body's acid-base levels. Now, I didn't discover this, but it helped me find the questions I was looking for. Read this paragraph over and over and over again, as it forms the basis for the remainder of this book.

Acid is not only waste-product of cellular energy production, but is produced in the metabolism of food. The amount of acids generated by the normal adult Western diet will eventually exceed the kidney's ability to eliminate these acids. Coupled with your normal decline in kidney function with age, the result is that you're at risk for an increased acidosis.

Practitioners of traditional Chinese medicine have always recommended that we increase our consumption of fruits and vegetables. Fruits and vegetables have been associated with increased health and longevity, most likely due to the increased vitamin and mineral content found in these foods. The bicarbonate precursors found in these foods also raise pH, by contributing to the buffering capacity of the body. The increased consumption of fruits and vegetables, is unfortunately, not typical of today's modern diet, which consists of high amounts of animal proteins, grains, legumes, and salt.

Hunter-gatherers consumed diets free of salt, and rich in fruits and vegetables. They showed an increased immunity to age-related degenerative diseases via the alkalizing effects of their diets.

Rural Cretans, found in Greece, have the lowest recorded rates of degenerative conditions and exceptional longevity. Researchers speculate that this has to do with the composition of their diet. They consume 2lbs of fresh fruits and vegetables; 1lb of grains, 3 ounces of meat, fish, eggs, and only 1 ounce of legumes. In other words, 2/3 of their diet comes from fruits and vegetables. Their diet remains alkaline, or at least, neutral.

The Okinawans, also known for their longevity, consume many vegetables, the most notable being sweet potatoes. Despite increased longevity, there is an increased risk of cardiovascular disease due to a reduction in fruit consumption, and increased salt intake.

Dr. Henry Lu, quoted by Jia Han, in the book entitled, *Chinese Food for Longevity*, stated that those who grow on mountains eat only sweet potatoes. This, he saw, as reason for their increased longevity. In the Nei Jing, increased salt has been associated with weakened bone, atrophy of muscles, and stagnation of heart qi.

Finally, Dr. Loren, author of the best-selling book, The Paleo Diet, recommends eating in a way similar to our ancestors. He claims that our ancestors' diets consisted of lean meats, fish, plants, fruits and nuts. And its because of this, he attributes their good health, virtually absence of degenerative diseases.

All foods upon digestion ultimately must report to the kidney as either acid or base. When the diet yields a net acid load (such as low-carbohydrate fad diets that restrict consumption of fruits and vegetables), the acid must be buffered by the alkaline stores in the body, such as the calcium found in bone. The highest acid-producing foods are hard cheeses, cereal grains, salted foods, meats, and legumes, whereas the only alkaline or base-producing foods are fruits and vegetables. Because the average North American diet is overloaded with grains, cheeses, salted processed foods, and fatty meats at the expense of fruits and vegetables, it produces a net acid load. By replacing hard cheeses, cereal grains, and processed foods with plenty of green vegetables and fruits, the body comes back into acid-base balance.

Let's take a look now at each of the macronutrients affects acid-alkaline balance.

Protein

Proteins, by their very nature, are acid forming. In the absence of sufficient fruit and vegetables, increased dietary protein has been shown to increase calcium loss from bone and at the kidneys. It has been demonstrated that for every 10g increase in dietary protein, calcium loss at the kidneys increases by 16mg. Dietary protein has also been shown to reduce bicarbonate concentration. Sulphuric acid, found in many sources of dietary protein, along with phosphoric acid and hydrochloric acid, is so

Nutrition and Acidosis

strong and destructive that it must be immediately neutralized by the buffer system.

We know that our Paleolithic ancestors had a more alkaline diet than our current diet, but also consumed far more protein than we currently do. For example, their diet consisted of approximately 251g protein per day, of which 191g and 60g were animal and plant-based, respectively. Today, we average 125g of protein per day, of which only 85 grams is animal based and 40g is plant based. Why, despite their increased protein intake, was the diet of our ancestors a more alkaline one? There are a few reasons for this.

First, protein increases the ability of the kidneys to eliminate acid in the form of ammonia. The next mechanism by which protein counteracts its own acid forming potential is the increased *glomerular filtration rate* (GFR) at the kidneys. GFR is simply the volume of blood filtered at the kidney per unit time. Finally, our ancestors consumed more alkaline minerals, in the form of fruits and vegetables, to offset the acid load from dietary protein, to be discussed later.

Grains

Since the advent of industrial scale food production, our diets have shifted from that of our hunter-gatherer forefathers to one rich in simple sugars, saturated fats, and salt. Subsequently, our diets are also now low in magnesium and potassium. These dietary changes are thought to be risk factors to a number of diseases, including atherosclerosis, hypertension, type 2 diabetes, osteoporosis and some cancers.

According to researchers, this switch from net base to net acid production is attributed to the replacement of alkaline-rich plant foods, such as roots, leafy green vegetables and fruit, with cereal grains and energy-dense, nutrient poor foods such as refined sugars and saturated fats. The latter foods are not net-alkaline producing, and therefore do not compensate for the net acid-producing portions of today's diet, namely animal foods such as meat, cheese, milk, yogurt and eggs.

Cereal grains, which are net acid-producing, account for 38 percent of the acid load in the present day diet. According to the recent report, when plant foods in two pre-agricultural-type diets (made up of varying animal and plant food ratios) were replaced by cereal grains, the result was a switch from a net alkalizing-producing diet to a net acid-producing one. However, when cereal grains were removed from the contemporary diet, acidity decreased.

Grains are touted as great sources of iron, magnesium, fibre and B-vitamins. They do indeed contain reasonable amounts of those nutrients, but

Nutrition and Acidosis

if you compare the amount of nutrients in grains with the amount of nutrients in fruit or vegetables, grains do not come close.

However, a grain that is getting a lot of good press lately is quinoa, for all the right reasons. Not only does quinoa have a lower glycemic index, and full of nutrients, it is also neutral with respect to acidity.

Fruits and Vegetables

The consumption of fruits and vegetables is paramount when alkalizing one's diet. This is due to their high concentration of alkalizing minerals: calcium, potassium, sodium, and magnesium. Not only do fruits and vegetables prevent metabolic acidosis, but they're also known to combat and prevent many of the degenerative diseases we see today.

Current evidence has shown us that consumption of fruits and vegetables reduces free radical damage, but is also associated with improved health, reduced risk of major degenerative diseases, and a possible delayed onset of age-related indicators.

Your body is alkaline by design and acid by function. That is a very important concept. *Alkaline by design; acidic by function.* Cellular produced acid is a lot weaker than acid produced from the breakdown of ash-producing foods. Ash-producing foods, such as meats and grains, leave an acid residue after they get into the body. Self-produced cellular acid doesn't need to be neutralized by vital minerals before it is sent out of the body as it easily eliminated through your lungs when you breathe and when you talk.

You also get acid from foods, such as oranges and lemons that are acid in their own right. In fact, they are so acid that many people can't eat them without suffering discomfort. Furthermore, fruits and vegetables have more built-in acid than do high-protein acid ash-producing foods. However, this acid is also different from the acid you get from protein sources foods. The organic or natural acid found in fruits and vegetables is completely decomposed during metabolism, and is easily eliminated through breathing. On the other hand, the acid from acid ash-producing foods is different. It must be weakened and neutralized before it is eliminated from the body via the kidneys and intestines.

Fruits, especially citrous fruits are abundantly stuffed with organically bound alkaline minerals. We are not able to sense them but they are responsible for the alkaline effect in our bodies. When metabolized, these organically bound minerals consume acid, thereby decreasing total acid load.

Just as high-protein foods leave a residual acidic ash, fruits and

Nutrition and Acidosis

vegetables leave an alkali ash residue. It contains minerals that help alkalize your body. Let's take a closer look at these alkalizing minerals:

Fruits and vegetables are high in potassium. Potassium exerts its alkalizing effects through its alkali salts, potassium bicarbonate. Compared to our ancestors, we consume far less potassium. A reduction in dietary potassium is linked to cardiovascular disease, kidney dysfunction, and bone disorders.

The organic salt of magnesium has also been shown to reduce acidity. Like potassium, reduced magnesium levels have been correlated with degenerative conditions, such as cardiovascular disease. We also consume less magnesium than our ancestors.

While our consumption of potassium and magnesium has decreased, our sodium chloride, commonly known as table salt, intake has increased dramatically. We consume ten times as much chlorine as our ancestors did. Elevated sodium chloride is responsible for hypertension and calcium loss, as well as metabolic acidosis.

Summary

Meat sources, grains, hard cheeses, and salted and processed foods are all acid forming. Our only dietary line of defense in the onslaught of excess acidity is fruits and vegetables.

We're almost there. We now know what acids and bases are, and how our dietary choices can affect our pH levels. We're now going to look at how to grade your food with the use of a scale called the potential renal acid load or PRAL.

Nutrition and Acidosis

Nutritional Grading

Nutritionally speaking, our body's acid-base acid status is a reflection of the amounts of alkaline minerals in our diet such as sodium, potassium, calcium and magnesium, as well as the acid generating elements, phosphate, chloride, and sulphur. Whew, what a mouthful! Taking into account different intestinal absorption rates of these nutrients, a special scientific procedure, known as the potential renal acid load (PRAL) allows us to predict the respective amount of acid or base in 100g of a particular food.

Once digestion has occurred, every food will present to the kidneys as either an acid-forming or alkaline-forming food, Various methods of assessing acid-base status of a food are *ash analysis*, *NAE (net acid excretion)*, and the *PRAL (potential renal acid load)*.

Ash analysis involves the combustion of a food, and the subsequent analysis of the ash to see how much of the food was acidic and how much was alkaline. While a step in the right direction, the ash analysis does not take into account the bioavailability of the nutrients in a given food. As such, this method has its limitations.

The NAE is determined by measuring the acid and the ammonium appearing in the urine and then subtracting out the measured urinary bicarbonate. While more accurate than the ash analysis, this method reflects total acid and base load of a mixed diet, not for an individual food.

To more accurately predict the acid or base potential of a given food, another technique was needed, and the PRAL was born. Researchers, Remer and Manz, developed the food-rating values referred to as PRAL. The PRAL most accurately predicts the acid or base potential of a particular food. It accounts for the bioavailability of micronutrients and macronutrients, sulphur content, and obligatory diet-independent organic acid losses.

Using the PRAL

It should now be evident that many conditions seen today could benefit from dietary means of modifying one's acid-base status. There is a general consensus amongst the scientific community that diet can markedly affect acid-base status and a person's acid-base load can be manipulated by diet.

As described before, the PRAL provides an estimation of the body's acid production over alkali production (or vice versa) for a given amount of food ingested daily. The PRAL is physiologically based and takes into account different absorption rates of individualized minerals (calcium, potassium, phosphorus, and magnesium) and sulphur containing protein, as well as sulphur produced from metabolized proteins. This method of

Nutrition and Acidosis

determined acid load has been validated in healthy adults, and under controlled conditions.

Each of the foods listed in Appendix A (Adapted from Remer and Manz) represents the PRAL of a 100g portion of a particular food. Acid forming foods are represented as positive numbers, and alkaline forming foods are represented as negative.

The PRAL table in this chapter contains the foods that you're going to consume. The foods in this table include lean protein sources, fruits, vegetables, and fats. Common beverages and snacks are also found in this table.

Interpreting the table is quite simple. The PRAL values represent 100g of a chosen food. Negative values are alkaline; positive values are acidic. By following the plan described, each meal will have a negative score.

Nutrition and Acidosis
STEP 3: DETERMINE THE ACID-BASE STATUS OF YOUR DIET

The foods in the PRAL Density Tables* on the following pages have been selectively chosen as they will not only provide you with a favourable PRAL score, thereby lowering your acidity, but they are also nutrient dense, providing your body with needed vitamins, minerals, and other co-factors.

To determine the PRAL of your diet, follow these simple steps:

1. Determine the amount (in grams) of each food and multiply by the PRAL value found in the table.
2. Next, divide that number by 100 to determine its specific PRAL.
3. Continue doing this until you've calculated all the food in a particular meal, or over the course of a day.
4. Your PRAL score is determined by the sum of all the specific PRAL scores for each food. If the number is positive, then your diet is acidic; if the number is negative, then alkaline.

If your meal is deemed acidic, there are ways you can neutralize or alkalize it. Simply adding vegetables will do this. In fact, we recommend increasing your vegetable intake regardless of your PRAL score. Also, glutamine supplementation has been shown to neutralize acidosis.

What's great about using the PRAL as method to improve health and lose fat, is that the table includes many of the foods that may be restricted on other diets, such as wines, and fattier foods. In other words, you can enjoy meals at your favourite restaurants and need not be worried about following bland, tasteless diets.

A complete list of the PRAL scores for all foods can be found in Appendix A. In addition, *The Kick Acid Diet ® Calculator* is available for all iPhone, BlackBerry, and Android users.

Food values are taken from the from U.S. Department of Agriculture, Agricultural Research Service. 2009. USDA National Nutrient Database for Standard Reference, Release 22. Nutrient Data Laboratory Home Page,

Nutrition and Acidosis
PRAL Density Tables

High Alkaline Carbohydrate Foods

Food Description	Kcals	Protein	Fat	Carbs	PRAL	Alkali Density
Spinach, raw	23	3	0	4	-11.84	-2.96
Squash, zucchini, baby, raw	21	3	0	3	-6	-2
Arugula, raw	25	3	1	4	-7.86	-1.97
Celery, raw	16	1	0	3	-5.04	-1.68
Squash, summer	16	1	0	3	-4.14	-1.38
*Lettuce, red leaf	15	1	0	3	-3.57	-1.35
Beets, raw	43	2	0	4	-5.36	-1.34
Radishes, raw	16	1	0	3	-4.39	-1.28
Peppers, sweet, yellow/red, raw	27	1	0	3	-3.45	-1.15
Rhubarb, raw	21	1	0	5	-5.51	-1.10
Turnip greens	32	1	0	7	-7.20	-1.03
Tomatoes	18	1	0	4	-4.07	-1.02
Mushrooms, brown, portabella, Italian, or Crimini	27	3	0	4	-4.36	-0.98
Seaweed, agar, raw	26	1	0	7	-6.74	-0.96
Avocados, raw, California/commercial	164	2	15	9	-8.40	-0.94
*Cucumber, peeled/unpeeled, raw	14	1	0	3	-2.35	-0.87
Beans, snap, yellow, cooked, boiled, drained	35	1	0	6	-5.15	-0.86
Kale	50	2	1	10	-8.33	-0.83
Okra	31	2	0	7	-5.58	-0.80
*Cabbage	27	1	0	6	-4.49	-0.77
Squash, winter	34	1	0	9	-6.76	-0.75
Avocados, raw, Florida	120	2	10	8	-5.55	-0.69
Melon balls, frozen	33	1	0	8	-5.51	-0.69
Peppers, sweet, green/red, cooked, boiled, drained	27	1	0	4	-2.74	-0.69
*Onions, raw	28	2	0	7	-4.83	-0.69
Rutabagas	36	1	0	8	-5.55	-0.69
Collards	30	3	0	6	-4.09	-0.68
*Cauliflower, raw	28	3	0	6	-3.86	-0.67
Eggplant	24	1	0	6	-3.89	-0.65
Pickles, cucumber, dill or kosher dill	12	1	0	3	-1.92	-0.64
Potatoes, raw, skin	58	3	0	12	-6.99	-0.58
Broccoli, raw	34	3	0	7	-3.96	-0.57
Carrots, raw	41	1	0	10	-5.71	-0.57
Peppers, hot chili, green/red	40	2	0	9	-5.34	-0.57

Nutrition and Acidosis
PRAL Density Tables

High Alkaline Carbohydrate Foods (continued)

Food Description	Kcals	Protein	Fat	Carbs	PRAL	Alkali Density
Melons, cantaloupe, raw	34	1	0	9	-5.06	-0.56
Peppers, jalapeno	30	1	1	6	-3.33	-0.56
Papayas, raw	39	1	0	10	-5.48	-0.55
Asparagus	22	2	0	4	-2.19	-0.55
Turnips	28	1	0	6	-3.24	-0.54
Yam	118	2	0	28	-15.11	-0.54
Melons, casaba, raw	28	1	0	7	-3.52	-0.50
Melons, honeydew, raw	36	1	0	9	-4.45	-0.49

High Alkaline Beverages

Food Description	Kcals	Protein	Fat	Carbs	PRAL	Alkali Density
Tea, instant, unsweetened, powder, decaffeinated	315	20	0	59	-116.70	-1.98
Coffee, instant, regular, powder	241	12	0	41	-67.38	-1.64
Coffee, instant, decaffeinated, powder	224	12	0	43	-67.16	-1.56
Coffee, instant, regular, powder, half the caffeine	350	14	0	71	-66.29	-0.93
Wine, table, red	85	0	0	3	-2.19	-0.73
Wine, table, all	84	0	0	3	-1.69	-0.56
Cream, half and half, fat free	59	3	1	9	0.87	0.29

High Alkaline Nuts and Sauces

Food Description	Kcals	Protein	Fat	Carbs	PRAL	Alkali Density
Nuts						
Coconut water	19	1	0	4	-5.11	-1.28
Pine nuts	629	12	61	19	-12.41	-0.65
Beechnuts	576	6	50	33	-18.33	-0.56
Coconut milk	197	2	21	3	-1.50	-0.50
Sauces						
Sauce, ready-to-serve, pepper, TABASCO	12	1	1	1	-1.67	-1.67
Salsa	27	2	0	6	-5.07	-0.85
Soup, cream of mushroom, canned, condensed, reduced sodium	52	1	2	8	-5.67	-0.71
Soup, vegetable, canned, low sodium, condensed	65	2	1	12	-7.26	-0.61
USDA Commodity, spaghetti sauce, meatless, canned	48	1	1	9	-5.21	-0.58
Butter, salted/unsalted	717	1	81	0	0.43	0.43

Nutrition and Acidosis
PRAL Density Tables

High Alkaline Spices and Herbs

Food Description	Kcals	Protein	Fat	Carbs	PRAL	Alkali Density
Spices, dill seed	305	4	15	4	-33.19	-8.30
Spices, cloves, ground	323	0	1	4	-31.58	-7.90
Horseradish, prepared	48	1	11	1	-4.87	-4.87
Spices, dill weed, dried	253	20	4	16	-74.51	-4.66
Spices, cinnamon, ground	261	0	0	6	-23.75	-3.96
Basil, fresh	27	3	1	3	-10.01	-3.34
Dill weed, fresh	43	3	1	7	-15.49	-2.21
Spices, chili powder	314	3	5	15	-31.05	-2.07
Spices, coriander leaf, dried	279	22	5	52	-99.48	-1.91
Spices, chervil, dried	237	23	4	49	-92.40	-1.89
Spices, parsley, dried	276	22	4	52	-81.49	-1.57
Vinegar, cider	21	0	0	1	-1.45	-1.45
Spices, basil, dried	251	14	4	61	-85.36	-1.40
Spices, tarragon, dried	295	23	7	50	-64.51	-1.29
Spearmint, fresh	44	3	1	8	-10.01	-1.25
Spearmint, dried	285	20	7	52	-55.42	-1.07
Spices, celery seed	392	18	25	41	-34.71	-0.85
Peppermint, fresh	70	4	1	15	-12.65	-0.84
Spices, fennel seed	345	16	15	42	-35.37	-0.84
Spices, marjoram, dried	271	13	7	61	-49.30	-0.81
Rosemary, fresh	131	3	6	21	-16.45	-0.78
Spices, oregano, dried	306	11	10	64	-49.76	-0.78
Spices, sage, ground	315	11	13	61	-46.49	-0.76
Spices, savory, ground	272	7	6	69	-51.11	-0.74
Spices, cumin seed	375	18	22	44	-31.97	-0.73
Spices, turmeric, ground	354	8	10	65	-46.66	-0.72
Vinegar, red wine	19	0	0	1	-0.68	-0.68
Vanilla extract, imitation, alcohol	237	0	0	2	-1.35	-0.68
Spices, paprika	289	15	13	56	-36.33	-0.65
Thyme, fresh	101	6	2	24	-15.56	-0.65
Spices, rosemary, dried	331	5	15	64	-37.43	-0.58
Spices, thyme, dried	276	9	7	64	-35.48	-0.55
Spices, pepper, red or cayenne	318	12	17	57	-31.44	-0.55
Spices, curry powder	325	13	14	58	-26.10	-0.45
Spices, coriander seed	298	12	18	55	-23.21	-0.42
Spices, pepper, black	255	11	3	65	-25.39	-0.39

Nutrition and Acidosis
PRAL Density Tables

High Alkaline Spices and Herbs (continued)

Food Description	Kcals	Protein	Fat	Carbs	PRAL	Alkali Density
Spices, anise seed	337	18	16	50	-18.17	-0.36
Spices, ginger, ground	347	9	6	71	-24.55	-0.35
Spices, poultry seasoning	307	10	8	66	-22.11	-0.34
Spices, cardamom	311	11	7	68	-22.57	-0.33
Spices, pumpkin pie spice	342	6	13	69	-19.13	-0.28
Spices, caraway seed	333	20	15	50	-13.33	-0.27
Vanilla extract	288	0	0	13	-3.31	-0.25
Spices, bay leaf	313	8	8	75	-17.16	-0.23
Spices, mace, ground	475	7	32	50	-9.87	-0.20
Capers, canned	23	2	1	5	-0.69	-0.14
Spices, onion powder	347	10	1	81	-10.15	-0.13
Spices, poppy seed	533	18	45	24	-1.87	-0.08
Spices, nutmeg, ground	525	6	36	49	-3.75	-0.08
Spices, garlic powder	332	17	1	73	-2	-0.03
Spices, fenugreek seed	323	23	6	58	-1.20	-0.02
Vanilla extract, imitation, no alcohol	56	0	0	14	-0.05	0
Vinegar, distilled	18	0	0	1	0	0
Spices, pepper, white	296	10	2	69	4.29	0.06
Mustard, prepared, yellow	67	4	4	5	1.13	0.23
Spices, mustard seed, yellow	469	25	29	35	14.49	0.41
Salt, table	0	0	0	0	-0.50	
Vinegar, balsamic	88	0	17	0	-2.07	

Nutrition and Acidosis

PRAL Density Tables

Low Acidity Protein Foods

Food Description	Kcals	Protein	Fat	Carbs	PRAL	Acid Density
Dairy						
Yogurt, fruit variety, nonfat	94	4	0	19	0.11	0.03
Yogurt, plain, skim milk, 13 grams protein per 8 ounce	56	6	0	8	0.18	0.03
Yogurt, vanilla, low fat, 11 grams protein per 8 ounce	85	5	1	14	0.17	0.03
Egg, white, raw, fresh	52	11	0	1	2.09	0.19
Egg substitute, liquid	84	12	3	1	2.5	0.21
Egg, white, dried	382	81	0	8	17.12	0.21
Egg substitute, powder	444	56	13	22	23.32	0.42
Lamb, Veal Game						
*Lamb, raw	140	21	6	0	9.48	0.47
*Veal, lean only, raw	118	20	4	0	9.606	0.48
Finfish and Shellfish						
Grouper	92	19	1	0	4.19	0.22
*Mackerel	202	19	13	0	6.28	0.33
*Cod, Atlantic/Pacific	82	18	1	0	6.27	0.35
Snapper, mixed species	100	21	1	0	7.37	0.35
Herring, Pacific	195	16	14	0	5.67	0.35
Pike, walleye	93	19	1	0	6.77	0.36
Yellowtail, mixed species	146	20	4	0	7.24	0.36
*Tuna, fresh, cooked, dry heat	136	29	1	0	10.82	0.38
*Halibut	148	18	8	0	6.48	0.39
Bass	114	19	4	0	7.34	0.39
Flatfish (flounder/sole species)	91	19	1	0	7.41	0.39
Lobster, northern	90	19	1	0	7.43	0.39
Oyster, eastern, farmed	59	5	2	6	1.96	0.39
*Salmon	156	21	8	0	8.72	0.42
*Trout, rainbow	129	21	4	0	8.88	0.43
Haddock	87	19	1	0	8.24	0.43
*Crab	88	18	1	0	7.72	0.44
Tilapia	96	20	2	0	8.95	0.45
Scallop, mixed species	88	17	1	2	7.79	0.46
Catfish, channel, wild	95	16	3	0	7.46	0.47
Shrimp, cooked, moist heat	99	21	1	0	10.10	0.48
*Perch, raw	106	22	2	0	10.68	0.49
Tuna, light, canned in water, drained solids	116	26	1	0	12.70	0.49
Beef						
Beef, top sirloin	168	21	9	0	9.78	0.47
Beef, ribs	161	20	8	0	9.01	0.44
Beef, lean, raw	150	21	7	0	9.75	0.46
Beef, flank	149	22	6	0	10.08	0.46
Beef, bottom sirloin, tri-tip roast	163	21	9	0	9.62	0.46
Beef, tenderloin	158	22	7	0	10.30	0.47
Beef, ground, 95% lean meat / 5% fat, raw	137	21	5	0	9.86	0.47
Beef, round	155	22	7	0	10.32	0.48
Pork						
*Pork, fresh, loin	154	21	6	0	8.98	0.42

Nutrition and Acidosis
PRAL Density Tables

Low Acidity Protein Foods (continued)

Food Description	Kcals	Protein	Fat	Carbs	PRAL	Acid Density
Sausage Luncheon Meats						
Turkey, pork, and beef sausage, low fat, smoked	101	8	3	11	1	0.13
Turkey breast meat	104	17	2	4	7.36	0.43
Sausage, Italian, sweet, links	149	16	8	2	7	0.44
Ham, sliced, extra lean	110	19	3	1	8.62	0.45
Honey loaf, pork, beef	125	11	4	10	5.15	0.47
Turkey roll, light and dark meat	149	18	7	2	8.55	0.48
Turkey sausage, fresh, raw	155	19	8	0	9.51	0.50
Poultry						
*Turkey, meat only, raw	143	21	6	1	9.83	0.46
Chicken, Cornish game hens, meat raw	116	20	3	0	9.38	0.47
*Chicken, meat only, raw	145	19	8	0	9.20	0.48

Putting it All Together

The *Kick Acid Diet* is not only focused on reducing the overall acidity of your diet, but it gives you a blueprint for a healthier lifestyle. Remember from the previous sections, we learned how to measure our body's pH using either saliva or urine. I also provided you with a hormone screen that you can use at your convenience. I strongly recommend that you consult with your healthcare professional if hormone screen shows signs of hormonal dysfunction.

The next step in the *Kick Acid Diet* is calculating the PRAL values of your meals. This step will give the acid-base status of your diet. Fortunately, I've included both a recipe section, with tasty alkaline meals.. There are over 3000 foods included in the PRAL tables found in the Appendix. In conjunction with step 3, step 4 involves using the *Kick Acid Diet* Meal Planner.

The final steps of the *Kick Acid Diet*, which will be discussed in the next chapter, are the Step 5: Biomarker Health Assessment and Step 6: *The Kick Acid Diet* Workout Program.

Nutrition is your best way of maintaining a healthy, lean body, free of unwanted fat! Exercise is important, but consuming the right foods, at the right times, and in the right amounts and proportions will make profound changes in your body composition...in a short amount of time!

The great thing about eating right is you don't need to starve yourself, nor do you have to consume foods you don't like. Armed with the right information, you can enjoy eating healthily. Furthermore, if you understand the methods outlined in this book, you can enjoy dining out at your favourite restaurants.

Nutrition and Acidosis

The first step in understanding nutrition is to understand the role of the following macronutrients – proteins, fats, and carbohydrates. They are important because they supply the body with energy and building blocks for growth and repair. Although they are found in all foods, the relative compositions may differ.

Macronutrient	Calories per gram
Protein	4
Fat	9
Carbohydrates	4
Water	0
Alcohol	7

Even though it has no caloric value, water is extremely important. Alcohol, on the other hand, at seven calories per gram is known as an empty calorie. This simply means that alcohol does not contain the nutrients required to break itself down into useable energy.

Eat Every Three Hours

The next step in effective fat loss is to understand the role of the meal timing and frequency – when and why to eat at certain times.

Not only is what you eat important, but when you eat is also important. With every meal, certain physiological and biochemical changes take place. In the absence of foods or in a "fasting" state, as in between meals, predictable changes occur.

It seems that Western populations increasingly are moving away from regular meals, perhaps because more meals are being eaten outside the home and because the tradition of families dining together has been eroded by hectic schedules. The prevalence of irregular meal patterns is even greater amongst teens than it was during previous decades. Japanese studies also found that irregular snacking has become more common in children and may be responsible for both the rising obesity rates.

It has been shown that even if we do not account for what is actually in our meals, infrequent meals reduce *insulin sensitivity*, increase energy intake due to this lack of insulin sensitivity, and reduce our caloric expenditure. One of the keys to stabilizing blood sugar, and preventing obesity (and type II diabetes) is to control insulin levels.

If we now combine a regular eating pattern with the right foods, at the right time, and in the right amounts, we can guarantee fat loss. Anybody

Nutrition and Acidosis

who is interested in nutrition has heard about the glycemic index. The *glycemic index* is a measure of how quickly one's blood sugar level increases in response to carbohydrate dominant foods. Unfortunately, it doesn't adequately address fat and/or protein content. The *insulinemic index (II)* on the other hand, specifically refers to the rise in insulin that occurs after a meal. The II is somewhat of an intermediary between dietary intake and the glycemic index.

Protein and fats generally results in a minimal rise in blood sugar levels, due to a low insulinemic response. When combined with carbohydrates, protein and fats blunt this response, resulting in a steadier level of blood sugar levels.

When compared to a high glycemic index diet, people on a low-carbohydrate, high protein diet lost less lean mass, had a higher metabolic rate immediately after their meal, as well as ten hours later.

Why is this important? High levels of insulin can lead to obesity, diabetes, and metabolic syndrome or syndrome X. More important than drastically reducing carbohydrates is to include protein and fat with every meal.

Eat Breakfast Every Morning

Similarly, we have been missing breakfast more frequently in the recent decades. It has been shown that missing breakfast will increase a person's body fat and cholesterol levels. There seems to be a direct effect on eating breakfast and ones insulin sensitivity: eating breakfast will increase ones insulin sensitivity.

Our bodies conserve fat at the expense of muscle tissue if calories are not consumed upon wakening. Furthermore, in the fasting state, even transient, the body's production of thyroid hormone decreases, resulting in a 20% reduction in one's basal metabolic rate.

What about the notion that we burn more fat on an empty stomach? We may burn more fat on an empty stomach, except for the fact that during sleep, most of our glycogen stores are depleted. This means that when we exercise on an empty stomach, not only is our body burning fat, it turns to muscle tissue as a fuel source in order to sustain exercise.

Nutrition and Acidosis

Consume Protein with Every Meal

Proteins are molecules composed of amino acids. These amino acids found in protein serve as building blocks for muscle tissue, enzyme, hair, skin, and immune cells. The amino acid composition varies between protein sources and from dietary protein to that found in your body. Not to worry. Your body has a pretty neat strategy to make proteins that it can actually use. It breaks down dietary protein into its amino acid constituents and then rebuilds the protein that it needs! Problems arise when we do not consume adequate amounts of protein.

In extreme circumstances, protein is mobilized for energy, as in times of illness and disease. This is not ideal, as it results in the breakdown of muscle tissue and ketosis, an acidic state in your body. The ketones produced from the degradation of protein are toxic to your body.

Not all protein sources are considered equal. A simple classification of dietary protein is based on their ability to provide an individual with all of the essential amino acids in the right proportions. Without going into too much detail, the body can make certain amino acids from others. The ones that the body cannot produce must be ingested in the diet. Complete sources of dietary protein are the following:

Unfortunately, few of us ingest adequate amounts of protein. The reasons for this could range from time constraints, inability to consume large quantities of food, to being unaware of quality protein sources. Protein shakes are a great way to make up the rest of your daily protein intake.

The amount of protein we should consume varies depending on both your lean body weight and activity levels. We should consume at least *1g of protein per lb* of body weight. Many people claim that high protein intakes are hard on the kidneys. According to the research, high protein diets have only been shown to be detrimental to individuals with prior end-stage kidney disease.

So, how does protein help me lose fat? Good question! Protein aids in fat by increasing your metabolism (**thermic effect of food** and by increased muscle mass) and stabilizing your blood sugar levels.

Consume Fat with Every Meal

Much more is known about dietary fats within the past decade compared to the last century. We have many people to thank for this, especially a man I have had the pleasure of meeting on a few occasions, Udo

Nutrition and Acidosis

Erasmus. For a complete description about dietary fats, I'll refer you his book, *Fats That Heal, Fats That Kill*.

Fortunately, fats have come into favour. Despite their bad press, some members of the fat family are absolutely essential. Hence, essential fatty acids (EFA's). However, not all fats are good. The easiest way to tell the good from the bad is to look at the structure and metabolism of fats. Technically speaking, fats are solid at room temperature, while oils are liquid.

The Good

Unsaturated fats are liquid at room temperature. These are classified as mono- or polyunsaturated fatty acids. The greater the degree of unsaturation, the more fluid the molecule.

Unsaturated fatty acids are labelled as omega 3, omega 6, or omega 9. This number is extremely important. For example, omega 3 fatty acids reduce inflammation, while omega 6 fatty acids are potent pro-inflammatories.

The Bad

Saturated fat, the kinds you should limit in your diet, are solid at room temperature. Look at the fat hanging off the edge of as steak or a stick of butter. This is saturated fat. Too much of it is unhealthy as it clogs your arteries, increases bad cholesterol, and promotes inflammation. What's worse than saturated fat is **hydrogenated fat**. Margarine is high in hydrogenated fat. The process of hydrogenation takes a healthy, unsaturated fat and adds hydrogen molecules to it, thereby, saturating it. This process also increases the shelf life of the fat. This renders these fats more harmful than saturated fats because the hydrogen is placed in an unnatural *trans-position*. These unnatural fats are known as trans-fats. As such, your body cannot metabolize it, leading to accumulation in blood vessels and cell membranes.

Of all the nutrients, fats are the most interesting in terms of functions. Fats are used as building blocks, an energy source, hormone regulator, and modulator of inflammation.

Fat for Fat Loss

Incorporating essential fatty acids into your diet will help you shed body fat for the many reasons. Like proteins, essential fatty acids will blunt the insulin response, thereby lowering the glycemic or insulinemic index of

Nutrition and Acidosis

your meals. It has been well established that the higher the fat content of a meal, the lower the glycemic and insulin response.

With respect to quality of fats, the degree of saturation also has an effect. Polyunsaturated fatty acids result in slower rise in blood glucose concentration than did monounsaturated fats. These effects are not just immediate, but can affect one's glucose tolerance hours to days after ingestion.

Incorporation of fatty acids into your cell's membranes results in improved response of its receptors to many hormones, including insulin.

Finally, EFA's turn on the fat burning hormone, lipase.

The amount of fat you're consuming will equal that of the caloric intake from protein. To determine this, perform the following:

1. Multiply the grams of protein by 4 to determine its caloric value.
2. The number obtained is also the total amount of dietary fat in calories for the day.
3. Divide this number obtained in step #2 by 9 to calculate the daily grams of fat.
4. Divide the number obtained in step #3 into thirds.
5. Finally, the number in step #4 represents the amount of essential fatty acids, omega 9 fatty acids, and saturated fats that you need to consume each day.
6. Since protein contains saturated fat, do not add any saturated fat into your diet. Omega 9 fatty acids can be obtained from avocado, olive oils, and nuts. Omega 3 fatty acids can be obtained from fish and supplements.

As you'll see in the table, sources of omega 6 fatty acids are abundant. As such, the typical Western diet will provide ten times more omega-6 fatty acids than omega-3 fatty acids. The optimal ratio is 3 omega 6 fatty acids for every 1 omega 3 fatty acid, contributing to many health problems, ranging from heart disease to inflammation to depression, as was confirmed by scientists at the Ohio State University School of Medicine.

Nutrition and Acidosis

When choosing foods from this table, opt for those high in omega 3 fatty acids and omega 9 fatty acids. In fact, it is possible to obtain enough omega 9 fatty acids from 1-2 teaspoons of olive oil with each meal.

Similarly, calculate the PRAL of fatty foods and add it to the PRAL score from protein. The PRAL from fat is often negligible, but calculate it anyway.

Consume Fruits and Vegetables with Every Meal

The body's metabolic needs, exercise levels, lean body mass, and disease state all affect the amount of these nutrients required. The body uses a mixture of protein, fats, and carbohydrates for its energy requirements. Carbohydrates, however, are the body's main source of fuel. This depends on the intensity of physical activity being performed and the composition of the food ingested.

Carbohydrates are not only important as fuel sources, but they also provide the body with many essential vitamins and alkalizing minerals. Reducing your intake of fruits and vegetables puts you at risk of developing many deficiencies. Humans only have approximately 500g of carbohydrates for 24 hours.

Finally, calculate the PRAL required to offset that from protein (and fats). Once you have this number, increase it by 50%. That's the total PRAL you should consume from fruits and vegetables. Using Appendix A, incorporate carbohydrates that total this PRAL value. As a guideline, you should consume no more than twice the amount of calories from carbohydrates as from protein and fat combined. Remember, life, stress, and physical activity make your body acidic. We need to combat this with fruits and vegetables.

You may have noticed that grains aren't included in this diet. That's right. Grains are acid producing, and you can obtain all the nutrients and fibre from fruits and vegetables.

Drink at Least 2 Litres of Water Every Day

Even though water does not affect the PRAL or our body's acidity directly, it is vital. As mentioned earlier, the body is made up of 60% water. All of our biochemical processes depend on water and without it, we could not survive. We can go weeks without food, but only days without water.

Nutrition and Acidosis

In fact, water is ranked second only to oxygen as the most important nutrient for the body. Our bodies are so sensitive to changes in water levels that a dehydration of 3% can result in fatigue, weakness, and loss of coordination. Furthermore, since our muscles consist of approximately 70% water, dehydration will prevent us from gaining lean mass. And without lean muscle mass, our metabolism slows down.

Water also aids in protecting the joints, digestion, lubricating the skin, and is important for proper mental functioning.

Supplementation

One of the questions I am asked often is about dietary supplementation. In an ideal world, free of pollution, healthy soil conditions, and clean food, would supplementation even be necessary? We have no way of ever really answering this question, do we?

Supplementation is necessary if we desire optimal health and performance. There are many supplements that I recommend, but I will only go into detail on the alkalizing supplements. For all others, I will include my recommendations.

<u>Alkalizing Supplements</u>

Glutamine

Glutamine not only helps the body build lean muscle tissue, it helps the body maintain the correct acid-alkaline balance.. Glutamine also helps promote a healthy digestive tract. Finally, glutamine has been used to curb the desire to consume sugar and alcohol.

<u>Recommended Dosage:</u>
- 5g daily

Magnesium Citrate

Magnesium citrate is a chemical agent used medicinally as a laxative. Once in the intestine, magnesium citrate can attract enough water into the intestine to stimulate bowel mobility. Magnesium citrate, as a supplement in pill form, is also cited as useful for the prevention of kidney stones due to its alkalizing effects.

<u>Recommended Dosage:</u>
- 350mg daily

Nutrition and Acidosis

Creatine Phosphate

Creatine has long been touted as one the most effective legal performance enhancing supplements on the market. Not only does it increases muscle mass and increases power output, it also reduces alkalinity.

<u>Recommended Dosage:</u>
- 1 teaspoon/5grams daily

Chlorophyll

Chlorophyll is a green pigment found in most plants and algae.. Chlorophyll is not soluble in water and is first mixed with a small quantity of oil to obtain the desired result. Chlorophyll is a rich source of vitamins, minerals, and protein. It plays an important role in regulating the acidity and alkalinity in our body.

<u>Recommended Dosage:</u>
- 1 tablespoon, 2-4 times daily

<u>Non-Alkalizing Supplements</u>

These supplements do not influence acidity directly, but are nevertheless, important. R

Omega 3 fatty acids

One third of your total fat intake should consist of omega 3 fatty acids or fish oil pills.

Multivitamin and mineral

To ensure that you're getting all of the required nutrients, supplementing with a multivitamin and mineral complex will help. Follow the instructions given.

Protein supplement

The amount of protein from supplement form will depend on the amount consumed from real food. Remember, our goal is 1g per pound of body weight.

Branched chain amino acids (BCAA)

BCAA's are essential in building and maintaining lean muscle tissue. The recommended daily dosage is 5-10g per day.

Nutrition and Acidosis

Vitamin C

Vitamin C is a water soluble vitamin that is constantly being used by the body. It is not only a powerful antioxidant, but has positive effects on the formation of collagen and on the immune system. It has been shown to have a positive, albeit, indirect effect on acidity. Recommended dosage is 1000mg per day in supplement form.

Vitamin B Complex

There isn't just one B vitamin, but rather they make up an entire complex of vitamins. Their main role is in energy metabolism and production. Like vitamin C, they are water soluble, and as such, your body requires a daily supply. Recommended dosage is 100mg per day in supplement form.

While supplements are important, they should not replace a balanced diet, high in low PRAL proteins, fruits and vegetables, and unsaturated fats.

Summary

- Eat every three hours
- Eat breakfast every day.
- Consume low-fat, low-PRAL protein with every meal
- Consume fat with every meal
- Consume fruits and vegetables with every meal
- Maintain a negative PRAL score every day.
- Consume at least 2 litres of water every day
- Supplement

Part V: The Kick Acid Diet Meal Planner

"The Lord hath created medicines out of the earth; and he that is wise will not abhor them. "
Ecclesiastes 38:4

The Kick Acid Diet Meal Planner

You should now be ready to incorporate the information from this book and customize your nutrition plan, based on your body build, personal tastes, and health goals. *The Kick Acid Diet* Meal Planner will guide you through each of the phases: Muscle Up; Fat Loss; Maintenance; Athletic Performance. To make the most out of the meal planning, it is best to coincide these phases with their corresponding phases in next chapters, *The Kick Acid Diet* Workout Program.

The Kick Acid Diet Meal Planner
STEP 4: USING THE KICK ACID DIET MEAL PLANNER

The meal planner is divided into two parts. The first part describes each phase and what is required for each phase. The second part of the meal planner consists the PRAL Density Table which contains foods that will be consuming in each phase. The great thing about the *Kick Acid Diet* Meal Planner is it's inclusive – not exclusive! You'll get to eat the foods you enjoy while reaching your health and fitness goals.

The first step involves describing how much protein, carbohydrates and fat you should eat per meal based on your goals and body weight. The goals of each phase will also be outlined to help your understanding and compliance.

PRAL Density

Next, look at the chart that describes the ***PRAL density*** of each food. The PRAL density is a measure of the alkalinity per gram of carbohydrate of carbohydrate-dominant foods. Similarly, the PRAL density measures the acidity per gram of protein of protein-dominant foods. The guidelines established ensure that you obtain the maximum amount of alkalinity per gram of carbohydrate, while minimizing the acidity per gram of protein.

You'll notice when you peruse the section on protein certain foods have a much more favourable PRAL density score, that is, a low acidity per gram of protein. However, these foods are not complete sources of protein. A complete source of protein provides the body with all of the essential amino acids. All of the recommended foods are complete protein sources.

All of your carbohydrate and protein sources can be found in Appendix A. While the amounts of carbohydrates and protein will differ based on your goals, your total fat intake will remain constant.

Using the Food Tables

Using the charts, calculate the amount of each food is required to ensure that you meet your meal requirement. You can obtain all your requirements from one food, or from a combination of foods, as long as you don't overshoot your requirements.

The Kick Acid Diet allows you to indulge in your favourite beverages. Refer to each phase for the type of beverage allowed during each phase.

Fortunately, the nuts and sauces listed in the tables are alkaline. However, they're also high in calories, so should you include them in your diet, use sparingly, being sure not to exceed your carbohydrate requirements.

The Kick Acid Diet Meal Planner

An easy way to alkalize your diet, not to mention, add some zest to your diet, is to add spices and herbs. I encourage the liberal use of herbs and spices, as they don't contribute a lot to total caloric intake, while providing an alkalizing boost.

Food Journal

Use *The Kick Acid Diet* Food Journal to make sure your meeting your protein, carbohydrate, fat, and PRAL requirements.

Start by writing in your protein, carbohydrate and fat requirements (using the daily requirement chart provided) in the top of the daily food journal. Record each meal, and place the values in the appropriate boxes. Tally up the numbers at the end of the day to see your final PRAL score.

Once you've reached your body composition goals, and have effectively learned how to alkalize your diet, feel free to include other foods from Appendix A, as long as your diet remains alkaline. I recommend that you complete each phase to maximize results.

Food Preparation and Mineral Loss

According to nutrition specialists, the amount of vitamin and mineral content loss varies widely with food preparation, Minerals are quite stable in cooking and their loss may be quite negligible. However, different vitamins are likely to be lost in varying proportions, depending on the duration of cooking the food. As we know, alkalinity depends on the mineral content of foods, and as such, we need not be concerned.

Since minerals are not lost due to heat, but are usually leached if boiled, I recommend that you steam your vegetables, whenever possible.

Why were these foods chosen?

The foods chosen are given in their raw form. Boiling them will reduce their alkalinity (refer to the Appendix to know exact values), but they remain alkaline enough to counteract the effects of acidity from protein sources.

Food Description	Kcals	Protein	Fat	Carbs	PRAL	Acid Density
Rutabagas, raw	36	1	0	8	-5.55	-0.69
Rutabagas, cooked, boiled, drained	39	1	0	9	-5.36	-0.60

Furthermore, foods in their various forms often have a different PRAL score, which is usually reflective a lower alkalinity. Once again, the

The Kick Acid Diet Meal Planner

foods chosen have a high enough alkalinity in their alternate forms to counteract the effects of acidity from protein sources.

Food Description	Kcals	Protein	Fat	Carbs	PRAL	Acid Density
Carrots, raw	41	1	0	10	-5.71	-0.57
Carrots, canned, regular pack, solids and liquids	23	1	0	5	-3.24	-0.65
Carrots, canned, drained solids	25	1	0	5	-3.09	-0.62
Carrots, canned, solids and liquids	23	1	0	5	-2.92	-0.58

You may notice if you refer to the Appendix, some protein foods with a low acidic density were left out. Similarly, certain carbohydrate foods with a high alkaline density were eliminated. The criteria for elimination were as follows:

1. Carbohydrates foods that had additives, such as saccharin
2. Protein foods that had a high amount of total fat, greater than 2/3 of protein content.
3. Smoked meats.

The Kick Acid Diet Meal Planner

Phase 1: Muscle Up

I purposely started with the Muscle Up phase as I feel building a solid foundation not only keeps you healthy, but makes fat loss more effective. Each pound of lean muscle has been shown to burn 30-50 calories a day. A 10lb increase in muscle mass translates to up to 500 calories a day, 3500 calories a week, or a pound of fat burnt every week to ten days! Experts have also found that regular weight training will boost metabolism by up to 15%.

A side effect of this phase is that you'll become stronger. Getting stronger will allow you to be more active, perform better and prevent injury.

Your dietary requirements for Phase 1 are as follows: Eat a minimum one gram of protein per pound of body weight. For example, a woman who weighs 120lbs will consume 120 grams of protein per day, or 20 grams of protein per meal. A 200lb man will consume at least 200 grams of protein per day, or approximately 35 grams of protein per meal.

Your carbohydrate intake will be a *minimum* of two grams per pound of body weight. Consuming this amount of carbohydrates serves two purposes. First, it provides the calories needed to perform strenuous workouts and to build muscle. Next, as the book suggests, it ensures an alkaline environment that ensures muscle hypertrophy occurs, as well as optimizing hormonal function.

Your protein choices will be "limited" to the foods listed in the table at the end of the chapter. Since you'll be consuming more carbohydrates to provide your body with adequate calories, the risk of acidifying your diet is low, and therefore, you'll have more leeway with your protein choices than in the fat loss phase.

To determine the amount of fat requires some math, or you can simply look at the daily requirement charts. Recall, your fat intake will remain the same for each phase.
The amount of fat calories will equal the amount of protein calories. Since the amount of calories per gram of fat is higher than that of protein, the actual amount of fat in grams will be less.

Let's take the example of the 120lb woman. Her protein intake is 120 grams per day, which is equal to 480 calories. To determine daily fat intake, simply divide the number of calories of protein, which is 480 in this case, and divide by nine, the number of calories in one gram of fat. For the woman in this example, the daily fat requirement is approximately 54 grams per day.

Now, divide the daily fat requirement by three. This will determine the relative amounts of each type of fat (saturated, omega 9 fats from olive

The Kick Acid Diet Meal Planner

oil and almonds, and from essential fats). In this example, your requirement for each type of fat is 18 grams per day.

Since you're consuming high protein foods, you will meet your requirement for saturated fats, so there is no need to purposely include these fats into your diet.

Omega 9 fatty acids, while non-essential, are important as they reduce cardiovascular disease and cancer risk, improve immunity, and help control blood sugar levels. Again, the requirement for the 120lb woman in this example is 18 grams per day. Fortunately, your body can convert other types of fat into these types if necessary. If your diet doesn't include avocadoes, you'll supplement your diet with one tablespoon per day of olive oil, sunflower oil or canola oil, which is equal to five grams.

Finally, the remaining third (18 grams from the example cited above), will come from essential fatty acids in the form of fish oil (salmon oil) or DHA/EPA capsules found in health foods stores. As mentioned above, these 18 grams will be divided into six equal meals, for three grams per meal.

The Kick Acid Diet Meal Planner

Body Weight (pounds)	Protein Grams Meal	Carbs from PRAL Density Tables	Other Carbs not found in PRAL Density Tables	Essential Fatty Acid Grams Meal
100	20	40	0	3
110	20	40	0	3
120	20	40	0	3
130	25	50	0	4
140	25	50	0	4
150	25	50	0	4
160	30	60	0	4
170	30	60	0	4
180	30	60	0	4
190	35	70	0	5
200	35	70	0	5
210	35	70	0	5
220	40	80	0	6
230	40	80	0	6
240	40	80	0	6
250	50	100	0	6

The Kick Acid Diet Meal Planner

Phase 2: Fat Loss

The next phase, Fat Loss, will build upon your body's increase muscle mass. First while you will you control the amount of calories that you consume, calories won't be restricted. Rather, as the premise of this book suggest, you'll achieve your fat loss goals through controlling acidity levels, and insulin sensitivity.

Your dietary requirements for phase two as follows: Eat at least one gram of protein per pound of body weight. Our 120lb will consume 120 grams of protein per day. Similarly, a 200lb man will consume at least 200 grams of protein per day.

Your carbohydrate intake will be a *maximum* of one gram per pound of body weight. Unlike the muscle up phase, there aren't as many carbohydrates consumed to offset the acid load from dietary protein. As such, this will be the most restrictive phase in terms of food choices.

By consuming carbohydrate foods, especially in the fat loss stage, that have a high negative PRAL density value, will allow to maintain the alkalinity of your body while reducing the amount of carbohydrates consumed.

Each protein source permitted in phase two has been carefully selected. Each one has a low acidic PRAL density. Similarly, carbohydrates have also been carefully selected as each food source as a high alkaline PRAL density. In order for this phase to be effective, eat only foods that are listed in the corresponding table.

Your fat intake will be identical to that of phase one.

The Kick Acid Diet Meal Planner

Body Weight (pounds)	Protein Grams Meal	Carbs from PRAL Density Tables	Other Carbs not found in PRAL Density Tables	Essential Fatty Acid Grams Meal
100	20	20	0	3
110	20	20	0	3
120	20	20	0	3
130	25	25	0	4
140	25	25	0	4
150	25	25	0	4
160	30	30	0	4
170	30	30	0	4
180	30	30	0	4
190	35	35	0	5
200	35	35	0	5
210	35	35	0	5
220	40	40	0	6
230	40	40	0	6
240	40	40	0	6
250	50	50	0	6

The Kick Acid Diet Meal Planner
Phase 3: Maintenance

The third phase is the maintenance phase. After all of your hard work and discipline gaining muscle and losing fat, in other words, getting the body you want, it's time to relax and give yourself a break!

In this phase you'll be allowed to eat more of the foods you like, as long as you consume enough protein, and maintain a negative or alkaline PRAL score. Again, your protein requirements will be at least one gram per pound of bodyweight. Similarly, your fat intake is identical to the other two phases.

Where this phase differs is your carbohydrate consumption. Your carbohydrate intake for foods in part one of the corresponding table (identical to those consumed during the fat loss phase) is limited to two grams per pound of body weight. Limit your carbohydrate intake from the foods in Appendix A to 0.5 grams per pound of bodyweight.

Overall your alkaline PRAL score derived from carbohydrate intake should be 1.5-2 times higher than your acidic PRAL score from your protein intake. That's it. The only restriction placed during this phase is on the amount of carbohydrates consumed from the foods in Appendix A (not found in the PRAL Density Tables).

The Kick Acid Diet Meal Planner

Body Weight (pounds)	Protein Grams Meal	Carbs from PRAL Density Tables	Other Carbs not found in PRAL Density Tables	Essential Fatty Acid Grams Meal
100	20	20	10	3
110	20	20	10	3
120	20	20	10	3
130	25	25	12.5	4
140	25	25	12.5	4
150	25	25	12.5	4
160	30	30	15	4
170	30	30	15	4
180	30	30	15	4
190	35	35	17.5	5
200	35	35	17.5	5
210	35	35	17.5	5
220	40	40	20	6
230	40	40	20	6
240	40	40	20	6
250	50	50	0	6

The Kick Acid Diet Meal Planner

Phase 4: Performance

With the exception of a few sports, such as wrestling, mixed martial arts, and boxing, maintaining weight, may aid in performance, but is not a necessity to compete. In some instances, following restrictive dietary practises may actually hinder performance.

Your body needs a constant supply of fuel in order to perform strenuous physical activity. The most readily available source of this fuel comes in the form of carbohydrates. Fortunately, as you serious athletes reading this know, that weight loss is often a nice side effect of heavy training, despite consuming a lot of calories. Remember the Michael Phelps example I used earlier?

Not only does your body need the fuel from carbohydrates, it needs the other vitamins and minerals found in these foods sources in order for its machinery to work properly. By limiting your carbohydrates, you're also limiting your body's ability to perform at high intensities or for long periods.

Your activity of choice will determine your dietary requirements. Your dietary requirements will be identical to the maintenance phase, but you're allowed up to one gram per pound of body of carbohydrates from the second part of this table

The Kick Acid Diet Meal Planner

Body Weight (pounds)	Protein Grams Meal	Carbs from PRAL Density Tables	Other Carbs not found in PRAL Density Tables	Essential Fatty Acid Grams Meal
100	20	20	20	3
110	20	20	20	3
120	20	20	20	3
130	25	25	25	4
140	25	25	25	4
150	25	25	25	4
160	30	30	30	4
170	30	30	30	4
180	30	30	30	4
190	35	35	35	5
200	35	35	35	5
210	35	35	35	5
220	40	40	40	6
230	40	40	40	6
240	40	40	40	6
250	50	50	50	6

The Kick Acid Diet Meal Planner

The Kick Acid Diet Food Journal

Sample for 120lb person

Body Weight Fat Loss	120lbs	Protein Grams	High Alkaline Grams	Moderate Alkaline Grams	Essential Fat Grams	PRAL
Daily Requirements		120 grams	120 grams	0 grams	18 grams	Negative
Meal 1						
Meal 2						
Meal 3						
Meal 4						
Meal 5						
Meal 6						
Total						

The Kick Acid Diet Meal Planner

The Kick Acid Diet Food Journal

Sample for 200lb person

Body Weight	200lbs	Protein Grams	High Alkaline Grams	Moderate Alkaline Grams	Essential Fat Grams	PRAL
Muscle Up						
Daily Requirements		420 grams	210 grams		30 grams	Negative
Meal 1						
Meal 2						
Meal 3						
Meal 4						
Meal 5						
Meal 6						
Total						

Part VI: The Kick Acid Diet Recipes

The art of healing comes from nature, not from the physician. Therefore the physician must start from nature, with an open mind."
Philippus Aureolus Paracelsus

Recipes
The Kick Acid Diet Recipes

I've provided you with all of the tools necessary to alkalize your diet in the previous chapter. I'm going to make this even easier in this chapter. The recipes found here will not only provide you with all of the essential nutrients, but each will have a negative PRAL value.

Below each recipe, you'll find the breakdown as follows:

- Calories
- Protein
- Carbohydrates
- Fat
- PRAL

Included with each recipe is the serving size.

Recipes

Chicken and White Beans   Serves 3

Ingredients

- 2 large fennel bulb, chopped into thin slices
- 1 tablespoon olive oil
- 2 chicken breasts, sliced into bite-sized pieces
- 1 teaspoon crushed rosemary
- 1 teaspoon pepper
- 2 cups chicken stock
- 1 can cannellini beans, rinsed and drained

Cooking instructions

1. Heat oil in a large pan. Add fennel slices and cook for 5 minutes, stirring.
2. Add chicken and rosemary, cooking another 5 minutes.
3. Add stock and bring to a boil. Cover and simmer 10 minutes.
4. Stir in beans, reduce heat, and simmer 10 minutes, until sauce thickens.

Nutrition Facts

	Per Meal	*Per Serving*
Grams	1169g	1390g
Calories	1200cal	400cal
Protein	71g	24g
Fat	29g	10g
Carbs	84g	28g
PRAL	-17.10	-5.7

Recipes

Scallops with Spinach and Arugula — Serves 2

Ingredients

- 16 large sea scallops, rinsed and dried
- Salt and pepper to taste
- 3 tablespoons canola oil
- 2 garlic cloves, sliced
- 7 ounces baby spinach
- 7 ounces baby arugula
- 1/4 teaspoon crush red-pepper flakes

Cooking Instructions

1. Pour two tablespoons of the oil into a large skillet over medium-high heat.
2. Season scallops with a pinch of salt and pepper and place them in the skillet. Cook for 6 to 7 minutes,
3. Flip them and then cook for 30 seconds. Remove and set aside.
4. Reduce the heat to medium, and pour in the rest of the oil. Add the garlic and cook, stirring rapidly, for about 15 seconds.
5. Add the spinach, arugula, red-pepper flakes, and another pinch of salt and pepper. Cook for 2 minutes, stirring often.
6. Serve the scallops with the greens.
7. Season with salt and pepper to taste

Nutrition Facts

	Per Meal	*Per Serving*
Grams	625g	313g
Calories	679 cal	340 cal
Protein	54g	27g
Fat	43g	22g
Carbs	22g	11g
PRAL	-18.42	-9.21

Recipes

Chicken with Zucchini and Squash — Serves 3

Ingredients

- 2 boneless, skinless chicken breast halves
- 1 (14.5 ounce) can stewed tomatoes
- 1 yellow squash, thinly sliced
- 1 medium zucchini, thinly sliced

Cooking Instructions

1. Pre-heat oven to 375 degrees F.
2. Lightly grease a medium baking dish.
3. Arrange chicken in the prepared baking dish, and top with the stewed tomatoes. Arrange squash and zucchini slices around the chicken.
4. Bake 45 minutes in the preheated oven.

Nutrition Facts

	Per Meal	*Per Serving*
Grams	1039g	346g
Calories	651 cal	217 cal
Protein	66g	22g
Fat	4g	1g
Carbs	68g	23g
PRAL	-1.56	-0.52

Recipes

Asian Steak   Serves 4

Ingredients

- 1 lb sirloin
- 3 tablespoons soy sauce
- 1 tablespoon honey
- 3 cloves garlic, finely chopped
- 1 tablespoon fresh ginger, finely chopped
- 1 tablespoon sesame oil
- 3 tablespoons olive oil, divided
- 3 tablespoons black sesame seeds
- 1 large Asian pear, cut into wedges
- 2 green onions
- 1.5 pound Chinese Broccoli

Cooking Instructions

1. Slice beef thinly, and lay in an overproof dish.
2. In a separate bowl, combine soy sauce, honey, sesame oil, 1 tablespoon of olive oil, and 1 tablespoon of sesame seeds. Pour over meat and mix thoroughly.
3. Refrigerate 30 minutes. Drain marinade and heat grill.
4. Brush grill with remaining oil.
5. Grill meat strips for 1-2 minutes per side.
6. Grill pear wedges for 2 minutes per side, until golden.
7. Steam Chinese broccoli and toss with scallions before serving.
8. Serve beef with pear and Chinese broccoli.

Nutrition Facts

	Per Meal	*Per Serving*
Grams	1549g	387g
Calories	1617 cal	404 cal
Protein	109g	27g
Fat	107g	27g
Carbs	84g	21g
PRAL	-8.61	-2.15

Recipes

Avocado Chicken Salad   Serves 4

Ingredients

- 3 tablespoons olive oil
- 2 boneless skinless chicken breasts
- 1 1 teaspoon chili powder
- Salt and pepper to taste
- 1/4cup chopped fresh coriander
- 2 tablespoons lime juice or cider vinegar
- 1/4teaspoon granulated sugar
- 1/4teaspoon hot pepper sauce
- 1 clove of garlic, minced
- 2 tablespoon light mayonnaise
- 2 cups cooked corn kernels
- 1 avocado, peeled and cubed
- 1 sweet red peppers, sliced
- 1/2 small red onions, sliced
- 1 head Boston lettuce, separated
- 4 hard-cooked eggs, quartered
- 2 tomatoes, cut in wedges

Cooking Instructions

1. Remove 2 teaspoon of the oil; brush over chicken. Sprinkle with chili powder and pinch each salt and pepper.
2. Place on greased grill over medium-high heat; close lid and cook, turning once for about 8 minutes.
3. Whisk together coriander, lime juice, sugar, hot pepper sauce, garlic and remaining oil, salt and pepper. Remove 2 tablespoon and mix with mayonnaise.
4. Toss corn, avocado, red pepper and onion with remaining dressing; mound on lettuce-lined platter.
5. Slice chicken and arrange over salad.
6. Surround with eggs and tomatoes; drizzle with mayonnaise mixture.

Recipes
Avocado Chicken Salad   **Serves 4**

Nutrition Facts

	Per Meal	*Per Serving*
Grams	1688g	422g
Calories	1502 cal	376 cal
Protein	85g	21g
Fat	85g	21g
Carbs	130g	33g
PRAL	-20.17	-5.04

Recipes
Broccoli, Salmon, and Cottage Cheese Bake   Serves 3

Ingredients

- 1 can wild red pacific salmon
- 5 cups steamed broccoli
- 2 cups cottage cheese
- 2 tablespoons pesto

Cooking Instructions

1. Combine all ingredients together
2. Place in an oiled baking dish.
3. Bake in preheated 350 degree oven for 20 minutes.

Nutrition Facts

	Per Meal	Per Serving
Grams	935g	322g
Calories	611 cal	204 cal
Protein	71g	24g
Fat	17g	6g
Carbs	51g	17g
PRAL	-2.72	-0.93

Recipes

Cooked Salmon with Onion   Serves 3

Ingredients

- 2 x 6oz. Salmon fillets
- Sea salt and fresh ground black pepper
- 1 cup lager beer (or vegetable/ fish stock)
- 1 tablespoon chopped fresh tarragon
- 2 tablespoons fresh lemon juice
- 1 cup sliced green onion
- 2 tablespoons olive oil

Cooking Instructions

1. Preheat oven to 225 F.
2. Season salmon with salt and pepper and lay it in an ovenproof dish.
3. Combine remaining ingredients in a pot and bring to a boil. Pour over salmon.
4. Bake 25 minutes, basting once, until slightly pink in the centre.
5. Reheat basting liquid until thickened (1/4 cup remaining). Drizzle over salmon.

Serve with steamed asparagus or bok choy.

Nutrition Facts

	Per Meal	Per Serving
Grams	745g	242g
Calories	897 cal	299 cal
Protein	78g	26g
Fat	18g	6g
Carbs	52g	17g
PRAL	-4.44	-1.45

Recipes
Steamed Chicken and Asparagus and Cauliflower — Serves 4

Ingredients

- 2 large boneless skinless chicken breast halves
- 500g of fresh asparagus
- Salt and pepper to taste
- 1 head of cauliflower
- 2-3 cloves of garlic, peeled and coarsely minced
- Lemon juice from half a lemon
- 1 tablespoon of Olive oil

Cooking Instructions

Chicken and Asparagus

1. Bring 1-2 cups of water to a boil.
2. Trim the asparagus by cutting off the tough stock.
3. Rinse the chicken in cold water and add salt and pepper to taste.
4. Place the chicken and the asparagus side by side on the food steamer rack and steam for 10 to 15 minutes until asparagus is crisp.

Cauliflower

1. Preheat oven to 400°F.
2. Cut cauliflower into florets and put in a single layer in an oven-proof baking dish.
3. Toss in the garlic.
4. Sprinkle lemon juice over cauliflower and drizzle each piece with olive oil.
5. Add salt and pepper to taste.
6. Place casserole in the hot oven, uncovered, for 25-30 minutes, or until the top is lightly brown.

Recipes

Steamed Chicken and Asparagus and Cauliflower   Serves 4

Nutrition Facts

	Per Meal	Per Serving
Grams	2040g	510g
Calories	781 cal	195 cal
Protein	92g	23g
Fat	15g	4g
Carbs	89g	22g
PRAL	-26.41	-6.6

Recipes

Seared Scallops with Arugula and Spinach   **Serves 1**

Ingredients

- 6 fresh, large sea scallops
- ½ teaspoon each of cumin and paprika
- Salt and pepper
- 2 tablespoons olive oil
- ¼ cup white wine
- 2 teaspoons each of resh lime juice and olive oil
- 1 cup each of arugula and baby spinach

Cooking Instructions

1. Place scallops in a small bowl. Sprinkle with cumin, paprika, salt and pepper.
2. Heat oil in a fry pan over medium-high heat. When hot, add scallops, cooking 3 minutes per side, until golden.
3. Add wine and reduce heat to medium-low. Cook 3 more minutes.
4. Whisk lime juice and 2 teaspoon olive oil in a small bowl. Place greens on 2 plates, drizzle with olive oil and lime mixture. Place 3 scallops on each. Serves 2.

Nutrition Facts

	Per Meal	Per Serving
Grams	316g	316g
Calories	437 cal	437 cal
Protein	16g	16g
Fat	28g	28g
Carbs	13g	13g
PRAL	-0.78	-0.78

Recipes
Orange Salmon with Ginger and Spinach — Serves 3

Ingredients

Salmon
- 1 orange, washed, peeled, and juiced.
- 1 tablespoon honey
- 2 tablespoons olive oil
- 1/2 teaspoon red pepper flakes
- 1 tablespoon fresh ginger, peeled and finely chopped.
- 2 x 6oz salmon fillets

Spinach
- (100g) 4 handfuls fresh spinach, washed and trimmed
- 1 glove garlic, finely chopped
- 1 teaspoon olive oil
- 1 tablespoon lemon juice
- Sea salt and fresh ground pepper

Cooking Instructions

1. Combine orange juice, honey, olive oil, ginger, and red pepper flakes.
2. Place salmon in a dish and pour liquid overtop. Marinate 30 minutes in fridge.
3. Grill salmon on a BBQ or indoor grill for 5 -7 minutes per side.
4. Just before salmon is finished, sauté spinach over medium heat, with 1 t olive oil and chopped garlic (careful not to burn garlic).
5. Place spinach on a plate, squeeze lemon overtop and season with salt and pepper. Place salmon fillet on top.

Nutrition Facts

	Per Meal	Per Serving
Grams	711g	237g
Calories	632 cal	211 cal
Protein	71g	24g
Fat	14g	5g
Carbs	26g	8.7g
PRAL	-2.42	-0.87

Recipes

Grilled Chicken with Pineapple — Serves 3

Ingredients

- 1/4 cup lemon juice
- 2 tablespoons lime juice
- 2 tablespoons orange juice
- 1 tablespoon canola oil
- 1/2 teaspoon oregano
- Salt and pepper to taste
- 2 chicken breasts
- 2 tomatoes - seeded, chopped
- 1 cup pineapple - chopped
- 1/2 cup red pepper - chopped
- 1/2 cup red onion - chopped
- 1 jalapeño - seeded, finely chopped
- 1/4 cup cilantro - chopped

Cooking Instructions

1. In a large re-sealable plastic bag, combine the first eight ingredients. Add chicken and seal bag; turn to coat. Refrigerate for at least 4 hours.
2. In a small bowl, combine remaining ingredients. Cover and refrigerate until serving.
3. Preheat grill to medium heat. Drain and discard marinade. Grill, covered, over medium heat for 5-6 minutes on each side or until chicken is no longer pink in the middle. Serve with salsa.

Nutrition Facts

	Per Meal	*Per Serving*
Grams	1102g	367g
Calories	715 cal	238 cal
Protein	64g	21g
Fat	15g	5g
Carbs	83g	28g
PRAL	-30.35	-10.12

Recipes
Ground Meat with Eggplant, Onions, and Pepper — Serves 2

Ingredients

- 1 eggplant
- 1/4 cup canola corn oil
- 1 cup lean ground beef
- 1/3 cup onions, sliced
- 1 ounce pine nuts
- Add salt and pepper to taste
- 1/4 cup minced parsley
- 1 small onion, sliced
- 1 green pepper, sliced
- 1 teaspoon salt
- 2 large tomatoes, sliced

Cooking Instructions

- Wash and stem the eggplants and pat dry.
- Sautee them in a skillet in the heated oil.
- Cut a pocket lengthwise in each eggplant.
- In the same oil sautee the ground meat for ten minutes.
- Stir in the one-third cup sliced onions and sautee ten more minutes.
- Add the pine nuts and cook for two to three minutes longer.
- Add salt and pepper to taste.
- Stir in the parsley.
- Cool slightly and fill the eggplants with the meat mixture.
- Arrange in a lightly oiled baking dish.
- Cover with the sliced onion, green pepper, salt and remaining oil from the pan.
- Arrange the tomatoes decoratively over the top.
- Bake at 350 degrees for about forty minutes, basting from time to time with some of the juices from the pan.

Recipes
Ground Meat with Eggplant, Onions, and Pepper — Serves 2

Nutrition Facts

	Per Meal	*Per Serving*
Grams	1625g	813g
Calories	1136 cal	568cal
Protein	45g	23g
Fat	80g	40g
Carbs	88g	44g
PRAL	-34.39	-17.2

Recipes

Beef and Kale Serves 2

Ingredients

- 1 cup lean ground beef
- 1 cup chopped onion
- 1 cup sliced crimini mushrooms
- Taco seasoning
- 1-2 teaspoons extra virgin olive oil
- 3 eggs
- 4 cups kale (rinsed, de-stemmed and coarsely chopped)
- 2 teaspoons of hot sauce

Cooking Instructions

1. Cook ground beef in large sauté pan over medium heat, stirring frequently.
2. After about 3 minutes, add onion. Continue to stir as cooking.
3. After 3 more minutes add mushrooms and sprinkle with seasoning.
4. Heat olive oil in separate skillet on medium heat. Once warm, crack eggs into skillet.
5. Add kale and stir frequently.
6. Skillet is ready when kale turns bright green.
7. Remove from skillet onto plates and top with egg and hot sauce.

Nutrition Facts

	Per Meal	*Per Serving*
Grams	767g	384g
Calories	686 cal	343 cal
Protein	54g	27g
Fat	33g	17g
Carbs	43g	22g
PRAL	-2.66	-1.33

Recipes

Spinach Omelette `Serves 1

Ingredients

- 2 eggs
- 4 cup torn baby spinach leaves
- 1 1/2 tablespoons grated Parmesan cheese
- 1/4 teaspoon onion powder
- 1/8 teaspoon ground nutmeg
- Salt and pepper to taste

Cooking Instructions

1. In a bowl, beat the eggs, and stir in the baby spinach and Parmesan cheese. Season with onion powder, nutmeg, salt, and pepper.
2. In a small skillet coated with cooking spray over medium heat, cook the egg mixture about 3 minutes, until partially set. Flip with a spatula, and continue cooking 2 to 3 minutes. Reduce heat to low, and continue cooking 2 to 3 minutes, or to desired doneness.

Nutrition Facts

	Per Meal	*Per Serving*
Grams	252g	252g
Calories	249 cal	249 cal
Protein	25g	25g
Fat	11g	11g
Carbs	15g	15g
PRAL	-4.66	-4.66

Recipes

Mushroom Spinach Omelette   Serves 1

Ingredients

- 1 egg
- 3 egg whites
- 1/4 teaspoon salt
- 1/8 teaspoon crushed red pepper flakes
- 1/8 teaspoon garlic powder
- 1/8 teaspoon pepper
- 1/2 cup sliced fresh mushrooms
- 2 tablespoons finely chopped green pepper
- 1 tablespoon finely chopped onion
- 1/2 teaspoon olive oil
- 2 cup torn fresh spinach

Cooking Instructions

1. In a small bowl, beat the egg and egg whites. Add cheeses, salt, pepper flakes, garlic powder and pepper; mix well. Set aside.
2. In an 8-in. nonstick skillet, sauté the mushrooms, green pepper and onion in oil for 4-5 minutes or until tender. Add spinach; cook and stir until spinach is wilted. Add egg mixture. As eggs set, lift edges, letting uncooked portion flow underneath. Cut into wedges. Serve immediately.

Nutrition Facts

	Per Meal	*Per Serving*
Total Grams	342g	342g
Total Calories	340 cal	340 cal
Protein	31g	31g
Fat	18g	18g
Carbohydrates	22g	22g
PRAL	-2.0	-2.0

Recipes

Kale and Potato Omelette   Serves 2

Ingredients

- 350g (12oz) medium waxy potatoes, diced
- 1 tablespoon olive oil
- 175g (6oz) onion, sliced
- 75g (3oz) kale, shredded
- 6 medium eggs, beaten
- 75ml (2 1/4fl oz) milk

Cooking Instructions

1. Boil the potatoes for 8-10 minutes until tender, then drain.
2. Meanwhile, heat the oil in a 24cm frying pan and fry the onion and kale for 7-8 minutes. Add the potatoes.
3. Mix together the eggs, milk and seasoning. Pour into the frying pan and cook gently, covered for 7-8 minutes, finishing under a preheated grill for 1-2 minutes until cooked throughout.

Nutrition Facts

	Per Meal	*Per Serving*
Total Grams	642g	321g
Total Calories	862 cal	431 cal
Protein	43g	22g
Fat	41g	21g
Carbohydrates	156g	78g
PRAL	-10.92	-5.96

Recipes

Swiss Chard with Lemon   Serves 1

Ingredients

- 1 tablespoon olive oil
- 12 cups Swiss chard (about 2 pounds)
- ½ teaspoon red pepper flakes
- 3 cloves garlic, minced
- 1 tablespoon fresh lemon juice
- ¼ teaspoon salt

Cooking Instructions

1. Heat oil in a large pan over medium heat. Add chard and sauté 1 minute.
2. Stir in pepper and garlic. Cook 4 minutes, until tender.
3. Uncover and cook until liquid evaporates. Add lemon juice and salt.(serves 4)

Nutrition Facts

	Per Meal	*Per Serving*
Grams	477g	477g
Calories	224 cal	224 cal
Protein	12g	12g
Fat	14g	4g
Carbs	17g	17g
PRAL	-35.78	-35.78

Recipes

Broccoli and Red Pepper with Ginger — Serves 1

Ingredients

- 1 tablespoon unrefined cold- processed sesame oil
- 2 cups broccoli, cut into florets, and the stem into thin slices
- 1 red pepper, cut into strips
- 1 inch ginger, cut into very thin slices
- ¼ cup water

Cooking Instructions

1. Heat a large pan over medium heat till hot.
2. Add oil and broccoli, frying for 2 minutes.
3. Add pepper, ginger and ¼ cup water.
4. Cover and cook for 3 minutes.

Nutrition Facts

	Per Meal	*Per Serving*
Grams	565g	565g
Calories	282 cal	282 cal
Protein	13g	13g
Fat	14g	14g
Carbs	31g	31g
PRAL	-22.33	-22.33

*High carbohydrate option – base serving size on bodyweight and phase

Recipes
Sautéed Bok Choy and Broccoli with Cashews — Serves 1

Ingredients

- 1 cup baby bok choy
- 1 small head broccoli, cut into florets, and stem cut into slices.
- 1 clove garlic, finely chopped
- 1 tablespoon olive oil
- 2 tablespoons chopped cashews

Cooking Instructions

1. Boil broccoli and bok choy for 1 minute in a pot of boiling water, covered.
2. Drain and set aside.
3. Sautee garlic in 1 T olive oil, preventing it from burning.
4. Add the greens and toss to heat through.
5. Serve topped with cashews.

Nutrition Facts

	Per Meal	*Per Serving*
Grams	391g	391g
Calories	384 cal	384 cal
Protein	15g	15g
Fat	26g	26g
Carbs	31g	31g
PRAL	-9.18	-9.18

High carbohydrate option – base serving size on bodyweight and phase

Recipes

Grilled Zucchini with Lemon and Dill — Serves 1

Ingredients

- 4 medium zucchini, sliced lengthwise
- 2 tablespoons olive oil
- Juice of 1 lemon
- 2 tablespoons chopped, fresh dill
- Salt and pepper to taste

Cooking Instructions

1. Preheat oven to 400.
2. Lay zucchini slices on a baking sheet, brushing both sides with olive oil.
3. Season with salt and pepper.
4. Grill for 10-15 minutes.
5. Squeeze lemon juice over top and add dill.

Nutrition Facts

	Per Meal	*Per Serving*
Grams	849g	849g
Calories	408 cal	408 cal
Protein	10g	10g
Fat	30g	30g
Carbs	37g	37g
PRAL	-37.12	-37.12

*High carbohydrate option – base serving size on bodyweight and phase

Recipes

Light Lemon Cauliflower   Serves 1

Ingredients

- ¼ cup fresh, chopped parsley
- 1 teaspoon lemon zest
- 6 cups (1 head) cauliflower florets
- 1 tablespoon olive oil
- 2 cloves garlic, minced
- 2 tablespoon fresh lemon juice
- ¼ cup goat's cheese (optional)

Cooking Instructions

1. Place 1 tablespoon parsley and lemon zest in 1 inch water. Place cauliflower in a steamer over top. Bring water to a boil over medium heat.
2. Cover and steam 15 minutes or until cauliflower is crisp – tender.
3. Heat olive oil in fry pan. Add garlic, cooking 2 minutes until soft. Stir in lemon juice and reserved water from steaming cauliflower.
4. Spoon sauce over cauliflower and top with remaining parsley and goat cheese. Serves 4.

Nutrition Facts

	Per Meal	*Per Serving*
Grams	677g	677g
Calories	295 cal	295 cal
Protein	13g	13g
Fat	14g	14g
Carbs	35g	35g
PRAL	-28.56	-28.56

Recipes
Cabbage and Red Peppers with Black Sesame Seeds — Serves 1

Ingredients

- 1 tablespoon black sesame seeds
- 1 tablespoon olive oil
- 5 cups thinly sliced Savoy cabbage
- 1 red pepper, thinly sliced
- 3 tablespoons brown rice vinegar
- 2 tablespoons soy sauce
- 1 teaspoon garlic minced
- 1 teaspoon chili paste
- 1 teaspoon sesame oil

Cooking Instructions

1. Heat oil in a large pan over medium heat. Add cabbage and peppers, cooking for 5 minutes.
2. Add vinegar, soy sauce, garlic, and chili paste. Reduce heat to low-medium and cook 5-7 minutes, stirring occasionally.
3. Remove from heat and stir in sesame seeds and sesame oil.

Nutrition Facts

	Per Meal	Per Serving
Grams	577g	577g
Calories	599 cal	599 cal
Protein	8g	8g
Fat	51g	51g
Carbs	30g	30g
PRAL	-16.82	-16.82

Part VII: The Kick Acid Diet Workout Program

"Absorb what is useful, discard what is not, add what is uniquely your own"
Bruce Lee

The Kick Acid Diet Workout Program

The *Kick Acid Diet* Workout Program is an easy to follow regime that will get you the body you desire. Resistance training is not only important if you want to be lean. It is also crucial to your health. Resistance training has also been shown to improve health by increasing bone density, improving mental health, and lowering blood pressure.

Since this book is about metabolism, let's talk about the relationship between resistance training, muscle mass, and fat loss. Our **basal metabolic rate** (BMR), that is, the amount of calories we burn at rest, accounts for the largest portion of energy expenditure, and muscle is the only part of BMR that is variable. The most effective way to burn more calories, is to increase your muscle mass.

Muscle increases fat loss in other ways, too. Strength-trained muscles are more responsive to insulin, improving insulin sensitivity, and thus, improving fat loss. In addition, muscle allows us to be more mobile, which in turn allows us to increase the amount of activity we can perform.

If you're an athlete whose goal is to improve performance, weight training is essential. Stronger muscles not only enhance one's performance, but will also prevent injury.

Finally, muscle gives both men and women the shape and curves desired.

The *Kick Acid Diet* Workout Program is a simple and effective program that can be performed anywhere. All you need to complete these workouts is a set of dumbbells, chin-up bar, bench, and a mat. If you're performing this workout at home, I highly recommend the use of selectorized dumbbells. A selectorized dumbbell set combines an entire set of adjustable weights into one compact unit. Most sets range in weight from 5lbs to 80lbs.

Whether you're a seasoned veteran or a weight-training rookie, this program will work for you. Each exercise is designed to move your body through a full range of motion, thus, not only increasing strength, but also increasing mobility. While you'll be pushing yourself to complete each workout, you will never reach total failure, or the point at which you cannot move the weight. .It's divided into three phases, each phase lasting six weeks. During each six week cycle, you will employ the principle of progressive overload. Increasing the resistance and/or reps each workout will force your body to change, increasing its muscle mass, as it accommodates to the increased stimulus. As your muscle mass increases, so will your body's ability to shed unwanted fat!

The Kick Acid Diet Workout Program

Each phase corresponds to the phases described in the previous chapter, the *Kick Acid Diet*. The goals are identical to the previous chapter – Muscle Up; Fat Loss; and Maintenance. The Performance Phase from the last chapter doesn't have a corresponding workout as it depends on what your training and competition goals are.

The *Kick Acid Diet* workouts are effective in helping you reach your goals. They are proven programs that many have used with success. What's more is that you don't need to belong to a gym in order to perform them. Each workout is designed so it can be performed in a gym or in the "comfort" of your own home. I use the word comfort loosely, as these workouts may be simple in design, they will challenge you to your limits.

Many of you reading this book already engage in a regular weight training program. That's great! The workouts are designed for those new to weight training or for those of you who are looking for some variety. Either way, the dietary recommendations given in the previous chapter will be more effective in conjunction with a weight training program – mine…or yours.

In order to determine the weights for your first workout of each phase, choose a weight that you can complete two additional reps compared to the prescribed rep range. For example, if you are starting the Muscle Up phase, choose a weight that you can do 12 reps with.

Another important point worth considering is how each rep is performed. To prevent the risk of injury, each rep should only be completed through a full range of motion. In addition (with the exception of abdominal crunches), a neutral spine, which involves a slight curvature in your lumbar spine should be maintained to avoid the risk of back injury.

Phase one is the Muscle Up phase. The muscle building phase is important as it lays the foundation for getting the body you desire and for life-long fat burning!

Phase Two is Fat Loss. The goal of this phase is to burn calories by following the *Kick Acid Diet* and utilizing your body's increased muscle mass gained during phase one.

Finally phase three is the Maintenance Phase. This phase emphasize a healthy lifestyle, which incorporates a regular weight training program, while making healthy eating choices that maintain the alkalinity of your body.

There's a full description of each exercise at the end of this chapter. Each description is accompanied by a picture and easy to follow instructions.

The Kick Acid Diet Workout Program

Before starting each workout, it is best to familiarize yourself with some common weight training terms that will be seen in this chapter.

First, a repetition is simply the performance of a complete cycle of an exercise, from start position to the end position, and returning to the starting position. A set is a series of repetitions, the number usually established in the parameters of the workout. A superset is a combination of two or more exercises in row, prior to a rest break.

The Kick Acid Diet Workout Program
STEP 5: BIOMARKER HEALTH ASSESSMENT

To know where you're going, you have to know where you're from. Before starting the *Kick Acid Diet Workout Program*, I recommend that you take the self-administered Biomarker Health Assessment.

This fitness assessment based on the Biomarkers of Aging concept. Researchers have determined that there are 10 markers that are more indicative of one's health than one's biological age. We'll focus on the biomarkers related to body composition: body mass index; percent body fat and lean body mass; and waist-to-hip ratio. For a full description of all the biomarkers and how to improve them with diet and exercise, refer to the Appendix or log onto to our website at www.thekickaciddiet.com

In order to perform the self-administered fitness assessment, you will need the following: Tanita ® bioelectrical impedance scale, cloth tape measure, and calculator.

Body Mass Index (BMI)

Body Mass Index is a ratio between a person's body weight and height. It is a mathematical formula that correlates somewhat with body fat. In general, if your BMI is high, you may have an increased risk of developing certain disease including hypertension, cardiovascular disease and others. BMI is a better predictor of disease risk than body weight alone. Competitive athletes, body builders, women who are pregnant or lactating, growing children or frail and sedentary elderly individuals should not use BMI as the basis for estimating their body fat content.

<u>Measurement</u>

1. Weigh yourself and record the number in kilograms
2. Using the cloth tape measure, record your height in metres.
3. Enter your numbers into the following formula to determine your BMI:

$$BMI = \frac{\text{weight (kg)}}{\text{height (m)} \times \text{height (m)}}$$

The Kick Acid Diet Workout Program

Percent Body Fat

Body Fat Mass is the body's less metabolically active storage tissue, technically known as "adipose tissue." With advancing age, even if our body weight doesn't change much, most of us tend to gain fat and lose heavier muscle tissue.

<u>Measurement</u>

1. Follow the directions on the unit.

Lean Body Mass (LBM)

Lean Body Mass consists of muscle, bone and other vital organ tissues of the body, in short, everything that is not fat. LBM is one of the most crucial components of the body to preserve and build. Protein provides the building blocks for the maintenance and growth of LBM, which determines approximately 90 percent of the Basal Metabolic Rate (BMR) of the body. Lean Body Mass is also known as Fat Free Mass (FFM).

<u>Measurement</u>

1. If you're using a Tanita ® scale, your lean body mass will be displayed.
2. Method two involves using the following formula:
   Lean Body Mass = Body Weight x (100-% Body Fat)

Waist Hip Ratio (WHR)

Your *waist to hip ratio (WHR)* is a measure of how fat is distributed throughout your body. Abdominal fat is related to an increased risk of many conditions, such as cardiovascular disease and diabetes.

<u>Measurement</u>

1. Using a cloth tape measure, measure the following points:
   - Waist: level of (umbilicus) belly button.
   - Hip: level of largest circumference at the buttocks or hip

2. Divide the waist circumference by the hip circumference to obtain the WHR.
   - WHR = waist circumference/hip circumference

The Kick Acid Diet Workout Program

Girth Measurements

Your girth measurements are not a component of the Biomarker of Aging method, but will give you a good indication of your progress. In addition to recording your waist-to-hip ratio, I recommend you record the girth measurements at the following points.

- Neck: Level of Adam's apple
- Chest (male): Level of nipples on full exhalation.
- Upper Arm: 2cm above the elbow crease with the arm in relaxed and vertical position.
- Mid Thigh: 4cm above the knee with leg in a relaxed position and foot on the floor.
- Calf: 4cm below the knee with leg in a relaxed position and foot on the floor.

Refer to the Appendix to see how your results measure up.

The Kick Acid Diet Workout Program
Kick Acid Diet Warm Up

The Kick Acid Diet Warm Up is not only important to prevent injury, but to have an effective workout. If you don't warm up properly, much of your actual workout serves as warm up, not allowing you to push yourself as hard as you need to.

The warm-up serves numerous functions. First, it increases blood flow, providing nutrients to the muscles. In the process, muscles become warm, allowing them to be more flexible.

An often overlooked benefit of a good warm up is it prepares your nervous system for the workout. Your nervous system is the control centre of your body, and in this case, controls proper movement of your muscles and joints. Priming your nervous system will increase the efficiency of movement, allowing you to increase the intensity of your workout.

Finally, the warm up serves as a mental prep for the upcoming workout.

The Kick Acid Diet Warm Up is what is known as a dynamic warm up. A dynamic warm up involves movement of the entire body, ensuring that all joints are moved through their full range of motion and at speeds similar to the exercises being performed.

The Kick Acid Diet Warm Up will be the same for each workout and will gradually increase in intensity. The warm up will last up to five minutes. If you're still feeling stiff after five minutes, feel free to repeat the circuit and you feel ready to go!

The first thing you'll notice is that there is no static stretching performed during the warm up. Static stretching has been actually shown to cause increased stiffness to muscles, increasing the risk of injury if performed prior to the workout. Static stretches can be done after the workout as long you remain injury free.

The Kick Acid Diet Workout Program

Circuit

Jumping Jacks   20 reps

Start with your arms at your sides and feet together. Next, jump so your legs are now spread apart, and your arms come together above your head. Return to the starting position with your arms at your sides and feet together.

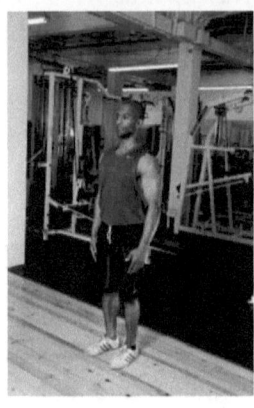 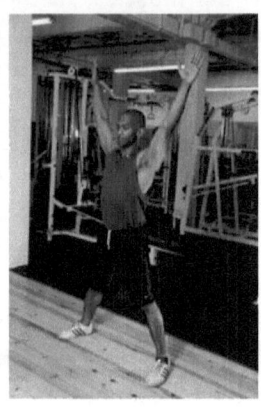 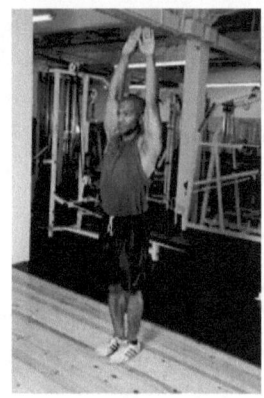

Arm Circles   10 reps each direction

Start with your feet shoulder width apart and arms at your side. Keeping your arms straight, swing your arms in full circles by bringing your arms behind your body and around to the starting position.

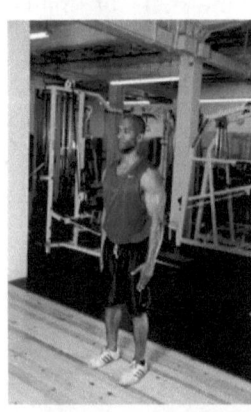 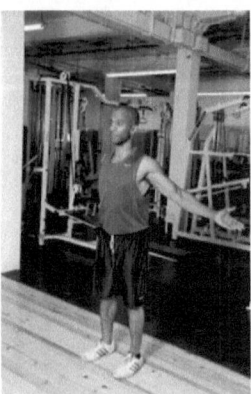 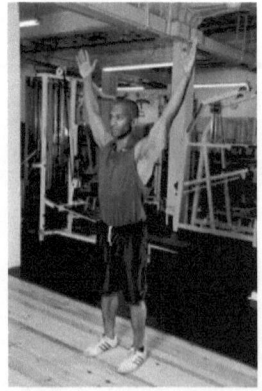

The Kick Acid Diet Workout Program

Bent Arm Swings   10 reps each arm

    Start with your feet shoulder with apart and arms to the sides with your elbows bent to 90 degrees. Swing your right arm forward so your upper arm is parallel to the ground. At the same time, swing your left arm back so your upper arm is parallel to the ground. Alternate sides.

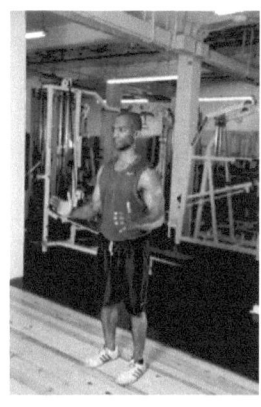 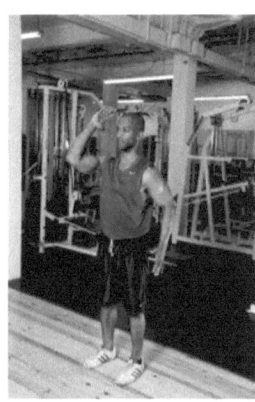

High Knee Skip   20 reps each leg

    Start with your feet shoulder width apart and elbows bent to 90 degrees. March by bringing your knee right knee up as high as possible and pointing your right foot up towards the ceiling. At the same time, swing your right arm back and left arm forward (as in Bent Arm Swing). Alternate.

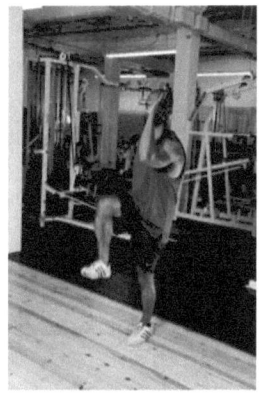

The Kick Acid Diet Workout Program

Butt Kicks   20 reps each leg

Start with your feet shoulder width apart and arms to your sides. March by bringing your knee right knee up as high as possible and pointing your right foot up towards the ceiling. At the same time, swing your right arm back and left arm forward (as in Bent Arm Swing). Alternate.

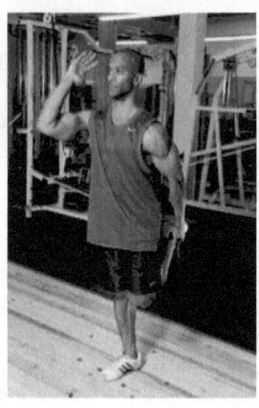

Body Weight Squats   20 reps

Start the exercise by standing with your feet shoulder width apart, and toes pointed slightly outward.

With your spine in neutral, inhale and tighten your abdominals, while lowering your body until the top of your thighs are parallel to the ground. Once, you reach this position, continue to hold your breath, and pushing with both the balls and heels of your feet, straighten your knees and your hips until you return to the start position, exhaling at the top.

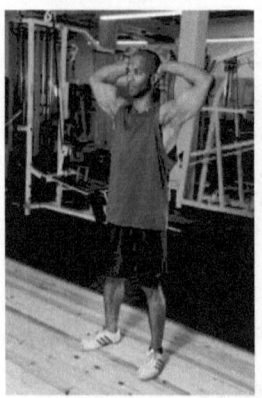 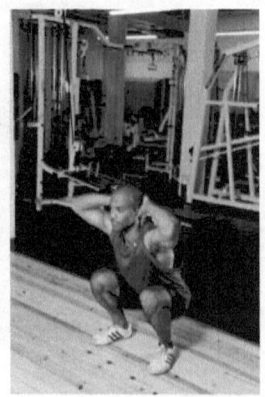

The Kick Acid Diet Workout Program

Walking Lunges   10 reps each leg

Start the movement stepping forward with one leg, bending it until the front thigh is parallel to ground and knee is bent to 90 degrees. The back knee should also be bent to 90 degrees. Bend forward at the hips while maintaining a neutral spine. Hold your breath at the bottom, return to the start position by straightening your stance leg at the knees and hips. Exhale at the top. Alternate legs while walking forward. *To be performed without dumbbells.*

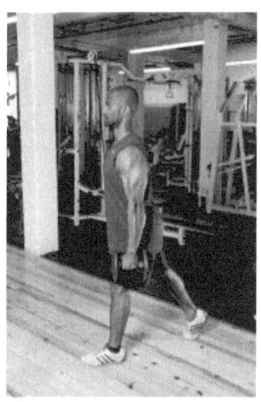 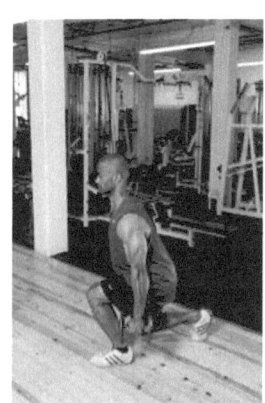

Low Lunge   10 reps each leg

Start the movement stepping forward with your leg, bending it until the right thigh is parallel to ground and knee is bent to 90 degrees. The back knee (left) should also be bent to 90 degrees. Bend forward at the hips while maintaining a neutral spine. Place your left elbow on the ground inside your right foot. Alternate legs.

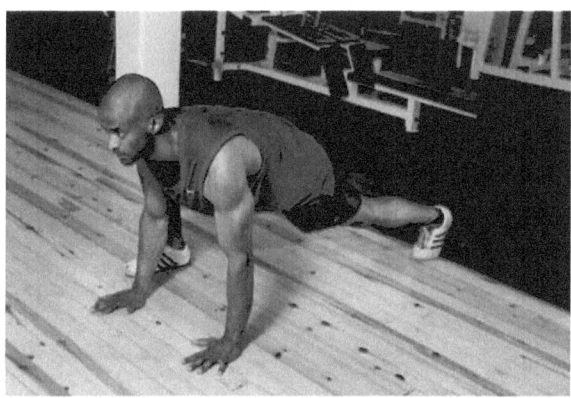

The Kick Acid Diet Workout Program

Phase 1: Muscle Up   6 weeks

Phase 1 involves four workouts a week divided into lower body and abdominals, and upper body. The workouts are based on successful bodybuilding routines designed to increase muscle size and definition.

Many people, especially women, are concerned that this type of training will result in bulky muscles. It is difficult to look like a bodybuilder, and the men and women dedicated to the sport of bodybuilding, have committed years, train with advanced methods, and have consumed a lot of calories to look the way they do.

There are two options with the muscle up phase. I recommend that beginners follow the workout program has planned, training four days a week. More advanced trainees can train six days a week, opting to include workout 3, arms and shoulders.

Workout 1

1. Squats
2. Deadlifts
3. Stiff-Leg Deadlifts
4. One Leg Standing Calf Raises

Workout 2

Superset 1
1.a. Dumbbell Bench Press
1.a. Chin Up

Superset 2
2.a. Incline Dumbbell Bench Press
2.b. Dumbbell Bent Over Row

Superset 3
3.a. One-Arm Dumbbell Row
3.b Decline Push-Ups

The Kick Acid Diet Workout Program
Workout 3

Superset 1
1.a. Dumbbell Shoulder Press
1.b. Dumbbell Skull Crusher

Superset 2
2.a. Dumbbell Bicep Curl
2.b. Lateral Dumbbell Raise

Superset 3
3.a. Tricep Bench Dip
3.b. Dumbbell Hammer Curl

<u>Notes</u>

Sets	3
Repetitions	10-12
Rest Interval	60 seconds
Tempo	1 second up; 2 seconds down

Progression
- Increase reps each workout, until you reach 12 reps
- Then, increase weight by 5lbs, and drop reps down to 10. Repeat

The Kick Acid Diet Workout Program
Phase 2:   Fat Loss   4 Weeks

Phase 2 employs a method of training known as metabolic conditioning. Metabolic conditioning, also known as interval training, is a method of training that allows individuals to train for both cardiovascular and strength endurance without sacrificing muscle. In turn, fat loss is increased during the workout and at rest.

This phase involves three workouts a week, with at least one day of rest between workouts. The large muscle groups will targeted during each workout. Advanced trainees can incorporate workout 3 (twice a week) from the Muscle Up phase.

The completion of each circuit is considered one set. This phase is demand which is why it only lasts four weeks. If you decide that you want to spend more time in this phase, increase the weight used by 5-10% for all exercises (where appropriate) and begin the cycle from the start.

Workout 1

Circuit
- One Leg Dumbbell Squat
- Dumbbell Bent Over Row
- Dumbbell Clean
- Dumbbell Bench Press
- Dumbbell Jump Squat

The weight is the same for all exercises
Perform each exercise consecutively without rest

Workout 2

Circuit
- Dumbbell Clean + Squat
- One Arm Clean (Alternate Arms)
- Burpee (Alternate: Burpee + Push Up)

The weight is the same for all exercises
Perform each exercise consecutively without rest

The Kick Acid Diet Workout Program
Workout 3

Circuit
- Lunges
- One Arm Snatch
- Standing Dumbbell Shoulder Press (alternate arms)

The weight is the same for all exercises
Perform each exercise consecutively without rest

<u>Notes</u>

Perform each workout once a week
Sets   4-5
Repetitions   8-10
Rest Interval   45-60 seconds

Progression

- Week One: 4 sets of each circuit x 8 reps; rest 60 seconds
- Week Two: 4 sets of each circuit x 10 reps; rest 60 seconds
- Week Three: 5 sets of each circuit x 8 reps; rest 45 seconds
- Week Four: 5 sets of each circuit x 10 reps; rest 45 seconds

The Kick Acid Diet Workout Program

Phase 3: Maintenance 6 weeks

The final phase is designed to prevent you from losing your hard-earned muscle and getting fat. It's a time to turn down the volume and give your body a much needed break, without completely falling off the wagon. In fact, some people continue to get stronger during this program, leading to future muscle gain and fat loss. Only perform each workout twice a week.

Workout 1

1. Squats

2. Dumbbell Cleans

Superset 1
3.a. Dumbbell Bent Over Row
3.b. Dumbbell Bench Press

Superset 2
4.a. Chin Ups
4.b. Incline Dumbbell Bench Press

Workout 2

1. Standing Dumbbell Shoulder Press

2. Front Dumbbell Raise

Superset 1
3.a. Dumbbell Bicep Curl
3.b. Dumbbell Skull Crusher

Superset 2
4.a. Dumbbell Hammer Curl
4.b. Tricep Bench Dip

The Kick Acid Diet Workout Program

<u>Notes</u>

Perform each workout twice a week
Increase reps each workout, until you reach 8 reps
Then, increase weight by 5lbs, and drop reps down to 6. Repeat

Sets	4
Repetitions	6-8
Rest Interval	90 seconds

The Kick Acid Diet Workout Program
Core Workout

The great thing about the *Kick Acid Diet Workout* Program is your core will be activated even when you don't realize it! The leg exercises are also designed to strengthen your abdominals and low back.

For those of you who are gluttons for punishment, I've included some abdominal exercise to supplement the rest of the routine.

Exercises

- Abdominal Crunches
- Reverse Crunch
- Plank

Notes

- Perform each core workout on non-consecutive days
- Increase reps by one each workout for exercises one and two, until you reach 15 reps
- Increase time by five seconds each workout for exercise three.

Sets   4
Repetitions   10/20 seconds
Rest Interval   30 seconds

The Kick Acid Diet Workout Program
Squats

This exercise is considered by many experts to be the best overall exercise, not only for one's legs, but for their entire body.

Start the exercise by standing with your feet shoulder width apart, and toes pointed slightly outward. To perform the dumbbell squat, hold the dumbbells with your palms facing your body.

With your spine in neutral, inhale and tighten your abdominals, while lowering your body until the top of your thighs are parallel to the ground. Once, you reach this position, continue to hold your breath, and pushing with both the balls and heels of your feet, straighten your knees and your hips until you return to the start position, exhaling at the top. A simple modification involves resting the dumbbells on your shoulder, while supporting the dumbbells with your hands.

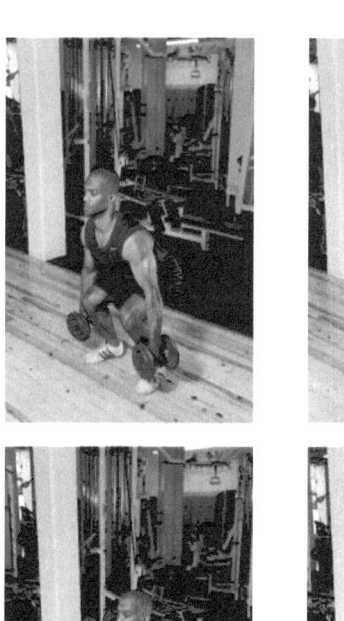
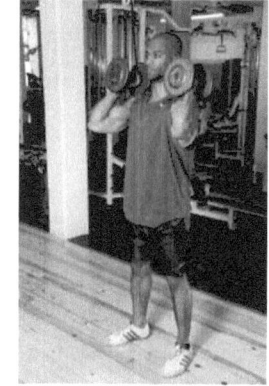

The Kick Acid Diet Workout Program
Deadlifts

This exercise is very similar to the squat in that it works both your upper and lower body.

Start the exercise by standing with your feet shoulder width apart, and toes pointed slightly outward. Assume the squat position, and grab the dumbbell with your arms in front of your body. At this point, your knees should be slightly over the dumbbells and your toes.

With your arms locked out, and spine in neutral, straighten the knees and the hips, while maintaining a neutral spine throughout the entire movement. Inhale and tighten your abdominals at the bottom and continue holding your breathe until you reach the top, then exhale.

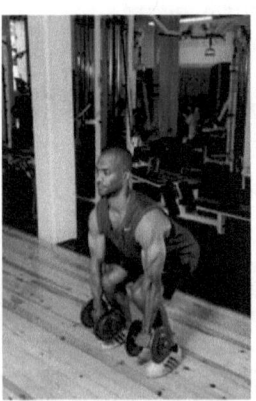 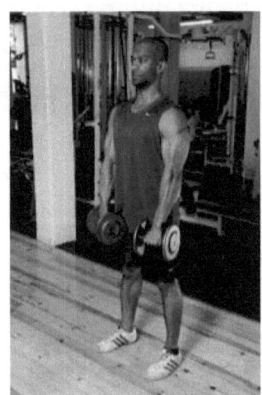

The Kick Acid Diet Workout Program
Dumbbell Cleans

This exercise is very similar to the squat and deadlift in that it works both your upper and lower body. Start the exercise by standing with your feet shoulder width apart, and toes pointed slightly outward. Assume the squat position, and grab the dumbbell with your arms in front of your body. At this point, your knees should be slightly over the bar and your toes. With your arms locked out, and spine in neutral, straighten the knees and the hips, while maintaining a neutral spine throughout the entire movement.

During the ascent, pull the weight up, using your arms, keeping the elbows pointed to the sides.

As your standing straight up, tuck your elbows into the sides of your body so the dumbbells rest upon your shoulders.

Inhale and tighten your abdominals at the bottom and continue holding your breathe until you reach the top, then exhale.

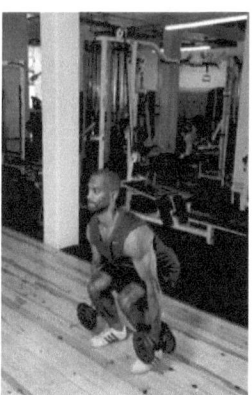 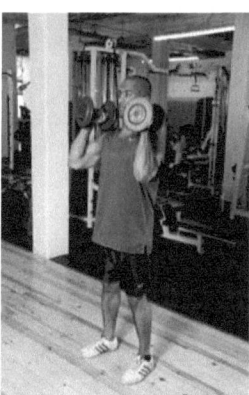 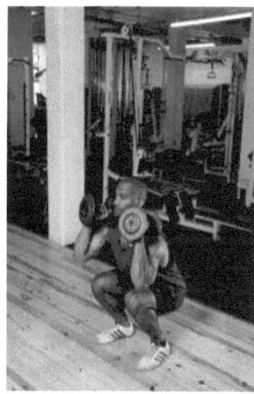

Stiff Leg Deadlifts

The stiff leg deadlift is similar to the deadlift with respect to arm and dumbbell placement, but is performed without movement in the knees. Begin, by bending your knees slightly, and holding the bar in front with a relaxed, neutral grip. With your spine in neutral, inhale, slowly lower the bar as low as possible by pushing your hips backward until you feel as if you cannot maintain neutral spine. At the bottom of the movement, continue inhaling, and return to the start position, by pushing your hips forward. Exhale at top.

Body weight should remain on heels throughout the entire movement.

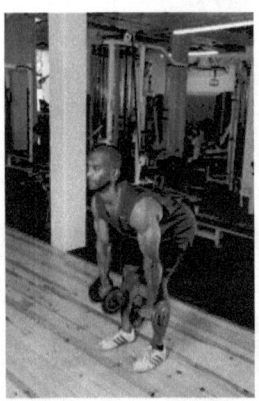
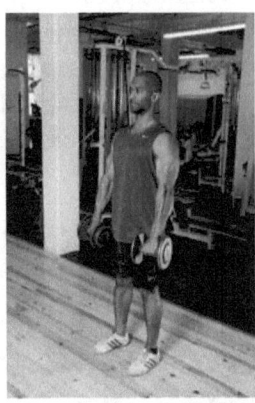

The Kick Acid Diet Workout Program
Lunges

Stand with both legs side by side, holding a dumbbell in each hand.. Start the movement stepping forward with one leg, bending it until the front thigh is parallel to ground and knee is bent to 90 degrees. The back knee should also be bent to 90 degrees. Bend forward at the hips while maintaining a neutral spine. Hold your breath at the bottom, return to the start position by straightening your stance leg at the knees and hips. Exhale at the top. Alternate legs.

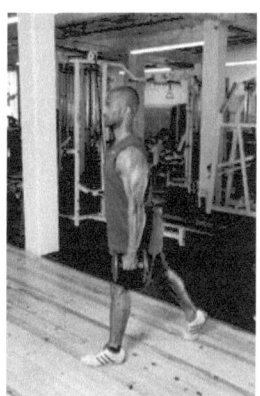 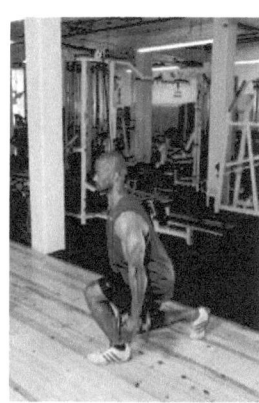

The Kick Acid Diet Workout Program
One-Leg Squats

Stand on one leg and place the opposite the leg on a bench which is situated behind you. The stance leg should lie directly beneath your hips (not in front, as in a lunge). Holding a dumbbell in each hand, slowly bend the stance leg, and bend forward at the hips while maintaining a neutral spine. Holding your breath at the bottom, return to the start position by straightening your stance leg at the knees and hips. Exhale at the top.

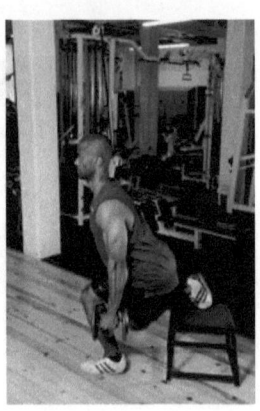 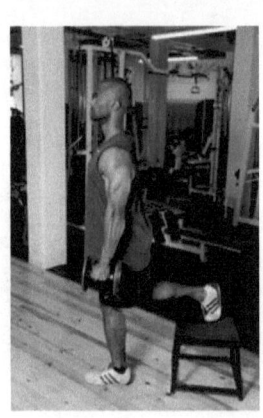

The Kick Acid Diet Workout Program
DB Jump Squat

Start the exercise by standing with your feet shoulder width apart, and toes pointed slightly outward. To perform the dumbbell, hold the dumbbells with your palms facing your body.

With your spine in neutral, inhale and tighten your abdominals, while lowering your body until the top of your thighs are parallel to the ground.

Once, you reach this position, continue to hold your breath, and pushing with both the balls and heels of your feet, straighten your knees and your hips, jumping as high as you can.

Land on the balls of feet and repeat.

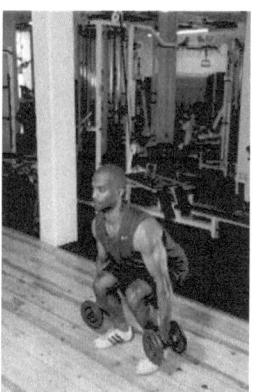
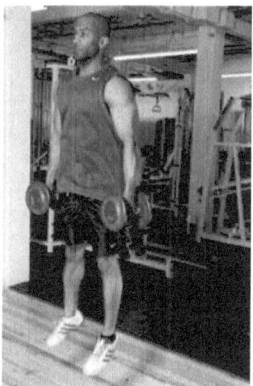

The Kick Acid Diet Workout Program
DB Hamstring Curl

This is a variation to a common exercise performed in many gyms. All you need is a bench and a dumbbell, however. Begin by laying face down on a bench, with your knees situated just off the far end of the bench. Either pick up the dumbbell with your feet or have a partner place the dumbbell between the insteps. Start with you knees straight, and slowly bend the knees, raising the weights until the soles of the feet face the ceiling. Exhale through the lifting phase and inhale as you lower the weight.

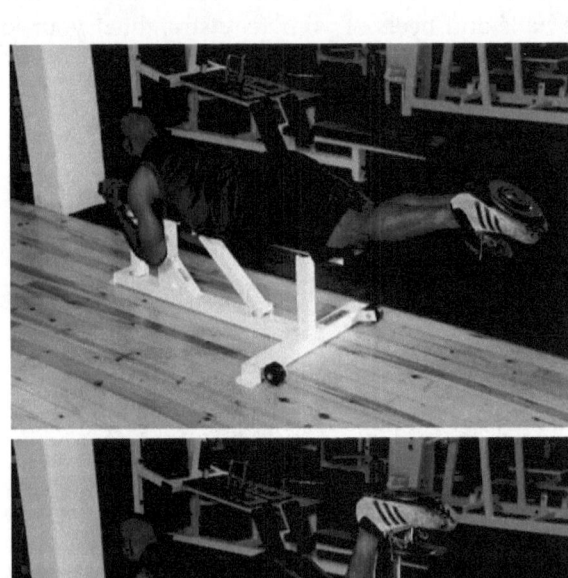

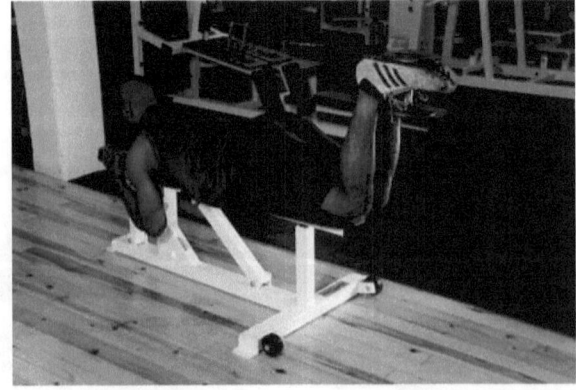

The Kick Acid Diet Workout Program
One Leg Standing Calf Raises

The calf is mainly compromised of two muscles, the gastrocnemius, and the deeper soleus. To work both of these muscles effectively, and in one exercise, the one leg standing calf raise is ideal. Start by holding a dumbbell in one hand, preferably on the same side of the calf that you're working on.

Standing on the edge of a bench, or elevated surface, put your weight on the balls of your feet (not your toes), and slowly lower your body until you can feel a slight stretch in the calf. Pushing on the balls of your feet, raise your body up, being sure to avoid bending your knee.

Hold on to a wall or another support with your opposite hand.

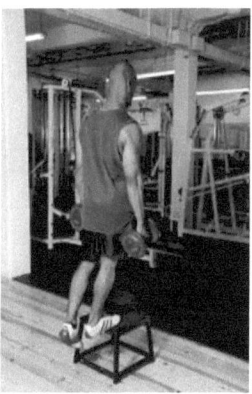 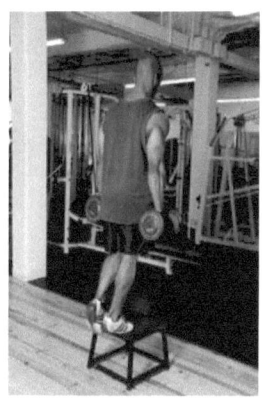

The Kick Acid Diet Workout Program

Bent Over Row

The bent over row is a great exercise for targeting the lats, rhomboids, and other muscles of your back. Begin by holding the dumbbells with the palms facing your body. Bend your knees slightly, and push your hips back until your torso is at approximately 45 degrees to the ground. Maintain a neutral spine, pull the dumbbell to the waistline, initiating the movement with your elbows to ensure that you're recruiting the proper muscles. Keep your elbows close to your body, and avoid locking the elbow at the bottom of the movement.

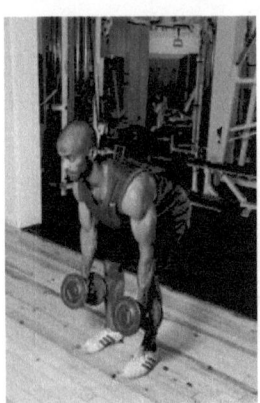 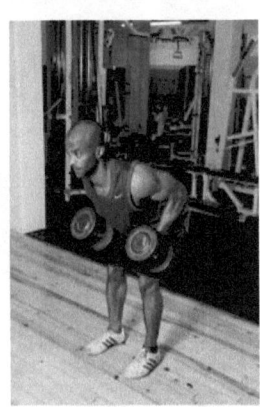

The Kick Acid Diet Workout Program
One Arm Dumbbell Row

Begin by placing one knee and the same arm on a bench so that your knee and hips are at 90 degrees, and your elbow is slightly bent. Maintain a neutral spine, and grab a dumbbell with your opposite hand. On the exhale, pull your elbow back towards your hips until your upper arm is parallel to the ground. Inhale, and slowly lower the weight to the start position.

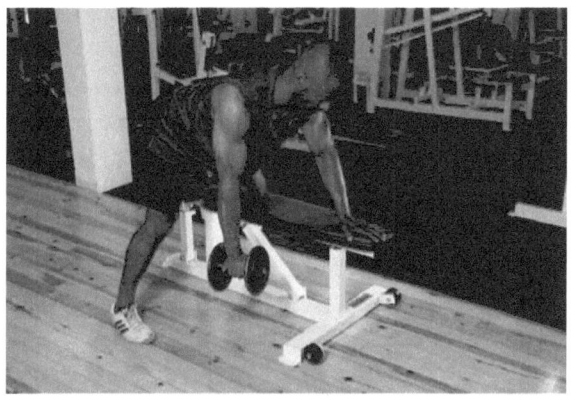

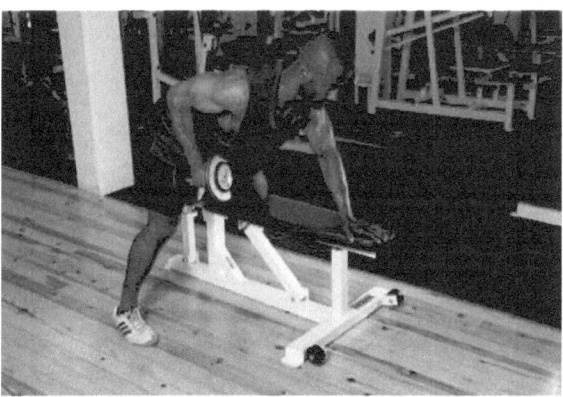

Chin Ups

The chin up and its variations are amongst the best back and upper body exercises. When performing the chin up, be sure to maintain a proper posture, as doing so will effectively target your core and stabilizing muscles. Begin by grabbing a bar with an underhand grip, and with your elbows shoulder width apart. Elbows should be facing forward when you begin the exercise. Start by flexing your knees to ninety degrees, and cross your feet at the ankles.

Maintain a neutral spine, and pull your body up towards the bar until your eyes are at bar level and slowly lower your body to the start position. Exhale as you pull your body upwards, and inhale on the descent.

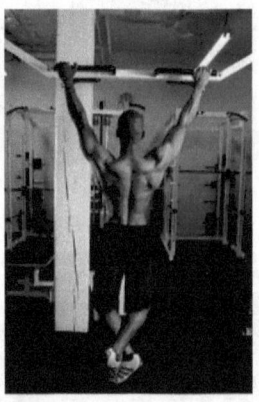
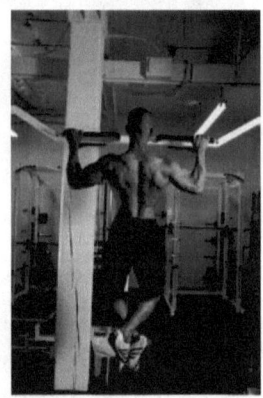

The Kick Acid Diet Workout Program
Push Ups

Start with your palms flat on the floor, your elbows and shoulders at ninety degrees and toes firmly on the ground. Maintain a neutral spine and lower your body until your chest touches the ground. Once you reach the bottom position, raise your body by extending your elbows and until they are just shy of locking out.

The pushup can be performed with your hands and feet flat on the floor, your upper body elevated on a bench, or your feet elevated on a bench.

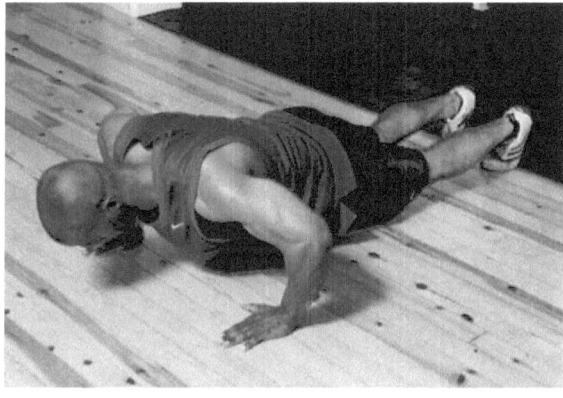

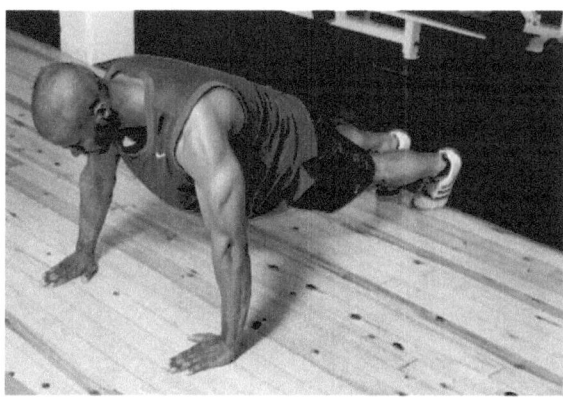

Bench Press

The bench press not only works the pectorals, but also places considerable stress on the triceps as well. Begin by laying on the floor or on a bench. Grip the dumbbells so that when your upper arms are parallel to the floor, the elbows form a ninety degree angle. The upper arms should also form a straight line from elbow to elbow.

When performing this exercise on a bench, slowly lower the arms so they drop down just below parallel, while avoiding arching your lower back. Hold your breath as you raise the weights, just stopping short of locking the elbows at the top. Exhale at the top of the movement, and inhale as you lower the bar to the starting position.

The bench press can be performed with either dumbbells or barbells, and can be performed on either a flat, incline or decline bench.

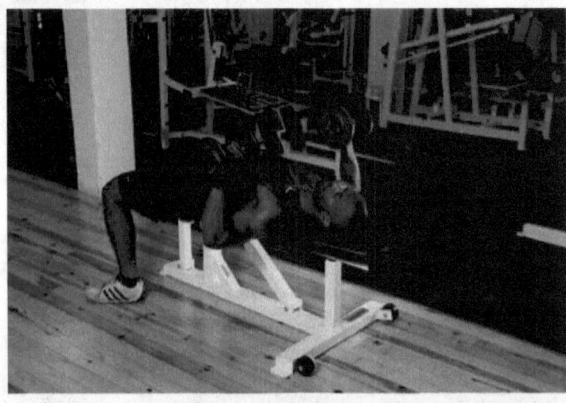

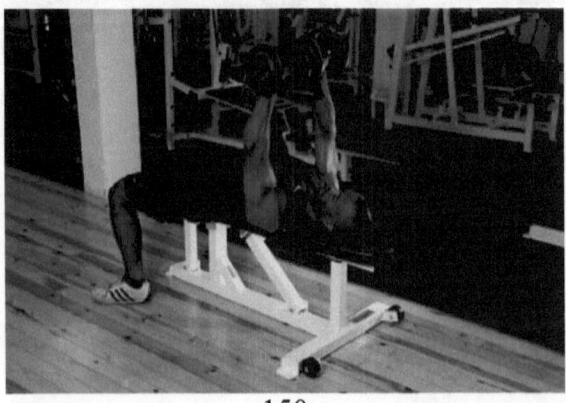

The Kick Acid Diet Workout Program
Dumbbell Shoulder Press

The dumbbell shoulder is performed seated or standing. Unlike the similar push press, there is no movement of the hips or knees.

Grip the dumbbells so that when your upper arms are parallel to the floor, the elbows form a ninety degree angle. The upper arms should also form a straight line from elbow to elbow.

When performing this exercise, slowly lower the arms so they drop down just below parallel. Hold your breath as you bring the dumbbells together at the top, just stopping short of locking the elbows at the top. Exhale at the top of the movement, and inhale as you lower the dumbbells to the starting position.

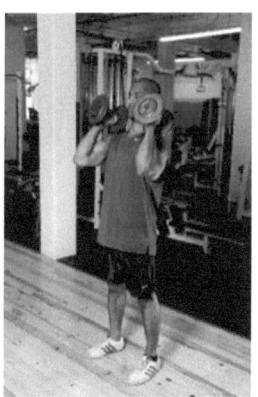 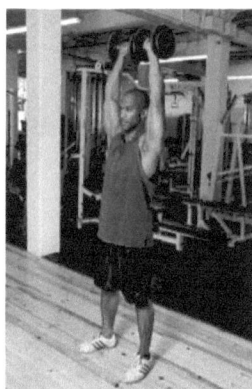

The Kick Acid Diet Workout Program
Lateral Dumbbell Raise

The lateral dumbbell raise can be either performed standing or seated. In either option, maintain a neutral spine. Begin by gripping a dumbbell in each hand, palms facing towards the body and raise the weights to your side. To achieve maximum effectiveness, raise the arms as high as possible, while turning the palms up as the arms get higher. Lower the weights slowly by reversing the rotation of the palms.

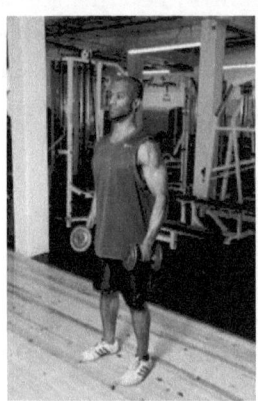 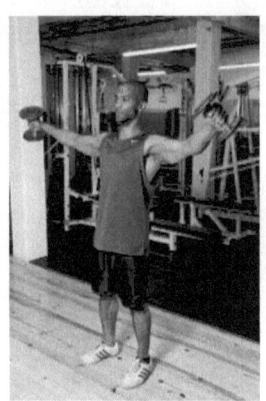

The Kick Acid Diet Workout Program
Front Dumbbell Raise

The front dumbbell raise can be either performed standing or seated. In either option, maintain a neutral spine. Begin by gripping a dumbbell in each hand, palms facing backward and raise the weights to your front. To achieve maximum effectiveness, raise the arms as high as possible.

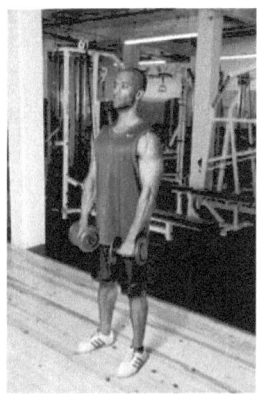
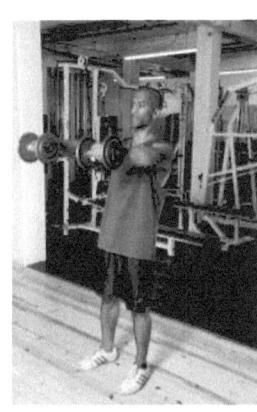

The Kick Acid Diet Workout Program
Bent Over Dumbbell Raise

Begin by gripping a dumbbell in each hand, palms facing towards the body. Bend your knees slightly, and push your hips back until your torso is at approximately 45 degrees to the ground. Maintaining a neutral spine, raise the arms until the entire arm is parallel to the floor. Keep your elbows locked in one position during the entire movement.

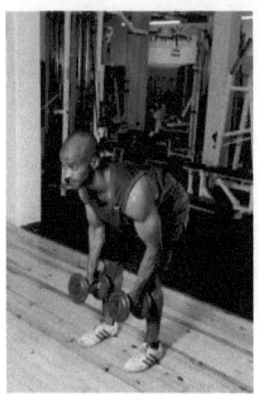
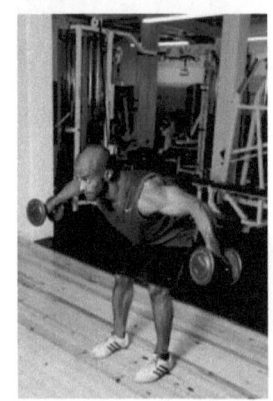

The Kick Acid Diet Workout Program
Tricep Bench Dips

Place the palms of your hands on a bench shoulder width apart behind you. Place your heels on the ground, so your knees are locked out. Begin the movement with your elbows pointing straight back and situated at ninety degrees. Straighten your arms while exhaling until your elbows are just short of locking out.

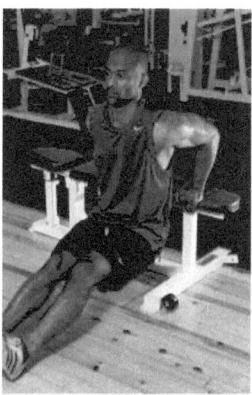 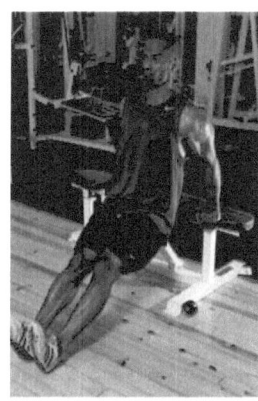

The Kick Acid Diet Workout Program
Skull Crushers

Begin by laying on the floor or on a bench. Grip the dumbbells so that when your forearms are parallel to the floor, the shoulders and elbows form a ninety degree angle. The upper arms should also be firmly pressed against your body and the dumbbells should rest at the level of your chest.

When performing this exercise on a bench, slowly lower the arms so they drop down just below parallel, while avoiding arching your lower back. Hold your breath as you raise the weights, just stopping short of locking the elbows at the top. Exhale at the top of the movement, and inhale as you lower the bar to the starting position.

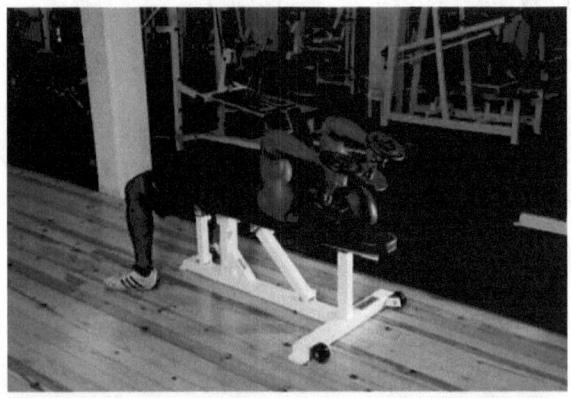

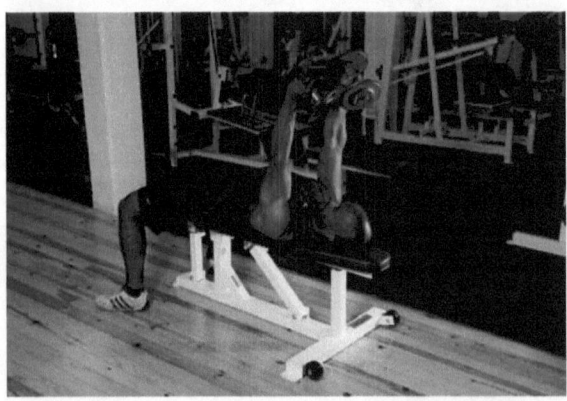

The Kick Acid Diet Workout Program
Dumbbell Bicep Curls

The dumbbell bicep curl can be either performed standing or seated. In either option, maintain a neutral spine. Begin by gripping a dumbbell in each hand, palms facing front body and raise the weights to the front by bending your elbows. Lower the weights slowly, keeping your elbows at close to your sides.

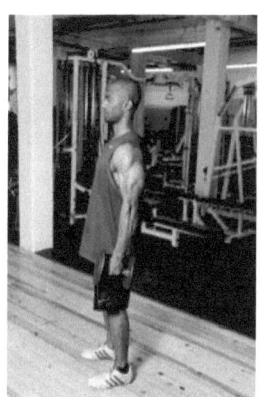 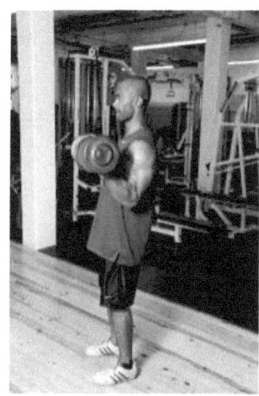

The Kick Acid Diet Workout Program
Dumbbell Hammer Curls

The dumbbell bicep curl can be either performed standing or seated. In either option, maintain a neutral spine. Begin by gripping a dumbbell in each hand, palms facing towards the body and raise the weights to the front by bending your elbows. Lower the weights slowly, keeping your elbows at close to your sides.

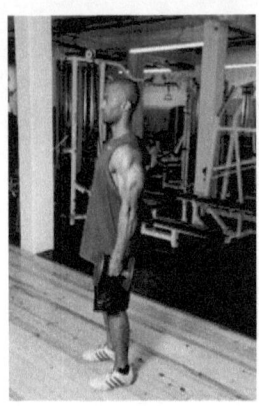 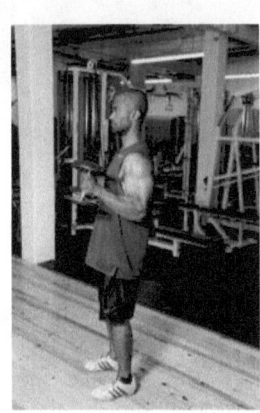

The Kick Acid Diet Workout Program
Dumbbell Clean + Squat

This movement combines two exercises – the dumbbell clean and modified squat (with dumbbells resting on shoulders).

Perform the dumbbell clean. Instead of returning to the start position, squat down with the dumbbells resting on your shoulders.

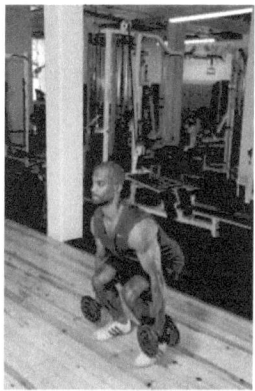 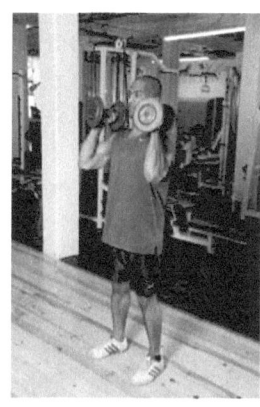 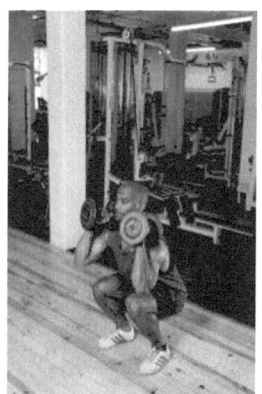

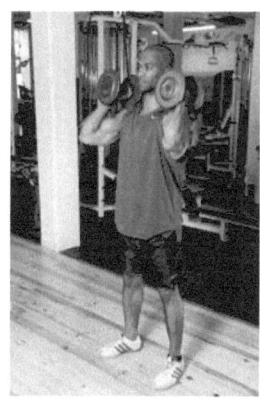

One Arm Clean

This exercise is very similar to the squat and deadlift in that it works both your upper and lower body. Start the exercise by standing with your feet shoulder width apart, and toes pointed slightly outward. Assume the squat position, and grab one dumbbell (situated between your legs). At this point, your knees should be slightly over the dumbbell and your toes.

With your arms locked out, and spine in neutral, straighten the knees and the hips, while maintaining a neutral spine throughout the entire movement. During the ascent, pull the weight up, using your arms, keeping the elbow pointed to the sides.

As your standing straight up, tuck your elbow into the side of your body so the dumbbell rest upon your shoulders. Alternate arms with each rep.

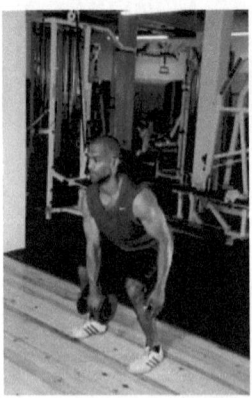 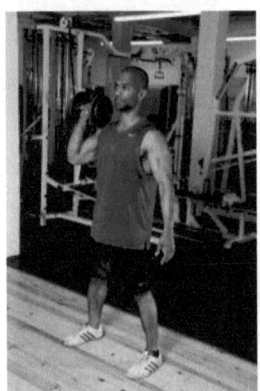 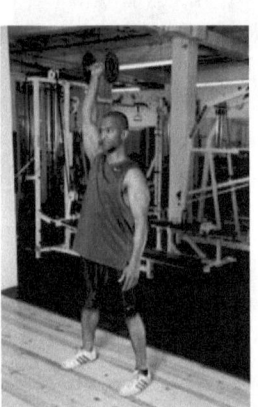

The Kick Acid Diet Workout Program
One Arm Snatch

This exercise is very similar to the one arm dumbbell clean in that it works both your upper and lower body. Start the exercise by standing with your feet shoulder width apart, and toes pointed slightly outward. Assume the squat position, and grab one dumbbell (situated between your legs). At this point, your knees should be slightly over the dumbbell and your toes. With your arms locked out, and spine in neutral, straighten the knees and the hips, while maintaining a neutral spine throughout the entire movement. During the ascent, pull the weight up, using your arms, keeping the elbow pointed to the sides.

As your standing straight up, tuck your elbow into the side of your body and raise the dumbbell straight overhead so you arm is completely straight. Alternate arms with each rep.

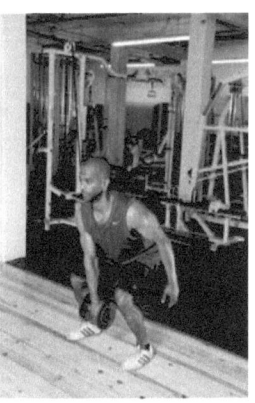 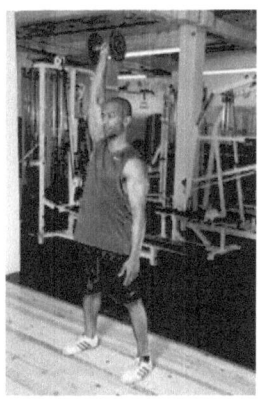

The Kick Acid Diet Workout Program
Burpee + Chin Up

A burpee can either be performed with a set of dumbbells or with just your body weight. Begin in a squat position with hands on the floor in front of you. Kick your feet back to a pushup position. Immediately return your feet to the squat position. Leap up as high as possible from the squat position.

In order to make the exercise more challenging, you can add a push up. To execute the burpee with a pushup, start off in a squat position with your hands on the floor (similar to the burpee). Kick your feet back to a pushup position. Instead of returning your feet or the squat position, perform a pushup first.

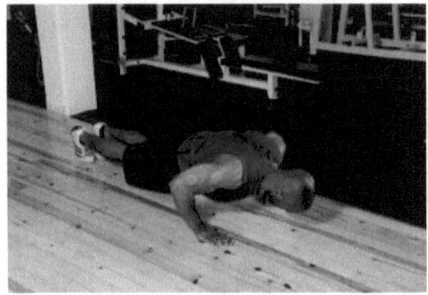 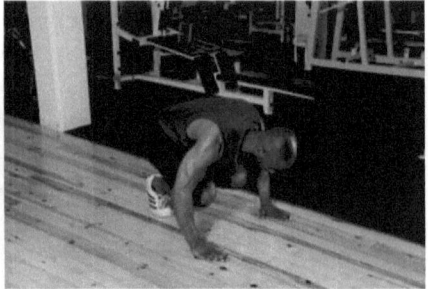

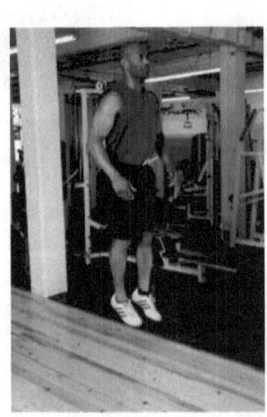

The Kick Acid Diet Workout Program
Abdominal Crunches

Start by lying on a mat or bench with your feet on the floor and knees at 90 degrees. Arch your back increasing the distance between your low back and the mat.

Hold a dumbbell directly over your face with your shoulders and elbows locked out.* Exhale as you flatten your lower back so it touches the mat, slowly raising your upper torso off the mat. Inhale as you return to the starting position.

*Contrary to popular belief, your abdominal muscles are not postural. In order to build a strong and chiseled mid-section, you need to train your abs with sufficient resistance and lower reps.

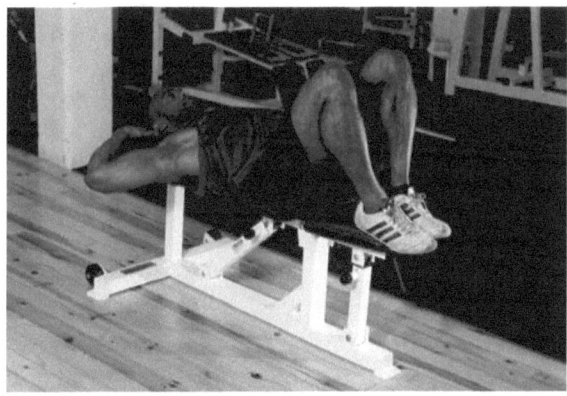

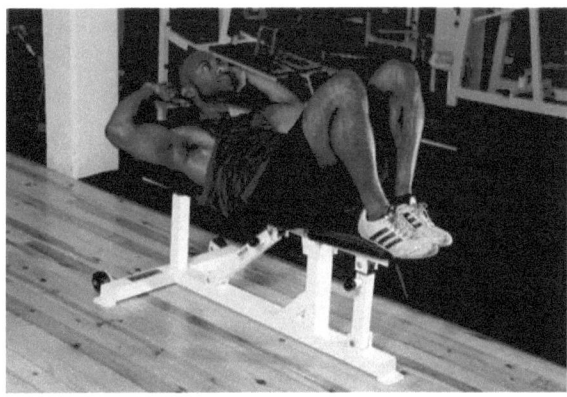

The Kick Acid Diet Workout Program
Reverse Crunches

Start by lying on a mat or bench with your hips and knees at 90 degrees. Arch your back increasing the distance between your low back and the mat. To make the movement more difficult, keep your knees locked out.

Exhale as you flatten your lower back so it touches the mat, slowly raising your lower body off the mat. Inhale as you return to the starting position.

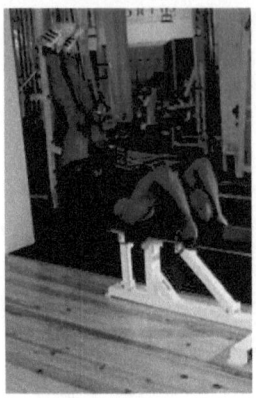 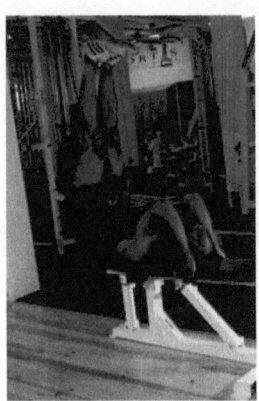

The Kick Acid Diet Workout Program
Plank

Lie face down on the mat with your forearms and palms resting on the floor. Your forearms should be parallel and shoulder width apart. Raise your body off the floor so you're now resting on your palms, forearms and toes.

Keep your spine in a neutral position, with a slight curve in your low back. Maintain an imaginary straight line through your ears, shoulders, hips, knees, and ankles.

Hold this position while inhaling and exhaling freely.

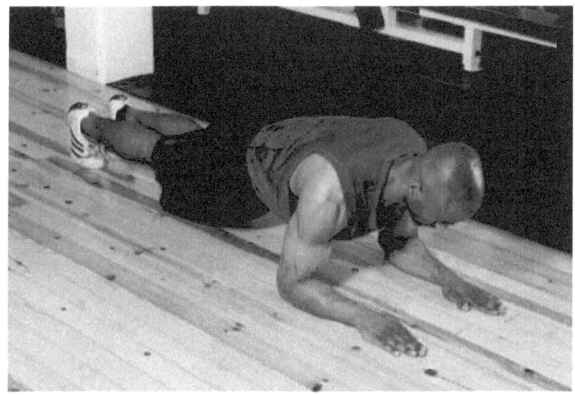

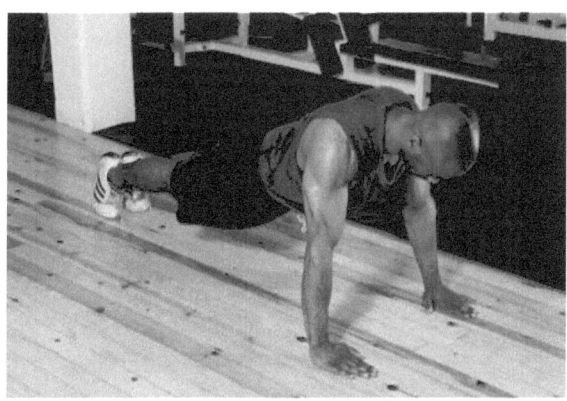

Conclusion and Acknowledgments

Conclusion and Acknowledgments
Conclusion

Congratulations! You're one step closer to reaching your goals. Simply follow the steps outlined in the Kick Acid Diet, and before you know it, you'll not only be healthy, but you'll have the body you've always desired.

I encourage you to read in depth the first section on acidity. Understanding how acidity can wreak havoc on your health is your first step in reducing it, ensuring long lasting fat loss. Use the steps outlined to measure your urinary pH or salivary pH.

To fully determine the extent of metabolic acidosis, use the hormone screen to see how your hormones have been affected. These screens are not a substitute for a consultation with a qualified healthcare professional.

Now that you know both your pH levels and the extent of damage to your various hormonal systems, it's time to make the necessary dietary changes to eliminate acidosis for good! The great thing about *The Kick Acid Diet* plan is it's not exclusive – it's inclusive. Eat the foods you enjoy and continue to shed fat!

Finally, in order to be healthy and strong…and lean, you need to engage in regular physical activity. *The Kick Acid Diet* Workout is a muscle building, metabolism boosting, energy filled, fun workout.

Remember the challenge I issued at the beginning of *The Kick Acid Diet*? In case you forgot, here it is,

I now offer you, the reader, a challenge. Challenge yourself to see your health as a gift. Your health is truly a gift that keeps giving. Only when you are healthy can you truly enjoy life. Health is a gift that must be cherished.

If you are serious about being healthy, getting fit, and performing at your peak, a well-balanced diet that provides all the vital nutrients and maintains an alkali environment is essential. It's time to kick some acid!

Are you up for the challenge?

Conclusion and Acknowledgments
Acknowledgments

The Kick Acid Diet grew out of an article I read by Dr. John Berardi in 2004, entitled, *Covering Your Nutritional Bases*. It was upon the reading of this piece that I originally saw on www.T-Nation.com, that I was not only motivated to research the topic, but was motivated to put pen to paper.

I owe special thanks to the many great minds who were responsible for the final product. First, I owe much gratitude to Candice Smith, academic and friend, who saw the potential from the first paragraph, giving me the blueprint to turn scientific jargon into a compelling, read for health professionals and the public alike. I also owe special thanks to Gail Raynor for putting her "special touch" on the first draft.

I would also like to thank Damian Box, Glen Grant, and Wil Nah for their artistic creations and vision, bringing this book to life. I would also like to thank Colin Vanion and Kevin Gonsalves for their web design, technological insights and web-savvy.

Finally, I would like to thank my patients, clients, and students, who have had faith in my skills and knowledge as a practitioner and educator, and have taught me the true art of healing.

Appendix A: PRAL Tables

Vegetables

Food Description	Kcals	Protein	Fat	Carbs	PRAL	Alkali Density
Alfalfa seeds, sprouted, raw	23	4	0.7	6.25	1.76	0.28
Amaranth leaves, cooked, boiled, drained, with salt	21	2	0	4	-13.91	-3.71
Amaranth leaves, cooked, boiled, drained, without salt	21	2	0	4	-13.91	-3.71
Amaranth leaves, raw	23	2	0	4	-14	-3.73
Arrowhead, cooked, boiled, drained, with salt	78	4	0	16	-10.37	-0.65
Arrowhead, cooked, boiled, drained, without salt	78	4	0	16	-10.37	-0.65
Arrowhead, raw	99	4	0	20	-11.76	-0.59
Arrowroot, raw	65	4	0	13	-4.55	-0.35
Artichokes, (globe or French), cooked, boiled, drained, with salt	50	3	0	12	-4.69	-0.39
Artichokes, (globe or French), cooked, boiled, drained, without salt	50	3	0	12	-4.69	-0.39
Artichokes, (globe or French), frozen, cooked, boiled, drained, with salt	45	3	0	9	-2.84	-0.32
Artichokes, (globe or French), frozen, cooked, boiled, drained, without salt	45	3	0	9	-2.84	-0.32
Artichokes, (globe or French), frozen, unprepared	38	3	0	8	-2.72	-0.34
Artichokes, (globe or French), raw	47	3	0	11	-4.97	-0.45
Arugula, raw	25	3	1	4	-7.86	-1.97
Asparagus, canned, drained solids	19	2	0	2	-1.44	-0.72
Asparagus, canned, no salt added, solids and liquids	15	2	0	2	-1.75	-0.88
Asparagus, canned, regular pack, solids and liquids	15	2	0	2	-1.75	-0.88
Asparagus, cooked, boiled, drained	22	2	0	4	-2.19	-0.55
Asparagus, cooked, boiled, drained, with salt	22	2	0	4	-2.19	-0.55
Asparagus, frozen, cooked, boiled, drained, with salt	18	3	0	2	-0.84	-0.42
Asparagus, frozen, cooked, boiled, drained, without salt	18	3	0	2	-0.84	-0.42
Asparagus, frozen, unprepared	24	3	0	4	-2.05	-0.51
Asparagus, raw	25	2	0	4	-1.91	-0.48
Balsam-pear (bitter gourd), leafy tips, cooked, boiled, drained, without salt	35	4	0	6	-11.01	-1.84
Balsam-pear (bitter gourd), leafy tips, cooked, boiled, drained, with salt	32	4	0	7	-11.01	-1.57
Balsam-pear (bitter gourd), leafy tips, raw	30	3	0	5	-9.81	-1.96
Balsam-pear (bitter gourd), pods, cooked, boiled, drained, with salt	19	1	0	4	-5.48	-1.37
Balsam-pear (bitter gourd), pods, cooked, boiled, drained, without salt	19	1	0	4	-5.48	-1.37
Balsam-pear (bitter gourd), pods, raw	17	1	0	4	-5.26	-1.32
Bamboo shoots, canned, drained solids	19	2	0	3	-0.12	-0.04
Bamboo shoots, cooked, boiled, drained, with salt	11	2	0	2	-9.93	-4.97
Bamboo shoots, cooked, boiled, drained, without salt	12	2	0	2	-9.93	-4.97
Bamboo shoots, raw	27	3	0	5	-7.98	-1.60

Vegetables

Food Description	Kcals	Protein	Fat	Carbs	PRAL	Alkali Density
Beans, fava, in pod, raw	88	8	0	18	0.34	0.02
Beans, kidney, mature seeds, sprouted, cooked, boiled, drained, with salt	33	5	0	5	-1.14	-0.23
Beans, kidney, mature seeds, sprouted, cooked, boiled, drained, w/o salt	33	5	0	5	-1.14	-0.23
Beans, kidney, mature seeds, sprouted, raw	29	4	0	4	-1.26	-0.32
Beans, lima, immature seeds, canned, regular pack, solids and liquids	71	4	0	4	-2.61	-0.65
Beans, mung, mature seeds, sprouted, canned, drained solids	12	1	0	2	0.88	0.44
Beans, navy, mature seeds, sprouted, cooked, boiled, drained, with salt	78	7	0	15	-2.47	-0.16
Beans, navy, mature seeds, sprouted, cooked, boiled, drained, without salt	78	7	0	15	-2.47	-0.16
Beans, navy, mature seeds, sprouted, raw	67	6	0	13	-2.55	-0.20
Beans, pinto, immature seeds, frozen, cooked, boiled, drained, with salt	162	9	0	31	-7.38	-0.24
Beans, pinto, immature seeds, frozen, cooked, boiled, drained, without salt	162	9	0	31	-7.38	-0.24
Beans, pinto, immature seeds, frozen, unprepared	170	10	0	32	-9.05	-0.28
Beans, pinto, mature seeds, sprouted, cooked, boiled, drained, with salt	20	9	0	26	-0.70	-0.03
Beans, pinto, mature seeds, sprouted, cooked, boiled, drained, without salt	22	9	0	26	-0.70	-0.03
Beans, pinto, mature seeds, sprouted, raw	62	5	0	12	-2.33	-0.19
Beans, shellie, canned, solids and liquids	30	2	0	6	-1.08	-0.18
Beans, snap, canned, all styles, seasoned, solids and liquids	16	1	0	3	-1.57	-0.52
Beans, snap, green variety, canned, regular pack, solids and liquids	15	1	0	4	-1.48	-0.37
Beans, snap, green, canned, no salt added, drained solids	20	1	0	5	-1.69	-0.34
Beans, snap, green, canned, no salt added, solids and liquids	15	1	0	5	-1.48	-0.30
Beans, snap, green, canned, regular pack, drained solids	20	1	0	4	-1.71	-0.43
Beans, snap, green, cooked, boiled, drained, with salt	35	2	0	8	-2.10	-0.26
Beans, snap, green, cooked, boiled, drained, without salt	35	2	0	8	-2.10	-0.26
Beans, snap, green, frozen, all styles, unprepared	33	2	0	8	-2.95	-0.37
Beans, snap, green, frozen, cooked, boiled, drained without salt	28	1	0	6	-2.57	-0.43
Beans, snap, green, frozen, cooked, boiled, drained, with salt	26	1	0	6	-2.57	-0.43
Beans, snap, green, raw	31	2	0	7	-3.22	-0.46
Beans, snap, yellow, canned, no salt added, drained solids	20	1	0	6	-1.69	-0.28
Beans, snap, yellow, canned, no salt added, solids and liquids	15	1	0	6	-1.61	-0.27
Beans, snap, yellow, canned, regular pack, drained solids	20	1	0	5	-1.69	-0.34
Beans, snap, yellow, canned, regular pack, solids and liquids	15	1	0	5	-1.61	-0.32
Beans, snap, yellow, cooked, boiled, drained, with salt	35	2	0	8	-5.15	-0.64

Vegetables

Food Description	Kcals	Protein	Fat	Carbs	PRAL	Alkali Density
Beans, snap, yellow, cooked, boiled, drained, without salt	35	1	0	6	-5.15	-0.86
Beans, snap, yellow, frozen, all styles, unprepared	33	2	0	8	-2.95	-0.37
Beans, snap, yellow, frozen, cooked, boiled, drained, with salt	26	1	0	6	-2.03	-0.34
Beans, snap, yellow, frozen, cooked, boiled, drained, without salt	28	1	0	6	-2.03	-0.34
Beans, snap, yellow, raw	31	2	0	7	-3.22	-0.46
Beet greens, cooked, boiled, drained, with salt	27	3	0	5	-19.56	-3.91
Beet greens, cooked, boiled, drained, without salt	27	3	0	5	-19.56	-3.91
Beet greens, raw	22	2	0	4	-16.74	-4.19
Beets, canned, drained solids	31	1	0	7	-2.67	-0.38
Beets, canned, no salt added, solids and liquids	28	1	0	7	-2.58	-0.37
Beets, canned, regular pack, solids and liquids	30	1	0	8	-3.12	-0.39
Beets, cooked, boiled, drained	44	2	0	10	-4.98	-0.50
Beets, cooked, boiled. drained, with salt	44	2	0	10	-4.98	-0.50
Beets, harvard, canned, solids and liquids	73	1	0	18	-3.04	-0.17
Beets, pickled, canned, solids and liquids	65	1	0	16	-2.62	-0.16
Beets, raw	43	2	0	4	-5.36	-1.34
Borage, cooked, boiled, drained, with salt	25	2	1	4	-10.06	-2.52
Borage, cooked, boiled, drained, without salt	25	2	1	4	-10.06	-2.52
Borage, raw	21	2	1	3	-9.58	-3.19
Broadbeans, immature seeds, cooked, boiled, drained, with salt	62	5	0	10	-0.04	0
Broadbeans, immature seeds, cooked, boiled, drained, without salt	62	5	0	10	-0.04	0
Broadbeans, immature seeds, raw	72	6	1	12	-0.26	-0.02
Broccoli raab, cooked	33	4	1	3	-4.52	-1.51
Broccoli raab, raw	22	3	0	3	-1.83	-0.61
Broccoli, Chinese, cooked	22	1	1	4	-5.17	-1.29
Broccoli, cooked, boiled, drained, with salt	28	2	0	7	-3.28	-0.47
Broccoli, cooked, boiled, drained, without salt	35	2	0	7	-3.57	-0.51
Broccoli, flower clusters, raw	28	3	0	5	-4.19	-0.84
Broccoli, frozen, chopped, cooked, boiled, drained, with salt	28	3	0	5	-0.41	-0.08
Broccoli, frozen, chopped, cooked, boiled, drained, without salt	28	3	0	5	-0.41	-0.08
Broccoli, frozen, chopped, unprepared	26	3	0	5	-2.42	-0.48
Broccoli, frozen, spears, cooked, boiled, drained, with salt	28	3	0	5	-1.40	-0.28
Broccoli, frozen, spears, cooked, boiled, drained, without salt	28	3	0	5	-1.40	-0.28
Broccoli, frozen, spears, unprepared	29	3	0	5	-2.51	-0.50
Broccoli, leaves, raw	28	3	0	5	-4.19	-0.84
Broccoli, raw	34	3	0	7	-3.96	-0.57

Vegetables

Food Description	Kcals	Protein	Fat	Carbs	PRAL	Alkali Density
Broccoli, stalks, raw	28	3	0	5	-4.19	-0.84
Brussels sprouts, cooked, boiled, drained, with salt	41	3	0	7	-4.32	-0.62
Brussels sprouts, cooked, boiled, drained, without salt	36	3	0	7	-4.32	-0.62
Brussels sprouts, frozen, cooked, boiled, drained, with salt	42	4	0	8	-3.04	-0.38
Brussels sprouts, frozen, cooked, boiled, drained, without salt	42	4	0	8	-3.04	-0.38
Brussels sprouts, frozen, unprepared	41	4	0	8	-4.48	-0.56
Brussels sprouts, raw	43	3	0	9	-5.10	-0.57
Burdock root, cooked, boiled, drained, with salt	88	2	0	21	-4.74	-0.23
Burdock root, cooked, boiled, drained, without salt	88	2	0	21	-4.74	-0.23
Burdock root, raw	72	2	0	17	-5.35	-0.31
Butterbur, (fuki), raw	14	0	0	4	-14.82	-3.71
Butterbur, cooked, boiled, drained, with salt	8	0	0	2	-8.03	-4.02
Butterbur, cooked, boiled, drained, without salt	8	0	0	2	-8.03	-4.02
Cabbage, Chinese (pak-choi), cooked, boiled, drained, with salt	12	2	0	2	-7.44	-3.72
Cabbage, Chinese (pak-choi), cooked, boiled, drained, without salt	12	2	0	2	-7.44	-3.72
Cabbage, Chinese (pak-choi), raw	13	1	0	2	-5.04	-2.52
Cabbage, Chinese (pe-tsai), cooked, boiled, drained, with salt	14	1	0	2	-3.22	-1.61
Cabbage, Chinese (pe-tsai), cooked, boiled, drained, without salt	14	1	0	2	-3.22	-1.61
Cabbage, Chinese (pe-tsai), raw	16	1	0	2	-4.67	-2.34
Cabbage, common (Danish, domestic, and pointed types), freshly harvest, raw	24	1	0	5	-4.72	-0.94
Cabbage, common (Danish, domestic, and pointed types), stored, raw	24	1	0	5	-4.72	-0.94
Cabbage, common, cooked, boiled, drained, with salt	23	1	0	6	-3.28	-0.55
Cabbage, cooked, boiled, drained, without salt	23	1	0	6	-3.28	-0.55
Cabbage, Japanese style, fresh, pickled	30	2	0	6	-16.47	-2.75
Cabbage, mustard, salted	28	1	0	6	-4.88	-0.81
Cabbage, Napa, cooked	12	1	0	2	-1.17	-0.59
Cabbage, raw	25	1	0	6	-2.81	-0.47
Cabbage, red, cooked, boiled, drained, with salt	29	2	0	7	-4.52	-0.65
Cabbage, red, cooked, boiled, drained, without salt	29	2	0	7	-4.52	-0.65
Cabbage, red, raw	31	1	0	7	-4.29	-0.61
Cabbage, Savoy, cooked, boiled, drained, with salt	24	2	0	5	-2.77	-0.55
Cabbage, Savoy, cooked, boiled, drained, without salt	24	2	0	5	-2.77	-0.55
Cabbage, Savoy, raw	27	1	0	7	-3.47	-0.50
Cardoon, cooked, boiled, drained, with salt	20	1	0	5	-9.06	-1.81

Vegetables

Food Description	Kcals	Protein	Fat	Carbs	PRAL	Alkali Density
Cardoon, cooked, boiled, drained, without salt	22	1	0	5	-9.06	-1.81
Cardoon, raw	17	1	0	4	-9.20	-2.30
Carrot juice, canned	40	1	0	9	-4.78	-0.53
Carrot, dehydrated	341	8	1	80	-42.39	-0.53
Carrots, baby, raw	35	1	0	8	-4.30	-0.54
Carrots, canned, no salt added, drained solids	25	1	0	5	-3.09	-0.62
Carrots, canned, no salt added, solids and liquids	23	1	0	5	-2.92	-0.58
Carrots, canned, regular pack, drained solids	25	1	0	5	-3.09	-0.62
Carrots, canned, regular pack, solids and liquids	23	1	0	5	-3.24	-0.65
Carrots, cooked, boiled, drained, with salt	35	1	0	8	-4.10	-0.51
Carrots, cooked, boiled, drained, without salt	35	1	0	8	-4.10	-0.51
Carrots, frozen, cooked, boiled, drained, with salt	37	1	1	8	-3.34	-0.42
Carrots, frozen, cooked, boiled, drained, without salt	37	1	1	8	-3.34	-0.42
Carrots, frozen, unprepared	36	1	0	8	-4.11	-0.51
Carrots, raw	41	1	0	10	-5.71	-0.57
Cassava, raw	160	1	0	38	-4.78	-0.13
Catsup	97	2	0	25	-6.67	-0.27
Catsup, low sodium	97	2	0	25	-6.67	-0.27
Cauliflower, cooked, boiled, drained, with salt	23	2	0	4	-1.33	-0.33
Cauliflower, cooked, boiled, drained, without salt	23	2	0	4	-1.33	-0.33
Cauliflower, frozen, cooked, boiled, drained, with salt	17	2	0	4	-1.69	-0.42
Cauliflower, frozen, cooked, boiled, drained, without salt	19	2	0	4	-1.69	-0.42
Cauliflower, frozen, unprepared	24	2	0	5	-2.37	-0.47
Cauliflower, green, cooked, no salt added	32	3	0	6	-3.14	-0.52
Cauliflower, green, cooked, with salt	32	3	0	6	-3.14	-0.52
Cauliflower, green, raw	31	3	0	6	-3.51	-0.59
Cauliflower, raw	25	3	0	6	-4.44	-0.74
Celeriac, cooked, boiled, drained, with salt	27	1	0	6	-1.37	-0.23
Celeriac, cooked, boiled, drained, without salt	27	1	0	6	-1.37	-0.23
Celeriac, raw	42	1	0	9	-2.38	-0.26
Celery flakes, dried	319	11	2	64	-84.46	-1.32
Celery, cooked, boiled, drained, with salt	18	1	0	4	-5.49	-1.37
Celery, cooked, boiled, drained, without salt	18	1	0	4	-5.49	-1.37
Celery, raw	16	1	0	3	-5.04	-1.68
Celtuce, raw	18	1	0	4	-6.30	-1.58
Chard, Swiss, cooked, boiled, drained, with salt	20	2	0	4	-12.37	-3.09
Chard, Swiss, cooked, boiled, drained, without salt	20	2	0	4	-12.37	-3.09

Vegetables

Food Description	Kcals	Protein	Fat	Carbs	PRAL	Alkali Density
Chard, Swiss, raw	19	2	0	4	-8.14	-2.04
Chayote, fruit, cooked, boiled, drained, with salt	22	1	0	5	-2.73	-0.55
Chayote, fruit, cooked, boiled, drained, without salt	24	1	0	5	-2.73	-0.55
Chayote, fruit, raw	17	1	0	5	-2.09	-0.42
Chicory greens, raw	23	2	0	5	-8.32	-1.66
Chicory roots, raw	73	1	0	18	-4.25	-0.24
Chicory, witloof, raw	17	1	0	4	-3.53	-0.88
Chives, freeze-dried	311	21	4	64	-59.81	-0.93
Chives, raw	30	3	1	4	-4.75	-1.19
Chrysanthemum leaves, raw	24	3	1	3	-10.61	-3.54
Chrysanthemum, garland, cooked, boiled, drained, with salt	20	2	0	4	-10.91	-2.73
Chrysanthemum, garland, cooked, boiled, drained, without salt	20	2	0	4	-10.91	-2.73
Chrysanthemum, garland, raw	24	3	1	3	-10.61	-3.54
Coleslaw, home-prepared	78	1	3	12	-2.83	-0.24
Collards, cooked, boiled, drained, with salt	26	2	0	5	-2.63	-0.53
Collards, cooked, boiled, drained, without salt	26	2	0	5	-2.63	-0.53
Collards, frozen, chopped, cooked, boiled, drained, with salt	36	2	0	5	-6.32	-1.26
Collards, frozen, chopped, cooked, boiled, drained, without salt	36	2	0	5	-6.32	-1.26
Collards, frozen, chopped, unprepared	33	3	0	6	-6.36	-1.06
Collards, raw	30	3	0	6	-4.09	-0.68
Coriander (cilantro) leaves, raw	23	2	1	4	-9.66	-2.42
Corn pudding, home prepared	131	4	5	17	0.96	0.06
Corn with red and green peppers, canned, solids and liquids	75	2	1	18	-0.49	-0.03
Corn, sweet, white, canned, cream style, no salt added	72	2	0	18	-0.55	-0.03
Corn, sweet, white, canned, cream style, regular pack	72	2	0	18	-0.55	-0.03
Corn, sweet, white, canned, vacuum pack, no salt added	79	2	0	18	-1.02	-0.06
Corn, sweet, white, canned, vacuum pack, regular pack	79	2	0	19	-1.02	-0.05
Corn, sweet, white, canned, whole kernel, drained solids	81	2	0	19	-0.99	-0.05
Corn, sweet, white, canned, whole kernel, no salt added, solids and liquids	64	2	0	15	-1.07	-0.07
Corn, sweet, white, canned, whole kernel, regular pack, solids and liquids	64	2	0	15	-1.07	-0.07
Corn, sweet, white, cooked, boiled, drained, with salt	108	3	1	25	-0.64	-0.03
Corn, sweet, white, cooked, boiled, drained, without salt	108	3	1	25	-0.64	-0.03
Corn, sweet, white, frozen, kernels cut off cob, boiled, drained, with salt	80	3	0	20	-0.17	-0.01
Corn, sweet, white, frozen, kernels cut off cob, boiled, drained, without salt	80	3	0	20	-0.17	-0.01

Vegetables

Food Description	Kcals	Protein	Fat	Carbs	PRAL	Alkali Density
Corn, sweet, white, frozen, kernels cut off cob, unprepared	88	3	0	20	-0.89	-0.04
Corn, sweet, white, frozen, kernels on cob, cooked, boiled, drained, with salt	94	3	1	22	-1.76	-0.08
Corn, sweet, white, frozen, kernels on cob, cooked, boiled, drained, without salt	94	3	1	22	-1.76	-0.08
Corn, sweet, white, frozen, kernels on cob, unprepared	98	3	1	24	-2.23	-0.09
Corn, sweet, white, raw	86	3	1	19	-1.78	-0.09
Corn, sweet, yellow, canned, brine pack, regular pack, solids and liquids	64	2	0	18	-1.07	-0.06
Corn, sweet, yellow, canned, cream style, no salt added	72	2	0	18	-0.55	-0.03
Corn, sweet, yellow, canned, cream style, regular pack	72	2	0	18	-0.55	-0.03
Corn, sweet, yellow, canned, no salt added, solids and liquids	64	2	0	15	-1.07	-0.07
Corn, sweet, yellow, canned, vacuum pack, no salt added	79	2	0	19	-1.02	-0.05
Corn, sweet, yellow, canned, vacuum pack, regular pack	79	2	0	19	-1.02	-0.05
Corn, sweet, yellow, canned, whole kernel, drained solids	81	3	0	25	-0.22	-0.01
Corn, sweet, yellow, cooked, boiled, drained, with salt	108	3	0	25	-0.64	-0.03
Corn, sweet, yellow, cooked, boiled, drained, without salt	108	3	0	25	-0.64	-0.03
Corn, sweet, yellow, frozen, kernels cut off cob, boiled, drained, without salt	81	3	1	21	-1.48	-0.07
Corn, sweet, yellow, frozen, kernels cut off cob, unprepared	88	3	1	21	-0.89	-0.04
Corn, sweet, yellow, frozen, kernels on cob, cooked, boiled, drained, with salt	93	3	1	21	-1.76	-0.08
Corn, sweet, yellow, frozen, kernels on cob, cooked, boiled, drained, without salt	93	3	1	21	-1.76	-0.08
Corn, sweet, yellow, frozen, kernels on cob, unprepared	98	3	1	24	-2.23	-0.09
Corn, sweet, yellow, frozen, kernels, cut off cob, boiled, drained, with salt	79	3	1	24	-1.48	-0.06
Corn, sweet, yellow, raw	86	3	1	19	-1.78	-0.09
Cornsalad, raw	21	2	0	4	-7.53	-1.88
Cowpeas (Blackeyes), immature seeds, cooked, boiled, drained, with salt	94	3	0	20	-8.35	-0.42
Cowpeas (Blackeyes), immature seeds, cooked, boiled, drained, without salt	97	3	0	20	-8.35	-0.42
Cowpeas (blackeyes), immature seeds, frozen, cooked, boiled, drained, with salt	132	3	0	20	-0.80	-0.04
Cowpeas (blackeyes), immature seeds, frozen, cooked, boiled, drained, without salt	132	3	0	20	-0.80	-0.04
Cowpeas (Blackeyes), immature seeds, frozen, unprepared	139	3	0	19	-2.11	-0.11
Cowpeas (blackeyes), immature seeds, raw	90	3	0	19	-8.60	-0.45
Cowpeas, leafy tips, cooked, boiled, drained, with salt	22	5	0	3	-6.03	-2.01
Cowpeas, leafy tips, cooked, boiled, drained, without salt	22	5	0	3	-6.03	-2.01
Cowpeas, leafy tips, raw	29	4	0	5	-9.15	-1.83
Cowpeas, young pods with seeds, cooked, boiled, drained, with salt	34	3	0	7	-2.81	-0.40

Vegetables

Food Description	Kcals	Protein	Fat	Carbs	PRAL	Alkali Density
Cowpeas, young pods with seeds, cooked, boiled, drained, without salt	34	3	0	7	-2.81	-0.40
Cowpeas, young pods with seeds, raw	44	2	0	7	-2.84	-0.41
Cress, garden, cooked, boiled, drained, with salt	23	2	1	4	-6.17	-1.54
Cress, garden, cooked, boiled, drained, without salt	23	2	1	4	-6.17	-1.54
Cress, garden, raw	32	3	1	6	-10.68	-1.78
Cucumber, peeled, raw	12	1	0	2	-2.28	-1.14
Cucumber, with peel, raw	15	1	0	4	-2.42	-0.61
Dandelion greens, cooked, boiled, drained, with salt	33	2	1	6	-4.78	-0.80
Dandelion greens, cooked, boiled, drained, without salt	33	2	1	6	-4.78	-0.80
Dandelion greens, raw	45	3	1	9	-7.93	-0.88
Dock, cooked, boiled, drained, with salt	20	2	1	3	-6.72	-2.24
Dock, cooked, boiled, drained, without salt	20	2	1	3	-6.72	-2.24
Dock, raw	22	2	1	3	-8.12	-2.71
Edamame, frozen, prepared	122	11	5	10	-0.05	-0.01
Edamame, frozen, unprepared	110	10	5	10	-1.50	-0.15
Eggplant, cooked, boiled, drained, with salt	35	1	0	9	-1.98	-0.22
Eggplant, cooked, boiled, drained, without salt	35	1	0	9	-1.98	-0.22
Eggplant, pickled	49	1	1	10	0.04	0
Eggplant, raw	24	1	0	6	-3.89	-0.65
Endive, raw	17	1	0	3	-6.01	-2
Epazote, raw	32	0	1	7	-16.67	-2.38
Eppaw, raw	150	5	2	32	-1.04	-0.03
Fennel, bulb, raw	31	1	0	7	-7.31	-1.04
Fiddlehead ferns, frozen, unprepared	34	0	4	6	0.74	0.12
Fiddlehead ferns, raw	34	5	0	6	-3.10	-0.52
Fireweed, leaves, raw	103	5	3	19	-13.70	-0.72
Fungi, Cloud ears, dried	284	9	1	73	-8.71	-0.12
Garlic, raw	149	6	0	33	-2.64	-0.08
Ginger root, raw	80	2	1	18	-7.89	-0.44
Gourd, dishcloth (towelgourd), cooked, boiled, drained, with salt	54	1	0	14	-8.68	-0.62
Gourd, dishcloth (towelgourd), cooked, boiled, drained, without salt	56	1	0	14	-8.68	-0.62
Gourd, dishcloth (towelgourd), raw	20	1	0	4	-1.77	-0.44
Gourd, white-flowered (calabash), cooked, boiled, drained, with salt	13	1	0	4	-3.39	-0.85
Gourd, white-flowered (calabash), cooked, boiled, drained, without salt	15	1	0	4	-3.39	-0.85
Gourd, white-flowered (calabash), raw	14	1	0	3	-2.98	-0.99
Grape leaves, canned	69	4	2	12	-1.38	-0.12

Vegetables

Food Description	Kcals	Protein	Fat	Carbs	PRAL	Alkali Density
Grape leaves, raw	93	6	2	17	-6.79	-0.40
Hearts of palm, canned	28	3	1	5	-1.81	-0.36
Horseradish-tree leafy tips, raw	64	9	1	8	-4.55	-0.57
Horseradish-tree, leafy tips, cooked, boiled, drained, with salt	60	5	1	11	-8.05	-0.73
Horseradish-tree, leafy tips, cooked, boiled, drained, without salt	60	5	1	11	-8.05	-0.73
Horseradish-tree, pods, cooked, boiled, drained, with salt	36	2	0	8	-8.11	-1.01
Horseradish-tree, pods, cooked, boiled, drained, without salt	36	2	0	8	-8.11	-1.01
Horseradish-tree, pods, raw	37	2	0	9	-8.36	-0.93
Hyacinth-beans, immature seeds, cooked, boiled, drained, with salt	50	3	0	9	-3.86	-0.43
Hyacinth-beans, immature seeds, cooked, boiled, drained, without salt	50	3	0	9	-3.86	-0.43
Hyacinth-beans, immature seeds, raw	46	3	0	9	-4.14	-0.46
Jerusalem-artichokes, raw	76	2	0	17	-5.76	-0.34
Jew's ear, (pepeao), raw	25	0	0	7	-1	-0.14
Jute, potherb, cooked, boiled, drained, with salt	37	4	0	7	-11.43	-1.63
Jute, potherb, cooked, boiled, drained, without salt	37	4	0	7	-11.43	-1.63
Jute, potherb, raw	34	5	0	6	-10.75	-1.79
Kale, cooked, boiled, drained, with salt	28	5	0	6	-4.22	-0.70
Kale, cooked, boiled, drained, without salt	28	5	0	6	-4.22	-0.70
Kale, frozen, cooked, boiled, drained, with salt	30	3	0	5	-6.57	-1.31
Kale, frozen, cooked, boiled, drained, without salt	30	3	0	5	-6.57	-1.31
Kale, frozen, unprepared	28	3	0	5	-6.85	-1.37
Kale, raw	50	2	1	10	-8.33	-0.83
Kale, scotch, cooked, boiled, drained, with salt	28	2	0	6	-6.61	-1.10
Kale, scotch, cooked, boiled, drained, without salt	28	2	0	6	-6.61	-1.10
Kale, scotch, raw	42	3	1	8	-10.73	-1.34
Kanpyo, (dried gourd strips)	258	9	1	65	-28.95	-0.45
Kohlrabi, cooked, boiled, drained, with salt	29	2	0	7	-5.41	-0.77
Kohlrabi, cooked, boiled, drained, without salt	29	2	0	7	-5.41	-0.77
Kohlrabi, raw	27	2	0	6	-5.62	-0.94
Lambsquarters, cooked, boiled, drained, with salt	32	3	1	5	-6.76	-1.35
Lambsquarters, cooked, boiled, drained, without salt	32	3	1	5	-6.76	-1.35
Lambsquarters, raw	43	4	1	7	-9.67	-1.38
Leeks, (bulb and lower leaf-portion), cooked, boiled, drained, with salt	31	1	0	8	-1.55	-0.19
Leeks, (bulb and lower leaf-portion), cooked, boiled, drained, without salt	31	1	0	8	-1.55	-0.19
Leeks, (bulb and lower leaf-portion), raw	61	1	0	14	-3.24	-0.23

Vegetables

Food Description	Kcals	Protein	Fat	Carbs	PRAL	Alkali Density
Leeks, (bulb and lower-leaf portion), freeze-dried	321	15	2	75	-39.01	-0.52
Lemon grass (citronella), raw	99	2	0	25	-12.95	-0.52
Lentils, sprouted, cooked, stir-fried, with salt	101	9	0	21	2.91	0.14
Lentils, sprouted, cooked, stir-fried, without salt	101	9	0	21	2.91	0.14
Lentils, sprouted, raw	106	9	1	22	2.74	0.12
Lettuce, butterhead (includes Boston and bibb types), raw	13	1	0	2	-3.90	-1.95
Lettuce, cos or romaine, raw	17	1	0	3	-4.26	-1.42
Lettuce, green leaf, raw	15	1	0	3	-3.14	-1.05
Lettuce, iceberg (includes crisphead types), raw	14	1	0	3	-2.19	-0.73
Lettuce, red leaf, raw	16	1	0	3	-2.98	-0.99
Lima beans, immature seeds, canned, no salt added, solids and liquids	71	4	0	13	-2.61	-0.20
Lima beans, immature seeds, cooked, boiled, drained, with salt	123	4	0	13	-6.16	-0.47
Lima beans, immature seeds, cooked, boiled, drained, without salt	123	4	0	13	-6.16	-0.47
Lima beans, immature seeds, frozen, baby, cooked, boiled, drained, with salt	105	7	0	19	-3.04	-0.16
Lima beans, immature seeds, frozen, baby, cooked, boiled, drained, without salt	105	7	0	19	-3.04	-0.16
Lima beans, immature seeds, frozen, baby, unprepared	132	8	0	25	-3.68	-0.15
Lima beans, immature seeds, frozen, fordhook, cooked, boiled, drained, with salt	103	6	0	19	-1.30	-0.07
Lima beans, immature seeds, frozen, fordhook, cooked, boiled, drained, without salt	103	6	0	19	-1.30	-0.07
Lima beans, immature seeds, frozen, fordhook, unprepared	106	6	0	20	-5.46	-0.27
Lima beans, immature seeds, raw	113	7	1	20	-3.37	-0.17
Lotus root, cooked, boiled, drained, with salt	66	2	0	16	-4.87	-0.30
Lotus root, cooked, boiled, drained, without salt	66	2	0	16	-4.87	-0.30
Lotus root, raw	74	3	0	16	-7.88	-0.49
Malabar spinach, cooked	23	3	1	3	-5.44	-1.81
Mountain yam, Hawaii, cooked, steamed, with salt	82	2	0	20	-8.43	-0.42
Mountain yam, Hawaii, cooked, steamed, without salt	82	2	0	20	-8.43	-0.42
Mountain yam, Hawaii, raw	67	1	0	16	-7.51	-0.47
Mung beans, mature seeds, sprouted, cooked, boiled, drained, with salt	19	7	0	19	-0.61	-0.03
Mung beans, mature seeds, sprouted, cooked, boiled, drained, without salt	21	7	0	19	-0.61	-0.03
Mung beans, mature seeds, sprouted, cooked, stir-fried	50	4	0	11	-0.59	-0.05
Mung beans, mature seeds, sprouted, raw	30	3	0	6	-0.35	-0.06
Mushroom, oyster, raw	35	3	0	6	-3.26	-0.54
Mushrooms, brown, Italian, or Crimini, raw	27	3	0	4	-4.21	-1.05
Mushrooms, canned, drained solids	25	2	0	5	0.11	0.02

Vegetables

Food Description	Kcals	Protein	Fat	Carbs	PRAL	Alkali Density
Mushrooms, cooked, boiled, drained, with salt	28	2	0	5	-3.58	-0.72
Mushrooms, cooked, boiled, drained, without salt	28	2	0	5	-3.58	-0.72
Mushrooms, enoki, raw	44	3	0	8	-2.87	-0.36
Mushrooms, Maitake, Raw	37	2	0	7	-0.86	-0.12
Mushrooms, portabella, grilled	35	4	1	5	-3.74	-0.75
Mushrooms, portabella, raw	26	3	0	5	-4.51	-0.90
Mushrooms, shiitake, cooked, with salt	54	2	0	14	-1.02	-0.07
Mushrooms, shiitake, cooked, without salt	56	2	0	14	-1.02	-0.07
Mushrooms, shiitake, dried	296	10	1	75	-20.21	-0.27
Mushrooms, shiitake, stir-fried	48	3	0	8	-1.56	-0.20
Mushrooms, straw, canned, drained solids	32	4	1	5	2.18	0.44
Mushrooms, white, microwaved	44	4	0	6	-4.07	-0.68
Mushrooms, white, raw	22	3	0	3	-2.25	-0.75
Mushrooms, white, stir-fried	26	4	0	4	-3.01	-0.75
Mustard greens, cooked, boiled, drained, with salt	15	2	0	2	-2.97	-1.49
Mustard greens, cooked, boiled, drained, without salt	15	2	0	2	-2.97	-1.49
Mustard greens, frozen, cooked, boiled, drained, with salt	19	2	0	2	-2.57	-1.29
Mustard greens, frozen, cooked, boiled, drained, without salt	19	2	0	2	-2.57	-1.29
Mustard greens, frozen, unprepared	20	2	0	3	-3.13	-1.04
Mustard greens, raw	26	3	0	5	-6.69	-1.34
Mustard spinach, (tendergreen), cooked, boiled, drained, with salt	16	2	0	3	-6.72	-2.24
Mustard spinach, (tendergreen), cooked, boiled, drained, without salt	16	2	0	3	-6.72	-2.24
Mustard spinach, (tendergreen), raw	22	2	0	4	-10.33	-2.58
New Zealand spinach, cooked, boiled, drained, with salt	12	1	0	2	-2.14	-1.07
New Zealand spinach, cooked, boiled, drained, without salt	12	1	0	2	-2.14	-1.07
New Zealand spinach, raw	14	1	0	3	-2.72	-0.91
Nopales, cooked, without salt	15	1	0	3	-6.19	-2.06
Nopales, raw	16	1	0	3	-7.64	-2.55
Okra, cooked, boiled, drained, with salt	22	2	0	5	-2.67	-0.53
Okra, cooked, boiled, drained, without salt	22	2	0	5	-2.67	-0.53
Okra, frozen, cooked, boiled, drained, with salt	28	2	0	5	-4.76	-0.95
Okra, frozen, cooked, boiled, drained, without salt	28	2	0	5	-4.76	-0.95
Okra, frozen, unprepared	30	2	0	7	-4.22	-0.60
Okra, raw	31	2	0	7	-5.58	-0.80
Onion rings, breaded, par fried, frozen, prepared, heated in oven	407	5	27	38	2	0.05

Vegetables

Food Description	Kcals	Protein	Fat	Carbs	PRAL	Alkali Density
Onion rings, breaded, par fried, frozen, unprepared	258	3	14	31	-1.59	-0.05
Onions, canned, solids and liquids	19	1	0	4	-1.62	-0.41
Onions, cooked, boiled, drained, with salt	42	1	0	10	-2.09	-0.21
Onions, cooked, boiled, drained, without salt	44	1	0	10	-2.09	-0.21
Onions, dehydrated flakes	349	9	0	83	-24.19	-0.29
Onions, frozen, chopped, cooked, boiled, drained, with salt	26	1	0	7	-1.55	-0.22
Onions, frozen, chopped, cooked, boiled, drained, without salt	28	1	0	7	-1.55	-0.22
Onions, frozen, chopped, unprepared	29	1	0	7	-1.80	-0.26
Onions, frozen, whole, cooked, boiled, drained, with salt	26	1	0	7	-2.25	-0.32
Onions, frozen, whole, cooked, boiled, drained, without salt	28	1	0	7	-2.25	-0.32
Onions, frozen, whole, unprepared	35	1	0	8	-2.42	-0.30
Onions, raw	40	1	0	9	-2.01	-0.22
Onions, spring or scallions (includes tops and bulb), raw	32	2	0	7	-4.98	-0.71
Onions, sweet, raw	32	1	0	8	-1.60	-0.20
Onions, welsh, raw	34	1	0	8	-2.54	-0.32
Onions, yellow, sautéed	132	1	11	8	-1.60	-0.20
Onions, young green, tops only	25	1	0	7	-4.67	-0.67
Palm hearts, raw	115	3	0	26	-31.91	-1.23
Parsley, freeze-dried	271	31	5	42	-108.64	-2.59
Parsley, raw	36	3	1	6	-11.12	-1.85
Parsnips, cooked, boiled, drained, with salt	71	1	0	17	-5.74	-0.34
Parsnips, cooked, boiled, drained, without salt	71	1	0	17	-5.74	-0.34
Parsnips, raw	75	1	0	18	-5.88	-0.33
Peas and carrots, canned, no salt added, solids and liquids	38	2	0	8	0	0
Peas and carrots, canned, regular pack, solids and liquids	38	2	0	8	0	0
Peas and carrots, frozen, cooked, boiled, drained, with salt	48	3	0	10	-0.70	-0.07
Peas and carrots, frozen, cooked, boiled, drained, without salt	48	3	0	10	-0.70	-0.07
Peas and carrots, frozen, unprepared	53	3	0	11	-1	-0.09
Peas and onions, canned, solids and liquids	51	3	0	9	0.84	0.09
Peas and onions, frozen, cooked, boiled, drained, with salt	45	3	0	9	-0.47	-0.05
Peas and onions, frozen, cooked, boiled, drained, without salt	45	3	0	9	-0.47	-0.05
Peas and onions, frozen, unprepared	70	4	0	14	-0.97	-0.07
Peas, edible-podded, boiled, drained, without salt	42	3	0	7	-2.62	-0.37
Peas, edible-podded, cooked, boiled, drained, with salt	40	3	0	7	-2.62	-0.37

Vegetables

Food Description	Kcals	Protein	Fat	Carbs	PRAL	Alkali Density
Peas, edible-podded, frozen, cooked, boiled, drained, with salt	50	3	0	7	-2.19	-0.31
Peas, edible-podded, frozen, cooked, boiled, drained, without salt	52	3	0	7	-2.19	-0.31
Peas, edible-podded, frozen, unprepared	42	3	0	7	-2.02	-0.29
Peas, edible-podded, raw	42	3	0	7	-2.05	-0.29
Peas, green, canned, no salt added, drained solids	69	3	0	10	0.31	0.03
Peas, green, canned, no salt added, solids and liquids	53	3	0	10	0.74	0.07
Peas, green, canned, regular pack, drained solids	69	3	0	10	0.31	0.03
Peas, green, canned, regular pack, solids and liquids	53	3	0	10	0.74	0.07
Peas, green, canned, seasoned, solids and liquids	50	3	0	10	0.36	0.04
Peas, green, cooked, boiled, drained, with salt	84	3	0	10	-0.10	-0.01
Peas, green, cooked, boiled, drained, without salt	84	3	0	10	-0.10	-0.01
Peas, green, frozen, cooked, boiled, drained, with salt	78	3	0	10	1.26	0.13
Peas, green, frozen, cooked, boiled, drained, without salt	78	3	0	10	2.17	0.22
Peas, green, frozen, unprepared	77	5	0	14	1.44	0.10
Peas, green, raw	81	5	0	14	0.34	0.02
Peas, mature seeds, sprouted, cooked, boiled, drained, with salt	98	7	1	17	-2.69	-0.16
Peas, mature seeds, sprouted, cooked, boiled, drained, without salt	98	7	1	17	-2.69	-0.16
Peas, mature seeds, sprouted, raw	128	9	1	28	0.49	0.02
Pepeao, dried	298	5	0	81	-13.47	-0.17
Pepper, ancho, dried	281	12	5	81	-41.11	-0.51
Pepper, banana, raw	27	2	0	5	-4	-0.80
Pepper, serrano, raw	32	2	0	8	-4.78	-0.60
Peppers, chili, green, canned	21	1	0	5	-2.18	-0.44
Peppers, hot chile, sun-dried	324	11	6	70	-31.07	-0.44
Peppers, hot chili, green, canned, pods, excluding seeds, solids and liquids	21	1	0	5	-3.31	-0.66
Peppers, hot chili, green, raw	40	2	0	9	-5.34	-0.59
Peppers, hot chili, red, canned, excluding seeds, solids and liquids	21	1	0	5	-3.31	-0.66
Peppers, hot chili, red, raw	40	2	0	9	-5.03	-0.56
Peppers, Hungarian, raw	29	1	0	7	-3.34	-0.48
Peppers, jalapeno, canned, solids and liquids	27	1	1	5	-3.62	-0.72
Peppers, jalapeno, raw	30	1	1	6	-3.33	-0.56
Peppers, pasilla, dried	345	12	16	51	-35.37	-0.69
Peppers, sweet, green, canned, solids and liquids	18	1	0	4	-2.75	-0.69
Peppers, sweet, green, cooked, boiled, drained, with salt	27	1	0	4	-2.74	-0.69
Peppers, sweet, green, cooked, boiled, drained, without salt	28	1	0	4	-2.74	-0.69

Vegetables

Food Description	Kcals	Protein	Fat	Carbs	PRAL	Alkali Density
Peppers, sweet, green, freeze-dried	314	18	3	69	-52.33	-0.76
Peppers, sweet, green, frozen, chopped, boiled, drained, without salt	18	1	0	4	-0.85	-0.21
Peppers, sweet, green, frozen, chopped, cooked, boiled, drained, with salt	16	1	0	4	-0.85	-0.21
Peppers, sweet, green, frozen, chopped, unprepared	20	1	0	4	-1.07	-0.27
Peppers, sweet, green, raw	20	1	0	4	-2.90	-0.73
Peppers, sweet, green, sautéed	127	1	12	4	-2.18	-0.55
Peppers, sweet, red, canned, solids and liquids	18	1	0	4	-2.75	-0.69
Peppers, sweet, red, cooked, boiled, drained, with salt	27	1	0	4	-2.74	-0.69
Peppers, sweet, red, cooked, boiled, drained, without salt	28	1	0	4	-2.74	-0.69
Peppers, sweet, red, freeze-dried	314	18	3	69	-52.33	-0.76
Peppers, sweet, red, frozen, chopped, cooked, boiled, drained, with salt	16	1	0	3	-0.85	-0.28
Peppers, sweet, red, frozen, chopped, cooked, boiled, drained, without salt	16	1	0	3	-0.85	-0.28
Peppers, sweet, red, frozen, chopped, unprepared	20	1	0	3	-1.07	-0.36
Peppers, sweet, red, raw	26	1	0	3	-3.38	-1.13
Peppers, sweet, red, sautéed	133	1	13	7	-3.09	-0.44
Peppers, sweet, yellow, raw	27	1	0	3	-3.52	-1.17
Pickle relish, hamburger	129	1	1	34	-0.89	-0.03
Pickle relish, hot dog	91	1	1	30	0.01	0
Pickle relish, sweet	130	0	0	35	0	0
Pickles, chowchow, with cauliflower onion mustard, sweet	121	1	1	27	-3.49	-0.13
Pickles, cucumber, dill or kosher dill	12	1	0	3	-1.92	-0.64
Pickles, cucumber, dill, low sodium	18	1	0	3	-1.75	-0.58
Pickles, cucumber, sour	11	1	0	3	0.09	0.03
Pickles, cucumber, sour, low sodium	11	1	0	3	0.09	0.03
Pickles, cucumber, sweet (includes bread and butter pickles)	80	1	0	21	-2.12	-0.10
Pickles, cucumber, sweet, low sodium	122	0	0	34	-0.20	-0.01
Pigeonpeas, immature seeds, cooked, boiled, drained, with salt	111	6	1	19	-3.86	-0.20
Pigeonpeas, immature seeds, cooked, boiled, drained, without salt	111	6	1	19	-3.86	-0.20
Pigeonpeas, immature seeds, raw	136	7	2	24	-5.67	-0.24
Pimento, canned	23	1	0	5	-2.38	-0.48
Poi	112	0	0	27	-3.04	-0.11
Pokeberry shoots, (poke), cooked, boiled, drained, with salt	20	2	0	3	-2.56	-0.85
Pokeberry shoots, (poke), cooked, boiled, drained, without salt	20	2	0	3	-2.56	-0.85
Pokeberry shoots, (poke), raw	23	2	0	3	-3.33	-1.11
Potato flour	357	7	0	83	-13.95	-0.17

Vegetables

Food Description	Kcals	Protein	Fat	Carbs	PRAL	Alkali Density
Potato pancakes	269	6	15	28	-6.70	-0.24
Potato puffs, frozen, oven-heated	190	2	9	28	-2.36	-0.08
Potato puffs, frozen, unprepared	175	2	8	26	-1.98	-0.08
Potato salad, home-prepared	143	3	1	11	-2.73	-0.25
Potato, baked, flesh and skin, without salt	93	3	0	21	-8.34	-0.40
Potato, flesh and skin, raw	77	2	0	18	-6.49	-0.36
Potatoes, au gratin, dry mix, prepared with water, whole milk and butter	93	2	3	13	-1.42	-0.11
Potatoes, au gratin, dry mix, unprepared	314	9	2	74	-7.18	-0.10
Potatoes, au gratin, home-prepared from recipe using butter	132	5	5	11	-3.72	-0.34
Potatoes, au gratin, home-prepared from recipe using margarine	132	5	4	11	-3.72	-0.34
Potatoes, baked, flesh and skin, with salt	93	3	0	21	-8.34	-0.40
Potatoes, baked, flesh, with salt	93	2	0	22	-6.11	-0.28
Potatoes, baked, flesh, without salt	93	2	0	22	-6.11	-0.28
Potatoes, baked, skin, with salt	198	4	0	46	-7.75	-0.17
Potatoes, baked, skin, without salt	198	4	0	46	-7.75	-0.17
Potatoes, boiled, cooked in skin, flesh, with salt	87	2	0	20	-6.05	-0.30
Potatoes, boiled, cooked in skin, flesh, without salt	87	2	0	20	-6.05	-0.30
Potatoes, boiled, cooked in skin, skin, with salt	78	3	0	17	-6.51	-0.38
Potatoes, boiled, cooked in skin, skin, without salt	78	3	0	17	-6.51	-0.38
Potatoes, boiled, cooked without skin, flesh, with salt	86	2	0	20	-5.19	-0.26
Potatoes, boiled, cooked without skin, flesh, without salt	86	2	0	20	-5.19	-0.26
Potatoes, canned, drained solids	60	1	0	14	-3.51	-0.25
Potatoes, canned, drained solids, no salt added	62	1	0	14	-3.51	-0.25
Potatoes, canned, solids and liquids	44	1	0	10	-3.77	-0.38
Potatoes, French fried, all types, salt added in processing, frozen, unprepared	147	2	1	25	-5.06	-0.20
Potatoes, French fried, all types, salt added in processing, frozen, home-prepared, oven heated	134	3	1	28	-5.41	-0.19
Potatoes, French fried, all types, salt not added in processing, frozen, as purchased	150	2	1	25	-5.06	-0.20
Potatoes, French fried, all types, salt not added in processing, frozen, oven-heated	172	3	1	29	-5.41	-0.19
Potatoes, French fried, crinkle or regular cut, salt added in processing, frozen, oven-heated	166	3	1	27	-5.96	-0.22
Potatoes, French fried, crinkle or regular cut, salt added in processing, frozen, as purchased	174	2	1	30	-5.36	-0.18
Potatoes, French fried, shoestring, salt added in processing, frozen, oven-heated	199	3	1	32	-5.84	-0.18
Potatoes, French fried, shoestring, salt added in processing, frozen, as purchased	167	2	1	27	-4.75	-0.18
Potatoes, French fried, steak fries, salt added in processing, frozen, oven-heated	152	3	1	27	-5.77	-0.21
Potatoes, French fried, steak fries, salt added in processing, frozen, as purchased	133	2	1	24	-5.10	-0.21

Vegetables

Food Description	Kcals	Protein	Fat	Carbs	PRAL	Alkali Density
Potatoes, frozen, French fried, par fried, cottage-cut, prepared, heated in oven, with salt	218	3	4	34	-6.69	-0.20
Potatoes, frozen, French fried, par fried, cottage-cut, prepared, heated in oven, without salt	218	3	4	34	-6.69	-0.20
Potatoes, frozen, French fried, par fried, cottage-cut, unprepared	153	2	3	24	-4.71	-0.20
Potatoes, frozen, French fried, par fried, extruded, prepared, heated in oven, without salt	333	4	6	40	-6.78	-0.17
Potatoes, frozen, French fried, par fried, extruded, unprepared	260	3	5	30	-5.37	-0.18
Potatoes, frozen, whole, cooked, boiled, drained, with salt	63	2	0	14	-4.47	-0.32
Potatoes, frozen, whole, cooked, boiled, drained, without salt	65	2	0	14	-4.47	-0.32
Potatoes, frozen, whole, unprepared	78	2	0	17	-5.35	-0.31
Potatoes, hashed brown, frozen, plain, prepared	218	3	4	28	-5.58	-0.20
Potatoes, hashed brown, frozen, plain, unprepared	82	2	0	18	-3.65	-0.20
Potatoes, hashed brown, frozen, with butter sauce, prepared	178	2	3	24	-5.07	-0.21
Potatoes, hashed brown, frozen, with butter sauce, unprepared	135	2	3	18	-3.83	-0.21
Potatoes, hashed brown, home-prepared	265	3	2	35	-9.12	-0.26
Potatoes, mashed, dehydrated, flakes without milk, dry form	354	8	0	81	-15.26	-0.19
Potatoes, mashed, dehydrated, granules with milk, dry form	358	11	0	78	-28.46	-0.36
Potatoes, mashed, dehydrated, granules without milk, dry form	372	8	0	85	-4.75	-0.06
Potatoes, mashed, dehydrated, prepared from flakes without milk, whole milk and butter added	97	2	3	11	-1.77	-0.16
Potatoes, mashed, dehydrated, prepared from granules with milk, water and margarine added	116	2	1	16	-0.81	-0.05
Potatoes, mashed, dehydrated, prepared from granules without milk, whole milk and butter added	108	2	3	14	-0.74	-0.05
Potatoes, mashed, home-prepared, whole milk added	83	2	0	18	-4.35	-0.24
Potatoes, mashed, home-prepared, whole milk and butter added	113	2	4	17	-4.16	-0.24
Potatoes, mashed, home-prepared, whole milk and margarine added	111	2	1	17	-4.87	-0.29
Potatoes, mashed, prepared from flakes, without milk, whole milk and margarine	113	2	1	15	-2.99	-0.20
Potatoes, mashed, prepared from granules, without milk, whole milk and margarine	108	2	1	14	-0.77	-0.06
Potatoes, microwaved, cooked in skin, flesh and skin, without salt	105	2	0	24	-5.15	-0.21
Potatoes, microwaved, cooked in skin, flesh, with salt	100	2	0	23	-4.28	-0.19
Potatoes, microwaved, cooked in skin, flesh, without salt	100	2	0	23	-4.28	-0.19
Potatoes, microwaved, cooked in skin, skin, without salt	132	4	0	30	-10.02	-0.33
Potatoes, microwaved, cooked, in skin, flesh and skin, with salt	105	2	0	24	-5.15	-0.21
Potatoes, microwaved, cooked, in skin, skin with salt	132	4	0	30	-10.02	-0.33

Vegetables

Food Description	Kcals	Protein	Fat	Carbs	PRAL	Alkali Density
Potatoes, O'Brien, frozen, prepared	204	2	3	22	-6.54	-0.30
Potatoes, O'Brien, frozen, unprepared	76	2	0	17	-3.15	-0.19
Potatoes, O'Brien, home-prepared	81	2	1	15	-3.52	-0.23
Potatoes, raw, skin	58	3	0	12	-6.99	-0.58
Potatoes, red, flesh and skin, baked	89	2	0	20	-8.49	-0.42
Potatoes, red, flesh and skin, raw	70	2	0	16	-7.07	-0.44
Potatoes, Russet, flesh and skin, baked	97	3	0	21	-8.64	-0.41
Potatoes, russet, flesh and skin, raw	79	2	0	18	-6.44	-0.36
Potatoes, scalloped, dry mix, prepared with water, whole milk and butter	93	2	3	13	-1.98	-0.15
Potatoes, scalloped, dry mix, unprepared	358	8	1	74	-10.24	-0.14
Potatoes, scalloped, home-prepared with butter	88	3	2	11	-5.43	-0.49
Potatoes, scalloped, home-prepared with margarine	88	3	1	11	-5.43	-0.49
Potatoes, white, flesh and skin, baked	94	2	0	21	-8.45	-0.40
Potatoes, white, flesh and skin, raw	69	2	0	17	-6.09	-0.36
Pumpkin flowers, cooked, boiled, drained, without salt	15	1	0	3	-1.56	-0.52
Pumpkin flowers, raw	15	1	0	3	-2.44	-0.81
Pumpkin leaves, cooked, boiled, drained, without salt	21	2	0	3	-6.48	-2.16
Pumpkin leaves, raw	19	3	0	2	-5.26	-2.63
Pumpkin pie mix, canned	104	1	0	26	-1.59	-0.06
Pumpkin, canned, with salt	34	1	0	8	-3.42	-0.43
Pumpkin, canned, without salt	34	1	0	8	-3.42	-0.43
Pumpkin, cooked, boiled, drained, with salt	20	1	0	5	-3.79	-0.76
Pumpkin, cooked, boiled, drained, without salt	20	1	0	5	-3.79	-0.76
Pumpkin, flowers, cooked, boiled, drained, with salt	15	1	0	3	-1.56	-0.52
Pumpkin, leaves, cooked, boiled, drained, with salt	21	3	0	3	-6.48	-2.16
Pumpkin, raw	26	1	0	6	-5.60	-0.93
Purslane, cooked, boiled, drained, with salt	18	1	0	4	-10.90	-2.73
Purslane, cooked, boiled, drained, without salt	18	1	0	4	-10.90	-2.73
Purslane, raw	16	1	0	3	-10.72	-3.57
Radicchio, raw	23	1	0	4	-4.74	-1.19
Radish seeds, sprouted, raw	43	4	1	4	2.43	0.61
Radishes, Hawaiian style, pickled	28	1	0	5	-5.87	-1.17
Radishes, oriental, cooked, boiled, drained, with salt	17	1	0	3	-5.22	-1.74
Radishes, oriental, cooked, boiled, drained, without salt	17	1	0	3	-5.22	-1.74
Radishes, oriental, dried	271	1	0	3	-74.55	-24.85
Radishes, oriental, raw	18	1	0	4	-4.38	-1.10

Vegetables

Food Description	Kcals	Protein	Fat	Carbs	PRAL	Alkali Density
Radishes, raw	16	1	0	3	-4.40	-1.47
Radishes, white icicle, raw	14	1	0	3	-4.89	-1.63
Rutabagas, cooked, boiled, drained, with salt	39	1	0	9	-5.36	-0.60
Rutabagas, cooked, boiled, drained, without salt	39	1	0	9	-5.36	-0.60
Rutabagas, raw	36	1	0	8	-5.55	-0.69
Salsify, (vegetable oyster), raw	82	3	0	19	-4.96	-0.26
Salsify, cooked, boiled, drained, with salt	68	3	0	15	-3.61	-0.24
Salsify, cooked, boiled, drained, without salt	68	3	0	15	-3.61	-0.24
Sauerkraut, canned, low sodium	22	1	0	4	-3.11	-0.78
Sauerkraut, canned, solids and liquids	19	1	0	5	-3.11	-0.62
Seaweed, agar, dried	306	6	0	81	-46.80	-0.58
Seaweed, agar, raw	26	1	0	7	-6.74	-0.96
Seaweed, irishmoss, raw	49	2	0	12	0.54	0.05
Seaweed, kelp, raw	43	2	0	10	-4.82	-0.48
Seaweed, laver, raw	35	6	0	5	-3.44	-0.69
Seaweed, spirulina, dried	290	57	3	24	-2.72	-0.11
Seaweed, spirulina, raw	26	6	0	2	-0.01	0
Seaweed, wakame, raw	45	3	0	9	-1.33	-0.15
Sesbania flower, cooked, steamed, with salt	21	1	0	5	-1.50	-0.30
Sesbania flower, cooked, steamed, without salt	22	1	0	5	-1.50	-0.30
Sesbania flower, raw	27	1	0	7	-2.68	-0.38
Shallots, freeze-dried	348	12	0	81	-22.75	-0.28
Shallots, raw	72	3	0	17	-4.59	-0.27
Soybeans, green, cooked, boiled, drained, with salt	141	12	1	11	-2.86	-0.26
Soybeans, green, cooked, boiled, drained, without salt	141	12	1	11	-2.86	-0.26
Soybeans, green, raw	147	13	1	11	-3.74	-0.34
Soybeans, mature seeds, sprouted, cooked, steamed	81	8	1	7	-0.63	-0.09
Soybeans, mature seeds, sprouted, cooked, steamed, with salt	81	8	1	7	-0.63	-0.09
Soybeans, mature seeds, sprouted, cooked, stir-fried	125	13	1	10	-1.05	-0.11
Soybeans, mature seeds, sprouted, cooked, stir-fried, with salt	125	13	1	10	-1.05	-0.11
Soybeans, mature seeds, sprouted, raw	122	13	1	10	-0.42	-0.04
Spinach soufflé	171	8	6	6	1.25	0.21
Spinach, canned, drained solids	23	3	0	3	-7.88	-2.63
Spinach, canned, no salt added, solids and liquids	19	2	0	3	-5.14	-1.71
Spinach, canned, regular pack, solids and liquids	19	2	0	3	-5.14	-1.71
Spinach, cooked, boiled, drained, with salt	23	3	0	4	-10.28	-2.57

Vegetables

Food Description	Kcals	Protein	Fat	Carbs	PRAL	Alkali Density
Spinach, cooked, boiled, drained, without salt	23	3	0	4	-10.28	-2.57
Spinach, frozen, chopped or leaf, cooked, boiled, drained, with salt	32	4	0	5	-6.64	-1.33
Spinach, frozen, chopped or leaf, cooked, boiled, drained, without salt	32	4	0	5	-6.64	-1.33
Spinach, frozen, chopped or leaf, unprepared	31	4	0	4	-7.87	-1.97
Spinach, raw	23	3	0	4	-11.84	-2.96
Squash, summer, all varieties, cooked, boiled, drained, with salt	20	1	0	4	-3.11	-0.78
Squash, summer, all varieties, cooked, boiled, drained, without salt	20	1	0	4	-3.11	-0.78
Squash, summer, all varieties, raw	16	1	0	3	-4.14	-1.38
Squash, summer, crookneck and straightneck, canned, drained, solid, without salt	13	1	0	3	-1.43	-0.48
Squash, summer, crookneck and straightneck, cooked, boiled, drained, with salt	20	1	0	4	-2.72	-0.68
Squash, summer, crookneck and straightneck, cooked, boiled, drained, without salt	20	1	0	4	-2.72	-0.68
Squash, summer, crookneck and straightneck, frozen, cooked, boiled, drained, with salt	25	1	0	6	-4.13	-0.69
Squash, summer, crookneck and straightneck, frozen, cooked, boiled, drained, w/o salt	25	1	0	6	-4.13	-0.69
Squash, summer, crookneck and straightneck, frozen, unprepared	20	1	0	5	-3.51	-0.70
Squash, summer, crookneck and straightneck, raw	19	1	0	4	-3.62	-0.91
Squash, summer, scallop, cooked, boiled, drained, with salt	16	1	0	3	-2.08	-0.69
Squash, summer, scallop, cooked, boiled, drained, without salt	16	1	0	3	-2.08	-0.69
Squash, summer, scallop, raw	18	1	0	4	-2.74	-0.69
Squash, summer, zucchini, includes skin, cooked, boiled, drained, with salt	16	1	0	4	-4.26	-1.07
Squash, summer, zucchini, includes skin, cooked, boiled, drained, without salt	16	1	0	4	-4.26	-1.07
Squash, summer, zucchini, includes skin, frozen, cooked, boiled, drained, with salt	15	1	0	3	-3.14	-1.05
Squash, summer, zucchini, includes skin, frozen, cooked, boiled, drained, without salt	17	1	0	3	-3.14	-1.05
Squash, summer, zucchini, includes skin, frozen, unprepared	17	1	0	4	-3.54	-0.89
Squash, summer, zucchini, includes skin, raw	16	1	0	3	-4.14	-1.38
Squash, summer, zucchini, Italian style, canned	29	1	0	7	-4.76	-0.68
Squash, winter, acorn, cooked, baked, with salt	56	1	0	15	-8.65	-0.58
Squash, winter, acorn, cooked, baked, without salt	56	1	0	15	-8.65	-0.58
Squash, winter, acorn, cooked, boiled, mashed, with salt	34	1	0	9	-5.21	-0.58
Squash, winter, acorn, cooked, boiled, mashed, without salt	34	1	0	9	-5.21	-0.58
Squash, winter, acorn, raw	40	1	0	10	-6.82	-0.68
Squash, winter, all varieties, cooked, baked, with salt	39	1	0	9	-8.39	-0.93
Squash, winter, all varieties, cooked, baked, without salt	37	1	0	9	-4.54	-0.50
Squash, winter, all varieties, raw	34	1	0	9	-6.76	-0.75

Vegetables

Food Description	Kcals	Protein	Fat	Carbs	PRAL	Alkali Density
Squash, winter, butternut, cooked, baked, with salt	40	1	0	10	-5.81	-0.58
Squash, winter, butternut, cooked, baked, without salt	40	1	0	10	-5.81	-0.58
Squash, winter, butternut, frozen, cooked, boiled, with salt	39	1	0	10	-2.15	-0.22
Squash, winter, butternut, frozen, cooked, boiled, without salt	39	1	0	10	-2.15	-0.22
Squash, winter, butternut, frozen, unprepared	57	2	0	14	-3.51	-0.25
Squash, winter, butternut, raw	45	1	0	12	-7.18	-0.60
Squash, winter, hubbard, cooked, baked, with salt	50	2	0	11	-6.24	-0.57
Squash, winter, hubbard, cooked, baked, without salt	50	2	0	11	-6.24	-0.57
Squash, winter, hubbard, cooked, boiled, mashed, with salt	30	1	0	6	-3.71	-0.62
Squash, winter, hubbard, cooked, boiled, mashed, without salt	30	1	0	6	-3.71	-0.62
Squash, winter, hubbard, raw	40	2	0	9	-5.63	-0.63
Squash, winter, spaghetti, cooked, boiled, drained, or baked, without salt	27	1	0	6	-2.17	-0.36
Squash, winter, spaghetti, raw	31	1	0	7	-2.12	-0.30
Squash, zucchini, baby, raw	21	3	0	3	-6	-2
Succotash, (corn and limas), canned, with cream style corn	77	3	0	18	-0.53	-0.03
Succotash, (corn and limas), canned, with whole kernel corn, solids and liquids	63	3	0	14	-0.75	-0.05
Succotash, (corn and limas), cooked, boiled, drained, with salt	111	5	0	24	-3.39	-0.14
Succotash, (corn and limas), cooked, boiled, drained, without salt	115	5	0	24	-3.39	-0.14
Succotash, (corn and limas), frozen, cooked, boiled, drained, with salt	93	4	0	20	-1.65	-0.08
Succotash, (corn and limas), frozen, cooked, boiled, drained, without salt	93	4	0	20	-1.65	-0.08
Succotash, (corn and limas), frozen, unprepared	93	4	0	4	-2.02	-0.51
Succotash, (corn and limas), raw	99	5	0	20	-2.58	-0.13
Swamp cabbage, (skunk cabbage), raw	19	3	0	3	-6.68	-2.23
Swamp cabbage, cooked, boiled, drained, with salt	20	2	0	4	-4.87	-1.22
Swamp cabbage, cooked, boiled, drained, without salt	20	2	0	4	-4.87	-1.22
Sweet potato leaves, cooked, steamed, with salt	34	2	0	7	-8.55	-1.22
Sweet potato leaves, cooked, steamed, without salt	34	2	0	7	-8.55	-1.22
Sweet potato leaves, raw	35	4	0	6	-7.50	-1.25
Sweet potato, canned, mashed	101	2	0	23	-2.53	-0.11
Sweet potato, canned, syrup pack, drained solids	108	1	0	25	-3.03	-0.12
Sweet potato, canned, syrup pack, solids and liquids	89	1	0	21	-2.93	-0.14
Sweet potato, canned, vacuum pack	91	2	0	21	-4.78	-0.23
Sweet potato, cooked, baked in skin, with salt	90	2	0	21	-8.18	-0.39

Vegetables

Food Description	Kcals	Protein	Fat	Carbs	PRAL	Alkali Density
Sweet potato, cooked, baked in skin, without salt	90	2	0	21	-8.18	-0.39
Sweet potato, cooked, boiled, without skin	76	1	0	18	-3.79	-0.21
Sweet potato, cooked, boiled, without skin, with salt	76	1	0	18	-3.79	-0.21
Sweet potato, cooked, candied, home-prepared	144	1	1	29	-3.20	-0.11
Sweet potato, frozen, cooked, baked, with salt	100	2	0	23	-6.45	-0.28
Sweet potato, frozen, cooked, baked, without salt	100	2	0	23	-6.45	-0.28
Sweet potato, frozen, unprepared	96	2	0	22	-6.21	-0.28
Sweet potato, raw, unprepared	86	2	0	20	-5.60	-0.28
Taro leaves, cooked, steamed, without salt	24	3	0	4	-8.96	-2.24
Taro leaves, raw	42	5	1	7	-11.50	-1.64
Taro shoots, cooked, without salt	14	1	0	3	-6.29	-2.10
Taro shoots, raw	11	1	0	2	-5.84	-2.92
Taro, cooked, with salt	142	1	0	35	-8.11	-0.23
Taro, cooked, without salt	142	1	0	35	-8.11	-0.23
Taro, leaves, cooked, steamed, with salt	24	3	0	4	-8.96	-2.24
Taro, raw	112	1	0	26	-9.98	-0.38
Taro, shoots, cooked, with salt	14	1	0	3	-6.29	-2.10
Taro, Tahitian, cooked, with salt	44	4	0	7	-11.82	-1.69
Taro, Tahitian, cooked, without salt	44	4	0	7	-11.82	-1.69
Taro, Tahitian, raw	44	3	0	7	-12.59	-1.80
Tomatillos, raw	32	1	0	6	-4.32	-0.72
Tomato and vegetable juice, low sodium	22	1	0	5	-3.55	-0.71
Tomato juice, canned, with salt added	17	1	0	4	-4.18	-1.05
Tomato juice, canned, without salt added	17	1	0	4	-4.18	-1.05
Tomato powder	302	13	0	75	-30.01	-0.40
Tomato products, canned, paste, with salt added	82	4	0	19	-17.66	-0.93
Tomato products, canned, paste, without salt added	82	4	0	19	17.66	0.93
Tomato products, canned, puree, with salt added	38	2	0	8	-7.76	-0.97
Tomato products, canned, puree, without salt added	38	2	0	9	-7.76	-0.86
Tomato products, canned, sauce	24	1	0	6	-5.92	-0.99
Tomato products, canned, sauce, Spanish style	33	1	0	7	-5.98	-0.85
Tomato products, canned, sauce, with herbs and cheese	59	2	1	10	-5.40	-0.54
Tomato products, canned, sauce, with mushrooms	35	1	0	8	-6.74	-0.84
Tomato products, canned, sauce, with onions	42	2	0	10	-7.18	-0.72
Tomato products, canned, sauce, with onions, green peppers, and celery	41	1	0	9	-7.20	-0.80
Tomato products, canned, sauce, with tomato tidbits	32	1	0	7	-6.28	-0.90

Vegetables

Food Description	Kcals	Protein	Fat	Carbs	PRAL	Alkali Density
Tomato sauce, no salt added	37	1	0	9	-6.64	-0.74
Tomatoes, crushed, canned	32	2	0	7	-5.12	-0.73
Tomatoes, green, raw	23	1	0	5	-3.08	-0.62
Tomatoes, orange, raw	16	1	0	3	-3.08	-1.03
Tomatoes, red, ripe, canned, packed in tomato juice	17	1	0	4	-3.55	-0.89
Tomatoes, red, ripe, canned, packed in tomato juice, no salt added	17	1	0	4	-3.55	-0.89
Tomatoes, red, ripe, canned, stewed	26	1	0	6	-3.91	-0.65
Tomatoes, red, ripe, canned, with green chilies	15	1	0	4	-1.93	-0.48
Tomatoes, red, ripe, cooked	18	1	0	4	-3.45	-0.86
Tomatoes, red, ripe, cooked, stewed	79	2	1	13	-3.54	-0.27
Tomatoes, red, ripe, cooked, with salt	18	1	0	4	-3.45	-0.86
Tomatoes, red, ripe, raw, year round average	18	1	0	4	-4.07	-1.02
Tomatoes, sun-dried	258	14	0	56	-58.35	-1.04
Tomatoes, sun-dried, packed in oil, drained	213	5	14	23	-27.96	-1.22
Tomatoes, yellow, raw	15	1	0	3	-4.06	-1.35
Tree fern, cooked, with salt	40	0	0	11	-0.04	0
Tree fern, cooked, without salt	40	0	0	11	-0.04	0
Turnip greens and turnips, frozen, cooked, boiled, drained, with salt	21	3	0	5	-1.14	-0.23
Turnip greens and turnips, frozen, cooked, boiled, drained, without salt	21	3	0	5	-1.14	-0.23
Turnip greens and turnips, frozen, unprepared	21	2	0	3	-1.57	-0.52
Turnip greens, canned, no salt added	19	1	0	3	-3.57	-1.19
Turnip greens, canned, solids and liquids	14	1	0	2	-3.57	-1.79
Turnip greens, cooked, boiled, drained, with salt	20	1	0	4	-4.98	-1.25
Turnip greens, cooked, boiled, drained, without salt	20	1	0	4	-4.98	-1.25
Turnip greens, frozen, cooked, boiled, drained, with salt	29	3	0	5	-4.45	-0.89
Turnip greens, frozen, cooked, boiled, drained, without salt	29	3	0	5	-4.45	-0.89
Turnip greens, frozen, unprepared	22	2	0	4	-3.89	-0.97
Turnip greens, raw	32	1	0	7	-7.20	-1.03
Turnips, cooked, boiled, drained, with salt	22	1	0	5	-2.27	-0.45
Turnips, cooked, boiled, drained, without salt	22	1	0	5	-3.07	-0.61
Turnips, frozen, cooked, boiled, drained, with salt	21	2	0	4	-2.89	-0.72
Turnips, frozen, cooked, boiled, drained, without salt	23	2	0	4	-2.89	-0.72
Turnips, frozen, unprepared	16	1	0	3	-2.18	-0.73
Turnips, raw	28	1	0	6	-3.24	-0.54
USDA Commodity, Potato wedges, frozen	123	3	1	26	-4.42	-0.17
Vegetable juice cocktail, canned	19	1	0	5	-3.54	-0.71

Vegetables

Food Description	Kcals	Protein	Fat	Carbs	PRAL	Alkali Density
Vegetables, mixed (corn, lima beans, peas, green beans, carrots) canned, no salt added	37	1	0	7	-1.50	-0.21
Vegetables, mixed, canned, drained solids	49	3	0	9	-4.05	-0.45
Vegetables, mixed, canned, solids and liquids	36	3	0	7	-1.49	-0.21
Vegetables, mixed, frozen, cooked, boiled, drained, with salt	60	3	0	13	-1.15	-0.09
Vegetables, mixed, frozen, cooked, boiled, drained, without salt	65	3	0	13	-1.15	-0.09
Vegetables, mixed, frozen, unprepared	64	3	0	13	-1.58	-0.12
Vinespinach, (basella), raw	19	2	0	3	-11.01	-3.67
Wasabi, root, raw	109	5	0	24	-10.07	-0.42
Waterchestnuts, Chinese, (matai), raw	97	1	0	24	-9.96	-0.42
Waterchestnuts, Chinese, canned, solids and liquids	50	1	0	12	-1.52	-0.13
Watercress, raw	11	2	0	1	-5.68	-5.68
Waxgourd, (Chinese preserving melon), cooked, boiled, drained, with salt	11	0	0	3	0.22	0.07
Waxgourd, (Chinese preserving melon), cooked, boiled, drained, without salt	14	0	0	3	0.22	0.07
Waxgourd, (Chinese preserving melon), raw	13	0	0	3	0.26	0.09
Winged bean leaves, raw	74	6	0	14	-1.61	-0.12
Winged bean tuber, raw	148	12	0	28	-5.97	-0.21
Winged bean, immature seeds, cooked, boiled, drained, with salt	37	5	0	3	-3.80	-1.27
Winged beans, immature seeds, cooked, boiled, drained, without salt	38s	5	0	3	-3.80	-1.27
Winged beans, immature seeds, raw	49	7	-	4	-1.88	-0.47
Yam, cooked, boiled, drained, or baked, with salt	114	1	0	27	-12.17	-0.45
Yam, cooked, boiled, drained, or baked, without salt	116	1	0	27	-12.17	-0.45
Yam, raw	118	2	0	28	-15.11	-0.54
Yambean (jicama), cooked, boiled, drained, with salt	36	1	0	9	-2.31	-0.26
Yambean (jicama), cooked, boiled, drained, without salt	38	1	0	9	-2.31	-0.26
Yambean (jicama), raw	38	1	0	9	-2.59	-0.29
Yardlong bean, cooked, boiled, drained, with salt	47	3	0	9	-4.40	-0.49
Yardlong bean, cooked, boiled, drained, without salt	47	3	0	9	-4.40	-0.49
Yardlong bean, raw	47	3	0	9	-3.27	-0.36
Yautia (tannier), raw	98	1	0	28	-10.69	-0.38
Yeast extract spread	158	28	0	12	-42.92	-3.58

Ethnic Foods

Food Description	Kcals	Protein	Fat	Carbs	PRAL	Alkali Density
Acorn stew (Apache)	95	7	1	9	2.82	0.40
Agave, cooked (Southwest)	135	1	0	32	-7.41	-7.41
Agave, dried (Southwest)	341	2	0	82	-29.29	-14.65
Agave, raw (Southwest)	68	1	0	16	-9	-9
Agutuk, fish/berry with seal oil (Alaskan ice cream) (Alaska Native)	353	3	38	13	1.61	0.54
Agutuk, meat-caribou (Alaskan ice cream) (Alaska Native)	258	22	19	1	11.40	0.52
Blackberries, wild, raw (Alaska Native)	52	1	1	10	-0.92	-0.92
Blueberries, wild, raw (Alaska Native)	61	1	1	10	-0.25	-0.25
Bread, kneel down (Navajo)	195	4	2	39	-0.04	-0.01
Buffalo, free range, top round steak, cooked (Shoshone Bannock)	146	33	2	0	16.38	0.50
Buffalo, free range, top round steak, raw (Shoshone Bannock)	99	21	1	0	9.84	0.47
Caribou, hind quarter meat, raw (Alaska Native)	122	22	3	0	12.13	0.55
Caribou, rump meat, partially dried (Alaska Native)	261	52	5	0	26.61	0.51
Caribou, shoulder meat, dried (Alaska Native)	271	59	4	0	30.64	0.52
Chilchen (Red Berry Beverage) (Navajo)	44	1	1	9	0.33	0.33
Chokecherries, raw, pitted (Shoshone Bannock)	156	3	1	34	-4.47	-1.49
Corn, dried (Navajo)	386	10	5	75	3.16	0.32
Corn, dried, Yellow, Yankton Sioux Reservation, SD - CY013ER (Plains)	419	14	11	67	-0.65	-0.05
Corn, white, steamed (Navajo)	386	10	5	75	1.75	0.18
Corned beef and potatoes in tortilla (Apache)	224	8	8	29	0.21	0.03
Cornmeal, blue (Navajo)	398	10	5	75	6.41	0.64
Cornmeal, white (Navajo)	398	11	1	77	3.04	0.28
Cornmeal, yellow (Navajo)	384	10	6	73	3.53	0.35
Elk, free range, ground, cooked patties (Shoshone Bannock)	143	29	3	0	14.46	0.50
Elk, free range, ground, raw (Shoshone Bannock)	103	20	2	2	9.60	0.48
Elk, free range, roast, eye of round, cooked (Shoshone Bannock)	151	31	3	1	15.22	0.49
Elk, free range, roast, eye of round, raw (Shoshone Bannock)	101	30	3	1	9.24	0.31
Fish, halibut, cooked, with skin (Alaska Native)	113	22	3	0	9.31	0.42
Fish, halibut, raw, with skin (Alaska Native)	108	21	3	0	8.72	0.42
Fish, salmon, chum, dried (Alaska Native)	338	62	14	0	31.67	0.51
Fish, Salmon, Chum, raw (Alaska Native)	116	21	3	0	10.11	0.48
Fish, salmon, Coho (silver), raw (Alaska Native)	145	21	3	0	11.16	0.53
Fish, salmon, king (Chinook), raw (Alaska Native)	190	20	12	1	8.67	0.43
Fish, salmon, king, with skin, kippered, (Alaska Native) - CY040CJ	209	22	13	2	11.69	0.53
Fish, salmon, red (sockeye), smoked (Alaska Native)	327	31	18	5	27.14	0.88
Fish, salmon, red, (sockeye), canned, smoked (Alaska Native)	206	35	7	0	18.41	0.53

Ethnic Foods

Food Description	Kcals	Protein	Fat	Carbs	PRAL	Alkali Density
Fish, salmon, red, canned, bones removed (Alaska Native)	161	27	6	0	14.03	0.52
Fish, sheefish, dried (Alaska Native)	161	27	6	0	14.03	0.52
Fish, whitefish, dried (Alaska Native)	371	62	13	0	11.34	0.18
Fish, whitefish, eggs (Alaska Native)	371	15	3	5	33.65	2.24
Frybread, made with lard (Apache)	104	8	10	74	13.13	1.64
Frybread, made with lard (Navajo)	309	7	12	48	5.50	0.79
Melon, banana (Navajo)	330	1	0	4	5	5
Moose, liver, braised (Alaska Native)	21	24	5	3	-2.62	-0.11
Moose, meat, raw (Alaska Native)	155	24	5	3	11.17	0.47
Mush, blue corn with ash (Navajo)	103	1	0	12	9.71	9.71
Mutton, cooked, roasted (Navajo)	54	33	11	0	-1.22	-0.04
Oil, bearded seal (Oogruk) (Alaska Native)	899	1	100	0	16.92	16.92
Oil, beluga, whale (Alaska Native)	900	0	100	0	0	High
Oil, spotted seal (Alaska Native)	900	0	100	0	0	High
Salmonberries, raw (Alaska Native)	896	0	100	0	0	High
Seal, bearded (Oogruk), meat, dried, in oil (Alaska Native)	378	35	25	3	-1.45	-0.04
Seal, bearded (Oogruk), meat, low quadrant, raw (Alaska Native)	378	35	25	3	16.93	0.48
Seal, bearded (Oogruk), meat, partially dried (Alaska Native)	194	62	2	0	11.85	0.19
Smelt, dried (Alaska Native)	270	56	18	1	27.54	0.49
Soup, fish, homemade (Alaska Native)	389	7	2	6	35.21	5.03
Squash, Indian, raw (Navajo)	72	1	0	6	4.60	4.60
Steelhead trout, boiled, canned (Alaska Native)	26	21	8	0	-3.98	-0.19
Steelhead trout, dried, flesh (Shoshone Bannock)	159	21	8	0	10.85	0.52
Stew, dumpling with mutton (Navajo)	382	9	4	8	34.56	3.84
Stew, hominy with mutton (Navajo)	101	7	2	9	4.48	0.64
Stew, moose (Alaska Native)	83	7	0	6	3.22	0.46
Stew, mutton, corn, squash (Navajo)	55	9	4	7	1.41	0.16
Stew, steamed corn (Navajo)	103	9	4	11	3.11	0.35
Stew/soup, caribou (Alaska Native)	112	4	1	5	3.65	0.91
Tamales (Navajo)	41	6	6	18	0.32	0.05
Tea, tundra, herb and Labrador combination (Alaska Native)	153	0	0	0	3.04	
Tennis Bread, plain (Apache)	258	9	1	53	-0.24	-0.03
Tortilla, includes plain and from mutton sandwich (Navajo)	258	9	1	53	6.63	0.74
Whale, beluga, meat, dried (Alaska Native)	237	70	5	0	5.36	0.08
Whale, beluga, meat, raw (Alaska Native)	111	27	0	0	35.82	1.33

Snacks

Food Description	Kcals	Protein	Fat	Carbs	PRAL	Alkali Density
Breakfast bar, corn flake crust with fruit	377	4	8	73	0.59	0.01
Breakfast bars, oats, sugar, raisins, coconut (include granola bar)	377	4	8	73	0.59	0.01
Cheese puffs and twists, corn based, low fat	464	8	12	72	4.79	0.07
Formulated Bar, MASTERFOODS USA, SNICKERS Marathon Energy Bar, all flavors	432	22	11	50	5.66	0.11
Formulated Bar, MASTERFOODS USA, SNICKERS MARATHON Protein Performance Bar, Caramel Nut Rush	389	25	10	53	2.15	0.04
Formulated bar, POWER BAR, chocolate	402	14	3	70	7.15	0.10
Granola bar, soft, milk chocolate coated, peanut butter	363	10	31	54	9.05	0.17
Popcorn, microwave, low fat and sodium	536	13	9	73	2.83	0.04
Popcorn, sugar syrup/caramel, fat-free	429	2	1	90	6.81	0.08
Potato chips, without salt, reduced fat	381	7	21	68	-0.23	0
Pretzels, soft	487	8	3	69	-28.59	-0.41
Rice cake, cracker (include hain mini rice cakes)	338	7	4	81	4.24	0.05
Snacks, banana chips	392	2	34	58	4.26	0.07
Snacks, beef jerky, chopped and formed	519	33	26	11	-10.26	-0.93
Snacks, beef sticks, smoked	410	22	50	5	17.20	3.44
Snacks, CHEX mix	550	11	17	65	10.36	0.16
Snacks, corn cakes, very low sodium	425	8	2	83	4.56	0.05
Snacks, corn-based, extruded, chips, barbecue-flavor	387	7	33	56	3.27	0.06
Snacks, corn-based, extruded, chips, barbecue-flavor, made with enriched masa flour	523	7	33	56	2.42	0.04
Snacks, corn-based, extruded, chips, plain	523	7	33	56	2.42	0.04
Snacks, corn-based, extruded, chips, unsalted	518	7	33	56	1.61	0.03
Snacks, corn-based, extruded, cones, nacho-flavor	557	7	33	56	2.72	0.05
Snacks, corn-based, extruded, cones, plain	536	7	33	56	2.29	0.04
Snacks, corn-based, extruded, onion-flavor	510	7	33	56	2.44	0.04
Snacks, corn-based, extruded, puffs or twists, cheese-flavor	500	5	30	51	2.32	0.05
Snacks, corn-based, extruded, puffs or twists, cheese-flavor, unenriched	559	6	36	54	1.40	0.03
Snacks, cornnuts, barbecue-flavor	558	9	14	72	1.40	0.02
Snacks, cornnuts, nacho-flavor	436	9	14	72	5.82	0.08
Snacks, crisped rice bar, chocolate chip	438	5	13	73	6.21	0.09
Snacks, DOO DADS snack mix, original flavor	404	10	18	64	2.40	0.04
Snacks, FRITOLAY, SUNCHIPS, Multigrain Snack, original flavor	456	8	21	67	7.66	0.11
Snacks, granola bar, fruit-filled, nonfat	491	6	1	78	5	0.06
Snacks, granola bar, with coconut, chocolate coated	342	5	32	55	1.44	0.03
Snacks, granola bars, hard, almond	531	8	26	62	0.91	0.01
Snacks, granola bars, hard, chocolate chip	495	6	20	75	3.95	0.05

Snacks

Food Description	Kcals	Protein	Fat	Carbs	PRAL	Alkali Density
Snacks, granola bars, hard, peanut butter	479	6	19	78	6.71	0.09
Snacks, granola bars, hard, plain	483	6	19	78	1.87	0.02
Snacks, granola bars, oats, fruits and nut	471	5	19	75	4.82	0.06
Snacks, granola bars, soft, coated, milk chocolate coating, chocolate chip	397	6	25	64	5.08	0.08
Snacks, granola bars, soft, coated, milk chocolate coating, peanut butter	466	6	25	64	0.57	0.01
Snacks, granola bars, soft, uncoated, chocolate chip	509	7	33	50	3.13	0.06
Snacks, granola bars, soft, uncoated, chocolate chip, graham and marshmallow	418	6	32	50	2.10	0.04
Snacks, granola bars, soft, uncoated, nut and raisin	427	6	32	50	1.68	0.03
Snacks, granola bars, soft, uncoated, peanut butter	454	6	32	51	1.14	0.02
Snacks, granola bars, soft, uncoated, peanut butter and chocolate chip	426	6	32	51	4.86	0.10
Snacks, granola bars, soft, uncoated, plain	432	6	32	51	3.25	0.06
Snacks, granola bars, soft, uncoated, raisin	443	6	32	51	2.02	0.04
Snacks, KELLOGG, KELLOGG'S Low Fat Granola Bar, Crunchy Almond/Brown Sugar	448	8	7	78	1.07	0.01
Snacks, KELLOGG, KELLOGG'S NUTRI-GRAIN Cereal Bars, fruit	390	7	7	70	5.15	0.07
Snacks, KELLOGG, KELLOGG'S RICE KRISPIES TREATS Squares	368	3	9	81	0.59	0.01
Snacks, KRAFT, CORNNUTS, plain	414	8	16	72	2.02	0.03
Snacks, M&M MARS, KUDOS Whole Grain Bar, chocolate chip	446	4	13	72	5.44	0.08
Snacks, oriental mix, rice-based	420	17	36	52	-11.92	-0.23
Snacks, popcorn, air-popped	506	13	5	78	7.51	0.10
Snacks, popcorn, air-popped, white popcorn	387	12	4	78	8.84	0.11
Snacks, popcorn, cakes	382	10	3	80	7.12	0.09
Snacks, popcorn, caramel-coated, with peanuts	384	6	8	81	3.88	0.05
Snacks, popcorn, caramel-coated, without peanuts	400	4	13	79	-2.55	-0.03
Snacks, popcorn, cheese-flavor	431	9	33	52	1.17	0.02
Snacks, popcorn, microwave, 94% fat free	526	10	7	76	8.59	0.11
Snacks, popcorn, oil-popped, microwave, regular flavor	410	7	44	45	7.01	0.16
Snacks, popcorn, oil-popped, unsalted	583	7	44	45	5	0.11
Snacks, popcorn, oil-popped, white popcorn	521	9	28	57	5.99	0.11
Snacks, popcorn, unpopped kernels	500	11	4	74	5.99	0.08
Snacks, pork skins, barbecue-flavor	375	58	32	2	7.37	3.69
Snacks, pork skins, plain	538	58	32	2	32.17	16.09
Snacks, potato chips, barbecue-flavor	545	8	32	53	29.83	0.56
Snacks, potato chips, cheese-flavor	491	8	32	53	-18.42	-0.35
Snacks, potato chips, fat free, salted	496	10	1	84	-19.74	-0.24
Snacks, potato chips, fat-free, made with olestra	379	8	1	65	-25.56	-0.39

Snacks

Food Description	Kcals	Protein	Fat	Carbs	PRAL	Alkali Density
Snacks, potato chips, made from dried potatoes, cheese-flavor	274	3	37	51	-16.37	-0.32
Snacks, potato chips, made from dried potatoes, fat-free, made with olestra	551	5	1	56	-1.34	-0.02
Snacks, potato chips, made from dried potatoes, light	253	6	26	65	-9	-0.14
Snacks, potato chips, made from dried potatoes, plain	501	6	26	65	-14.74	-0.23
Snacks, potato chips, made from dried potatoes, sour-cream and onion-flavor	558	6	26	65	-14.28	-0.22
Snacks, potato chips, plain, made with partially hydrogenated soybean oil, unsalted	536	7	35	53	-19.29	-0.36
Snacks, potato chips, plain, made with partially hydrogenated soybean oil, salted	547	7	35	53	-3.19	-0.06
Snacks, potato chips, plain, salted	536	7	35	53	-19.29	-0.36
Snacks, potato chips, plain, unsalted	547	7	35	53	-27.66	-0.52
Snacks, potato chips, reduced fat	536	7	35	53	-19.29	-0.36
Snacks, potato chips, sour-cream-and-onion-flavor	471	56	30	53	-28.59	-0.54
Snacks, potato chips, white, restructured, baked	531	5	18	71	-20.33	-0.29
Snacks, potato sticks	469	7	34	53	-5.29	-0.10
Snacks, pretzels, hard, confectioner's coating, chocolate-flavor	522	8	18	71	-18.22	-0.26
Snacks, pretzels, hard, plain, made with enriched flour, unsalted	458	9	4	79	2.28	0.03
Snacks, pretzels, hard, plain, made with unenriched flour, salted	381	9	4	79	4.19	0.05
Snacks, pretzels, hard, plain, made with unenriched flour, unsalted	381	9	4	79	4.19	0.05
Snacks, pretzels, hard, plain, salted	381	9	4	79	4.19	0.05
Snacks, pretzels, hard, whole-wheat	380	9	4	79	5.40	0.07
Snacks, rice cakes, brown rice, buckwheat	362	9	4	79	-0.11	0
Snacks, rice cakes, brown rice, buckwheat, unsalted	380	9	1	80	8.12	0.10
Snacks, rice cakes, brown rice, corn	380	9	1	80	8.12	0.10
Snacks, rice cakes, brown rice, multigrain	385	9	1	80	7.10	0.09
Snacks, rice cakes, brown rice, multigrain, unsalted	387	8	1	80	7.84	0.10
Snacks, rice cakes, brown rice, plain	387	8	1	80	7.84	0.10
Snacks, rice cakes, brown rice, plain, unsalted	387	8	1	80	7.69	0.10
Snacks, rice cakes, brown rice, rye	387	8	1	80	7.69	0.10
Snacks, rice cakes, brown rice, sesame seed	386	8	4	82	7.48	0.09
Snacks, rice cakes, brown rice, sesame seed, unsalted	392	8	4	82	7.81	0.10
Snacks, sesame sticks, wheat-based, salted	392	8	4	82	7.81	0.10
Snacks, sesame sticks, wheat-based, unsalted	541	8	4	82	3.35	0.04
Snacks, sweet potato chips	541	8	4	82	3.35	0.04
Snacks, taro chips	496	2	25	68	-14.95	-0.22
Snacks, tortilla chips, light (baked with less oil)	498	9	15	73	-12.84	-0.18
Snacks, tortilla chips, low fat, made with olestra, nacho cheese	465	8	4	65	5.72	0.09

Snacks

Food Description	Kcals	Protein	Fat	Carbs	PRAL	Alkali Density
Snacks, tortilla chips, low fat, unsalted	402	11	6	80	0.23	0
Snacks, tortilla chips, nacho cheese	416	8	26	62	6.85	0.11
Snacks, tortilla chips, nacho-flavor, made with enriched masa flour	514	8	26	62	4.56	0.07
Snacks, tortilla chips, nacho-flavor, reduced fat	498	8	16	62	4.27	0.07
Snacks, tortilla chips, plain, white corn	445	8	23	66	5.72	0.09
Snacks, tortilla chips, ranch-flavor	489	7	25	63	0.64	0.01
Snacks, tortilla chips, taco-flavor	501	7	25	63	3.40	0.05
Snacks, tortilla chips, unsalted, white corn	480	8	23	66	3.85	0.06
Snacks, trail mix, regular	488	14	29	45	0.64	0.01
Snacks, trail mix, regular, unsalted	462	14	29	45	0.02	0
Snacks, trail mix, regular, with chocolate chips, salted nuts and seeds	462	14	32	45	0.02	0
Snacks, trail mix, regular, with chocolate chips, unsalted nuts and seeds	484	14	32	45	2.06	0.05
Snacks, trail mix, tropical	484	6	17	66	2.06	0.03
Tortilla chips, low fat, baked without fat	407	11	6	80	-8.15	-0.10

Meals, Entrees, and Sidedishes

Food Description	Kcals	Protein	Fat	Carbs	PRAL	Alkali Density
Beef Macaroni, frozen entrée	88	6	1	14	1.12	0.08
Beef stew, canned entrée	95	5	5	7	0.28	0.04
Burrito, bean and cheese, frozen	243	7	6	32	-1.01	-0.03
Burrito, beef and bean, frozen	278	7	10	31	0.29	0.01
Chicken pot pie, frozen entrée	223	6	13	20	2.02	0.10
Chili con carne with beans, canned entree	121	7	5	11	0.06	0.01
Chili, no beans, canned entrée	118	8	7	6	1.74	0.29
Lasagna with meat & sauce, frozen entree	127	8	5	13	1.68	0.13
Lasagna with meat & sauce, low-fat, frozen entrée	101	7	2	13	-0.45	-0.03
Lasagna, Cheese, frozen, prepared	130	7	5	14	1.35	0.10
Macaroni and Cheese, canned entree	82	3	2	12	0.94	0.08
NESTLE, CHEF-MATE Chili with Beans, canned entrée	166	7	9	13	0.79	0.06
NESTLE, CHEF-MATE Chili without Beans, canned entrée	147	5	9	13	1.47	0.11
NESTLE, CHEF-MATE Corned Beef Hash, canned entrée	180	7	11	11	2.63	0.24
Pasta with meatballs in tomato sauce, canned entrée	103	4	4	12	-0.15	-0.01
Pasta with Sliced Franks in Tomato Sauce, canned entrée	104	4	5	12	-1.20	-0.10
Spaghetti with meat sauce, frozen entree	90	5	1	15	0.64	0.04
Spaghetti, no meat, canned	75	3	1	15	-1.57	-0.10
Spaghetti, with meatballs, canned	107	4	2	14	-1.29	-0.09
Tortellini, pasta with cheese filling	307	13	7	47	10.06	0.21
WORTHINGTON FOODS, MORNINGSTAR FARMS "Burger" Crumbles	150	19	4	9	10.45	1.16

Fastfood

Food Description	Kcals	Protein	Fat	Carbs	PRAL	Alkali Density
BURGER KING, Cheeseburger	286	15	15	26	6.85	0.26
BURGER KING, CHICKEN TENDERS	289	17	17	18	10.48	0.58
BURGER KING, Chicken WHOPPER Sandwich	216	12	11	19	6.46	0.34
BURGER KING, CROISSAN'WICH with Egg and Cheese	283	10	16	25	7.31	0.29
BURGER KING, CROISSAN'WICH with Sausage and Cheese	376	14	23	25	6.38	0.26
BURGER KING, CROISSAN'WICH with Sausage, Egg and Cheese	322	12	22	18	7.34	0.41
BURGER KING, DOUBLE WHOPPER, no cheese	252	14	15	16	5.98	0.37
BURGER KING, DOUBLE WHOPPER, with cheese	266	14	17	15	6.34	0.42
BURGER KING, French Fries	331	4	17	42	-3.82	-0.09
BURGER KING, French Toast Sticks	349	6	18	41	2.64	0.06
BURGER KING, Hamburger	275	14	12	28	6.24	0.22
BURGER KING, Hash Brown Rounds	369	3	24	35	-2.89	-0.08
BURGER KING, Original Chicken Sandwich	286	13	15	26	6.05	0.23
BURGER KING, Vanilla Shake	168	3	9	19	0.27	0.01
BURGER KING, WHOPPER, no cheese	233	11	13	20	4.06	0.20
BURGER KING, WHOPPER, with cheese	250	11	13	20	4.58	0.23
DOMINO'S 14" Cheese Pizza, Classic Hand-Tossed Crust	257	11	8	34	6.74	0.20
DOMINO'S 14" Cheese Pizza, Crunchy Thin Crust	315	13	17	28	10.06	0.36
DOMINO'S 14" Cheese Pizza, Ultimate Deep Dish Crust	274	11	10	34	7.02	0.21
DOMINO'S 14" EXTRAVAGANZZA FEAST Pizza, Classic Hand-Tossed Crust	244	10	11	26	6.17	0.24
DOMINO'S 14" Pepperoni Pizza, Classic Hand-Tossed Crust	270	12	11	32	6.59	0.21
DOMINO'S 14" Pepperoni Pizza, Ultimate Deep Dish Crust	288	12	12	32	7.60	0.24
Egg, Cheese and Bacon Griddle Cake Sandwich	272	12	13	26	14.13	0.54
Egg, Cheese and Sausage Griddle Cake Sandwich	291	12	13	26	11.99	0.46
Entrees, crab cake	266	19	17	9	12.03	1.34
Entrees, fish fillet, battered or breaded, and fried	232	15	12	17	5.93	0.35
Fast Food, Pizza Chain, 14" Pizza, cheese topping, regular crust	264	11	8	34	7.52	0.22
Fast Food, Pizza Chain, 14" Pizza, cheese topping, thick crust	272	11	8	34	7.53	0.22
Fast Food, Pizza Chain, 14" Pizza, cheese topping, thin crust	304	11	8	34	9.30	0.27
Fast Food, Pizza Chain, 14" pizza, meat and vegetable topping, regular crust	244	9	10	30	6.14	0.20
Fast Food, Pizza Chain, 14" pizza, pepperoni topping, regular crust	276	12	12	32	7.17	0.22
Fast Food, Pizza Chain, 14" Pizza, pepperoni topping, thick crust	284	12	12	32	7.31	0.23
Fast foods, bagel, with breakfast steak, egg, cheese, and condiments	282	16	14	23	10.53	0.46
Fast foods, bagel, with egg, sausage patty, cheese, and condiments	295	16	14	23	8.88	0.39
Fast foods, bagel, with ham, egg, and cheese	253	17	14	25	9.85	0.39

Fastfood

Food Description	Kcals	Protein	Fat	Carbs	PRAL	Alkali Density
Fast foods, biscuit with egg and steak	277	16	14	26	5.56	0.21
Fast foods, biscuit, with egg	274	9	16	23	9.90	0.43
Fast foods, biscuit, with egg and bacon	305	11	21	19	5.87	0.31
Fast foods, biscuit, with egg and ham	240	11	21	19	5.92	0.31
Fast Foods, biscuit, with egg and sausage	323	11	21	19	10.05	0.53
Fast foods, biscuit, with egg, cheese, and bacon	320	12	22	22	12.74	0.58
Fast foods, biscuit, with ham	342	12	10	39	17.91	0.46
Fast foods, biscuit, with sausage	391	10	7	30	12.99	0.43
Fast foods, brownie	405	5	17	65	3.47	0.05
Fast foods, burrito, with beans	206	6	6	33	-3.19	-0.10
Fast foods, burrito, with beans and cheese	203	8	4	30	-0.66	-0.02
Fast foods, burrito, with beans and chili peppers	202	8	7	28	-1.50	-0.05
Fast foods, burrito, with beans and meat	220	10	4	29	-0.47	-0.02
Fast foods, burrito, with beans, cheese, and beef	163	7	4	20	0.34	0.02
Fast foods, burrito, with beans, cheese, and chili peppers	197	10	3	25	1.06	0.04
Fast foods, burrito, with beef	238	12	5	27	0.33	0.01
Fast foods, burrito, with beef and chili peppers	212	11	4	25	1.28	0.05
Fast foods, burrito, with beef, cheese, and chili peppers	208	13	3	21	4.29	0.20
Fast foods, burrito, with fruit (apple or cherry)	312	3	13	47	-1.09	-0.02
Fast foods, cheeseburger, regular, double patty and bun, plain	305	30	11	30	6.27	0.21
Fast foods, cheeseburger; double, large patty, with condiments and vegetables	273	15	17	15	6.29	0.42
Fast foods, cheeseburger; double, large patty; with condiments	272	17	16	14	7.40	0.53
Fast Foods, cheeseburger; double, large patty; with condiments, vegetables and mayonnaise	253	15	16	14	6.82	0.49
Fast foods, cheeseburger; double, regular patty, with condiments and vegetables	251	13	13	21	5.62	0.27
Fast foods, cheeseburger; double, regular patty; plain	308	17	17	21	7.75	0.37
Fast foods, cheeseburger; double, regular patty; with condiments and special sauce	261	12	14	22	4.76	0.22
Fast foods, cheeseburger; double, regular patty; with condiments	274	15	15	20	6.13	0.31
Fast foods, cheeseburger; double, regular, patty and bun; with condiments and vegetables	285	13	15	23	7.08	0.31
Fast foods, cheeseburger; single, large patty; plain	305	17	17	21	8.07	0.38
Fast foods, cheeseburger; single, large patty; with condiments	269	15	14	20	6.53	0.33
Fast foods, cheeseburger; single, large patty; with condiments and vegetables	207	15	16	18	3.94	0.22
Fast foods, cheeseburger; single, large patty; with condiments and bacon	282	16	16	19	7.05	0.37
Fast foods, cheeseburger; single, large patty; with condiments, vegetables and mayonnaise	235	16	19	18	5.60	0.31
Fast foods, cheeseburger; single, large patty; with condiments, vegetables and ham	286	16	19	13	8.83	0.68

Fastfood

Food Description	Kcals	Protein	Fat	Carbs	PRAL	Alkali Density
Fast foods, cheeseburger; single, regular patty, with condiments	270	13	13	25	5.80	0.23
Fast foods, cheeseburger; single, regular patty, with condiments and vegetables	233	14	13	24	5.74	0.24
Fast foods, cheeseburger; single, regular patty; plain	303	15	13	30	6.27	0.21
Fast foods, cheeseburger; triple, regular patty; plain	310	18	19	16	8.53	0.53
Fast foods, chicken fillet sandwich, plain	283	13	16	21	6.23	0.30
Fast foods, chicken fillet sandwich, with cheese	277	13	17	18	7.87	0.44
Fast foods, chicken tenders	290	17	17	18	10.74	0.60
Fast foods, chicken, breaded and fried, boneless pieces, plain	297	16	19	16	12.01	0.75
Fast foods, chicken, breaded and fried, dark meat (drumstick or thigh)	291	20	18	11	8.66	0.79
Fast foods, chicken, breaded and fried, light meat (breast or wing)	303	22	18	12	9.32	0.78
Fast foods, chili con carne	101	10	3	9	1.10	0.12
Fast foods, chimichanga, with beef	244	11	11	25		0
Fast foods, chimichanga, with beef and cheese	242	11	13	21	4.26	0.20
Fast foods, chimichanga, with beef and red chili peppers	223	10	10	24	-1.29	-0.05
Fast foods, chimichanga, with beef, cheese, and red chili peppers	202	11	10	26	0.97	0.04
Fast foods, clams, breaded and fried	392	11	24	34	7.33	0.22
Fast foods, coleslaw	148	1	11	13	-2.38	-0.18
Fast foods, cookies, animal crackers	446	6	13	75	4.17	0.06
Fast foods, cookies, chocolate chip	423	5	22	66	1.71	0.03
Fast foods, corn on the cob with butter	106	3	2	22	-1.69	-0.08
Fast foods, croissant, with egg and cheese	290	10	10	19	9.25	0.49
Fast foods, croissant, with egg, cheese, and bacon	320	13	22	18	8.81	0.49
Fast foods, croissant, with egg, cheese, and ham	312	13	22	18	8.84	0.49
Fast foods, croissant, with egg, cheese, and sausage	327	13	24	14	7.63	0.55
Fast foods, Danish pastry, cheese	388	6	27	32	2.26	0.07
Fast foods, Danish pastry, cinnamon	397	5	19	53	2.53	0.05
Fast foods, Danish pastry, fruit	356	5	17	48	2.03	0.04
Fast foods, egg and cheese sandwich	233	11	13	18	7.79	0.43
Fast foods, egg, scrambled	212	10	12	18	11.54	0.64
Fast foods, enchilada, with cheese	196	8	12	18	-0.55	-0.03
Fast foods, enchilada, with cheese and beef	168	6	9	16	-2.68	-0.17
Fast foods, enchirito, with cheese, beef, and beans	178	8	10	17	0.31	0.02
Fast foods, English muffin, with butter	300	8	9	42	3.80	0.09
Fast foods, English muffin, with cheese and sausage	342	13	18	17	.16	0.01
Fast foods, English muffin, with egg, cheese, and Canadian bacon	211	14	18	18	8.34	0.46
Fast foods, English muffin, with egg, cheese, and sausage	295	13	18	17	7.11	0.42

Fastfood

Food Description	Kcals	Protein	Fat	Carbs	PRAL	Alkali Density
Fast foods, fish sandwich, with tartar sauce	273	11	14	26	4.46	0.17
Fast foods, fish sandwich, with tartar sauce and cheese	286	11	16	26	5.92	0.23
Fast foods, French toast sticks	364	6	18	41	2.99	0.07
Fast foods, French toast with butter	264	8	14	27	3.98	0.15
Fast foods, frijoles with cheese	135	7	5	17	-3.17	-0.19
Fast foods, ham and cheese sandwich	241	14	11	23	5.16	0.22
Fast foods, ham, egg, and cheese sandwich	243	14	11	24	10.07	0.42
Fast foods, hamburger, large, single patty, with condiments	248	16	12	22	4.80	0.22
Fast foods, hamburger, large, triple patty, with condiments	267	19	16	11	7.84	0.71
Fast foods, hamburger; double, large patty; with condiments and vegetables	239	14	16	15	6.12	0.41
Fast foods, hamburger; double, large patty; with condiments, vegetables and mayonnaise	252	15	16	15	5.98	0.40
Fast foods, hamburger; double, regular patty; with condiments	268	14	16	15	5.88	0.39
Fast foods, hamburger; double, regular, patty; plain	295	13	16	15	6.80	0.45
Fast foods, hamburger; single, large patty, with condiments and vegetables	235	12	13	18	4.05	0.23
Fast foods, hamburger; single, large patty; plain	311	17	14	24	7.50	0.31
Fast foods, hamburger; single, large patty; with condiments	256	17	15	24	5.68	0.24
Fast foods, hamburger; single, large patty; with condiments and vegetables	197	17	15	24	3.44	0.14
Fast foods, hamburger; single, large patty; with condiments, vegetables and mayonnaise	226	17	15	24	4.13	0.17
Fast foods, hamburger; single, regular patty; plain	295	11	15	14	5.34	0.38
Fast foods, hamburger; single, regular patty; with condiments	258	11	16	14	5.10	0.36
Fast foods, hamburger; single, regular patty; with condiments and special sauce	259	11	15	14	4.07	0.29
Fast foods, hamburger; single, regular patty; with condiments and vegetables	254	11	15	14	4.34	0.31
Fast foods, hotdog, plain	247	11	15	18	5.14	0.29
Fast foods, hotdog, with chili	260	12	12	27	8.50	0.31
Fast foods, hotdog, with corn flour coating (corndog)	263	10	11	32	4.05	0.13
Fast foods, hush puppies	329	6	15	45	5.34	0.12
Fast foods, ice milk, vanilla, soft-serve, with cone	159	4	6	23	1.07	0.05
Fast foods, Miniature cinnamon rolls	403	7	18	53	6.30	0.12
Fast foods, nachos, with cheese	306	8	17	32	5.37	0.17
Fast foods, nachos, with cheese and jalapeno peppers	298	8	12	22	2.82	0.13
Fast foods, nachos, with cheese, beans, ground beef, and peppers	223	8	12	22	2.75	0.13
Fast foods, nachos, with cinnamon and sugar	543	7	33	58	1.35	0.02
Fast foods, onion rings, breaded and fried	332	4	19	38	1.11	0.03
Fast foods, oysters, battered or breaded, and fried	265	9	13	29	6.18	0.21
Fast foods, pancakes with butter and syrup	224	4	6	39	5.80	0.15

Fastfood

Food Description	Kcals	Protein	Fat	Carbs	PRAL	Alkali Density
Fast foods, potato, baked and topped with cheese sauce	160	5	10	16	-3.79	-0.24
Fast foods, potato, baked and topped with cheese sauce and bacon	151	6	9	15	-2.90	-0.19
Fast foods, potato, baked and topped with cheese sauce and broccoli	119	4	6	14	-5.06	-0.36
Fast foods, potato, baked and topped with cheese sauce and chili	122	5	6	14	-2.89	-0.21
Fast foods, potato, baked and topped with sour cream and chives	130	5	6	14	-7.33	-0.52
Fast foods, potato, French fried in vegetable oil	319	4	17	38	-5.65	-0.15
Fast foods, potato, mashed	83	12	1	16	-3.74	-0.23
Fast foods, potatoes, hashed brown	326	3	22	32	-2.82	-0.09
Fast foods, roast beef sandwich, plain	249	15	10	24	8.09	0.34
Fast foods, salad, vegetable, tossed, without dressing	16	1	0	3	-2.01	-0.67
Fast foods, salad, vegetable, tossed, without dressing, with cheese and egg	47	4	3	2	-0.23	-0.12
Fast foods, salad, vegetable, tossed, without dressing, with chicken	48	4	3	2	1.89	0.95
Fast foods, salad, vegetable, tossed, without dressing, with pasta and seafood	91	6	10	11	0.18	0.02
Fast foods, salad, vegetable, tossed, without dressing, with shrimp	45	6	8	6	1.19	0.20
Fast foods, salad, vegetables tossed, without dressing, with turkey, ham and cheese	82	8	5	1	4.55	4.55
Fast foods, scallops, breaded and fried	268	11	13	27	7.84	0.29
Fast foods, shrimp, breaded and fried	277	12	15	24	9.77	0.41
Fast foods, submarine sandwich, with cold cuts	200	10	8	22	3.86	0.18
Fast foods, submarine sandwich, with roast beef	190	13	6	21	5.52	0.26
Fast foods, submarine sandwich, with tuna salad	228	12	11	22	4.93	0.22
Fast foods, sundae, caramel	196	5	6	32	1.12	0.04
Fast foods, sundae, hot fudge	180	5	6	32	-0.42	-0.01
Fast foods, sundae, strawberry	175	4	5	29	0.24	0.01
Fast foods, taco	217	12	12	16	1.76	0.11
Fast foods, taco salad	141	7	7	12	-0.41	-0.03
Fast foods, taco salad with chili con carne	111	7	5	10	0.55	0.06
Fast foods, tostada, with beans and cheese	155	7	7	18	-2.57	-0.14
Fast foods, tostada, with beans, beef, and cheese	148	7	7	8	-0.09	-0.01
Fast foods, tostada, with beef and cheese	193	7	9	19	-0.33	-0.02
LITTLE CAESARS 14" Cheese Pizza, Large Deep Dish Crust	263	13	10	30	7.39	0.25
LITTLE CAESARS 14" Cheese Pizza, Thin Crust	309	11	8	34	9.01	0.27
LITTLE CAESARS 14" Original Round Cheese Pizza, Regular Crust	265	12	9	32	7.78	0.24
LITTLE CAESARS 14" Original Round Meat and Vegetable Pizza, Regular Crust	243	12	11	32	6.70	0.21
LITTLE CAESARS 14" Original Round Pepperoni Pizza, Regular Crust	273	12	11	34	7.75	0.23
LITTLE CAESARS 14" Pepperoni Pizza, Large Deep Dish Crust	265	13	10	32	7.34	0.23

Fastfood

Food Description	Kcals	Protein	Fat	Carbs	PRAL	Alkali Density
McDonald's Bacon Egg & Cheese Biscuit	306	12	13	26	14.92	0.57
McDonald's, Bacon Ranch Salad without chicken	61	4	4	4	-1.60	-0.40
McDonald's, Baked Apple Pie	323	3	16	44	1.08	0.02
McDonald's, Barbeque Sauce	165	2	1	37	-2.74	-0.07
McDonald's, BIG BREAKFAST	279	10	20	17	9.22	0.54
McDonald's, BIG MAC	257	12	15	20	4.47	0.22
McDonald's, BIG MAC (without Big Mac Sauce)	234	13	12	21	4.88	0.23
McDonald's, Biscuit	346	6	16	35	15.74	0.45
McDonald's, Caesar Salad without chicken	44	3	2	4	-1.40	-0.35
McDonald's, Cheeseburger	263	13	12	28	4.64	0.17
McDonald's, Chicken McNuggets	264	16	15	16	13.95	0.87
McDonald's, Chicken SELECTS Premium Breast Strips	286	17	16	19	11.78	0.62
McDonald's, Chocolate TRIPLE THICK Shake	163	4	5	28	-1.05	-0.04
McDonald's, Creamy Ranch Sauce	468	1	52	3	-0.43	-0.14
McDonald's, Deluxe Breakfast	279	8	15	30	7.21	0.24
McDonald's, Deluxe Warm Cinnamon Roll	367	6	16	52	2.24	0.04
McDonald's, Double Cheeseburger	265	15	15	20	6.13	0.31
McDonald's, DOUBLE QUARTER POUNDER with Cheese	262	17	16	14	7.40	0.53
McDonald's, Egg McMuffin	215	13	9	21	7.01	0.33
McDonald's, English Muffin	285	9	8	44	1.89	0.04
McDonald's, FILET-O-FISH	284	11	15	29	3.81	0.13
McDonald's, FILET-O-FISH (without tartar sauce)	235	12	9	32	4.37	0.14
McDonald's, French Fries	337	3	18	41	-6.26	-0.15
McDonald's, Fruit 'n Yogurt Parfait	105	3	1	21	-0.54	-0.03
McDonald's, Fruit 'n Yogurt Parfait (without granola)	90	2	1	18	-1.07	-0.06
McDonald's, Hamburger	252	12	9	31	3.65	0.12
McDonald's, Hash Browns	257	2	17	25	-3.94	-0.16
McDonald's, Honey	351	0	0	86	-0.52	-0.01
McDonald's, Hot Caramel Sundae	188	2	5	33	0.02	0
McDonald's, Hot Fudge Sundae	186	2	5	33	-0.70	-0.02
McDonald's, Hot Mustard Sauce	190	3	7	29	0.60	0.02
McDonald's, Hotcakes (plain)	228	6	6	38	7.34	0.19
McDonald's, Hotcakes (with 2 pats margarine & syrup)	272	4	8	46	4.83	0.11
McDonald's, Hotcakes and Sausage	294	6	13	39	5.06	0.13
McDonald's, Low Fat Caramel Sauce	313	2	3	72	0.58	0.01
McDonald's, McChicken Sandwich	289	10	16	27	5.06	0.19
McDonald's, McChicken Sandwich (without mayonnaise)	240	11	9	29	5.44	0.19

Fastfood

Food Description	Kcals	Protein	Fat	Carbs	PRAL	Alkali Density
McDonald's, McDonaldLand Chocolate Chip Cookies	480	6	23	66	1.05	0.02
McDonald's, McDonaldLand Cookies	447	6	23	66	4.60	0.07
McDonald's, McFlurry with M&M'S CANDIES	177	4	6	27	-0.30	-0.01
McDonald's, McFlurry with OREO cookies	165	4	6	26	-0.14	-0.01
McDonald's, NEWMAN'S OWN Cobb Dressing	196	2	14	15	0.82	0.05
McDonald's, NEWMAN'S OWN Creamy Caesar Dressing	319	4	32	7	2.10	0.30
McDonald's, NEWMAN'S OWN Low Fat Balsamic Vinaigrette	86	0	6	25	-0.47	-0.02
McDonald's, NEWMAN'S OWN Ranch Dressing	313	4	32	7	0.49	0.07
McDonald's, Peanuts (for Sundaes)	640	28	53	16	8.27	0.52
McDonald's, Premium Crispy Chicken Classic Sandwich	217	12	8	26	5.80	0.22
McDonald's, Premium Grilled Chicken Classic Sandwich	183	14	4	22	8.15	0.37
McDonald's, QUARTER POUNDER	244	14	12	22	5.06	0.23
McDonald's, QUARTER POUNDER with Cheese	258	15	14	20	6.06	0.30
McDonald's, Sausage Biscuit	372	10	25	28	12.08	0.43
McDonald's, Sausage Biscuit with Egg	312	11	22	20	12.38	0.62
McDonald's, Sausage Burrito	262	12	15	21	8.09	0.39
McDonald's, Sausage McGriddles	312	8	18	31	11.58	0.37
McDonald's, Sausage McMuffin	333	13	21	25	4.82	0.19
McDonald's, Sausage McMuffin with Egg	274	13	18	17	6.20	0.36
McDonald's, Sausage Patty	405	15	40	1	6.28	6.28
McDonald's, Sausage, Egg & Cheese McGriddles	283	10	20	33	11.95	0.36
McDonald's, Scrambled Eggs	193	15	15	2	12.94	6.47
McDonald's, Spicy Buffalo Sauce	142	1	15	2	-1.70	-0.85
McDonald's, Strawberry Sundae	158	3	4	28	-0.41	-0.01
McDonald's, Strawberry TRIPLE THICK Shake	158	4	4	27	-0.34	-0.01
McDonald's, Sweet 'N Sour Sauce	170	1	1	39	-1.39	-0.04
McDonald's, Tangy Honey Mustard Sauce	167	1	6	29	0.33	0.01
McDonald's, Vanilla Reduced Fat Ice Cream Cone	162	4	5	26	0.11	0
McDonald's, Vanilla TRIPLE THICK Shake	156	3	4	27	-0.18	-0.01
McDonald's, Warm Cinnamon Roll	398	7	18	53	3.19	0.06
PAPA JOHN'S 14" Cheese Pizza, Original Crust	260	12	9	33	7.48	0.23
PAPA JOHN'S 14" Cheese Pizza, Thin Crust	295	11	8	32	8.06	0.25
PAPA JOHN'S 14" Pepperoni Pizza, Original Crust	275	12	30	12	7.39	0.62
PAPA JOHN'S 14" The Works Pizza, Original Crust	240	10	10	27	5.75	0.21
PIZZA HUT 12" Cheese Pizza, Regular Crust	271	12	11	31	8.13	0.26
PIZZA HUT 12" Cheese Pizza, Thick Crust	280	13	12	32	7.88	0.25

Fastfood

Food Description	Kcals	Protein	Fat	Carbs	PRAL	Alkali Density
PIZZA HUT 12" Cheese Pizza, THIN 'N CRISPY Crust	303	15	14	29	10.97	0.38
PIZZA HUT 12" Pepperoni Pizza, Regular Crust	280	13	11	32	7.40	0.23
PIZZA HUT 12" Pepperoni Pizza, Thick Crust	298	12	14	30	6.80	0.23
PIZZA HUT 12" Super Supreme Pizza, Regular Crust	243	11	11	26	5.57	0.21
PIZZA HUT 14" Cheese Pizza, Regular Crust	271	12	11	31	7.85	0.25
PIZZA HUT 14" Cheese Pizza, Thick Crust	280	13	12	32	8.14	0.25
PIZZA HUT 14" Cheese Pizza, THIN 'N CRISPY Crust	296	15	14	29	10.86	0.37
PIZZA HUT 14" Pepperoni Pizza, Regular Crust	287	13	11	32	7	0.22
PIZZA HUT 14" Pepperoni Pizza, Thick Crust	298	12	14	30	7.47	0.25
PIZZA HUT 14" Super Supreme Pizza, Regular Crust	248	11	11	26	6.01	0.23
Pizza, cheese topping, regular crust, frozen, cooked	268	10	12	29	5.58	0.19
Pizza, cheese topping, rising crust, frozen, cooked	260	12	9	33	8.21	0.25
Pizza, meat and vegetable topping, regular crust, frozen, cooked	276	13	12	29	5.20	0.18
Pizza, meat and vegetable topping, rising crust, frozen, cooked	271	13	12	29	7.31	0.25
Pizza, pepperoni topping, regular crust, frozen, cooked	296	13	12	28	6.40	0.23
Sandwiches and burgers, roast beef sandwich with cheese	269	15	10	24	11.34	0.47
Sandwiches and burgers, steak sandwich	225	15	10	23	6.08	0.26
Sausage Griddle Cake Sandwich	318	8	18	31	11.58	0.37
Side dishes, potato salad	114	2	6	14	-3.23	-0.23
TACO BELL, Bean Burrito	204	8	7	28	2.18	0.08
TACO BELL, BURRITO SUPREME with beef	189	8	8	21	1.97	0.09
TACO BELL, BURRITO SUPREME with chicken	179	8	7	20	3.35	0.17
TACO BELL, BURRITO SUPREME with steak	183	8	8	22	2.51	0.11
TACO BELL, Nachos	366	5	22	36	6.66	0.19
TACO BELL, Nachos Supreme	246	8	14	23	3.78	0.16
TACO BELL, Original Taco with beef	236	11	13	18	5.45	0.30
TACO BELL, Soft Taco with beef	219	12	10	20	5.98	0.30
TACO BELL, Soft Taco with chicken	202	14	7	20	8.39	0.42
TACO BELL, Soft Taco with steak	225	12	12	17	5.61	0.33
TACO BELL, Taco Salad	170	7	9	15	0.34	0.02
Tostada with guacamole	138	5	9	12	-2.42	-0.20
WENDY'S, Chicken Nuggets	334	16	23	16	12.53	0.78
WENDY'S, CLASSIC DOUBLE, with cheese	241	17	14	12	7.31	0.61
WENDY'S, CLASSIC SINGLE Hamburger, no cheese	213	13	11	17	4.99	0.29
WENDY'S, CLASSIC SINGLE Hamburger, with cheese	221	15	12	14	6.55	0.47
WENDY'S, French Fries	319	4	19	39	-6.17	-0.16

Fastfood

Food Description	Kcals	Protein	Fat	Carbs	PRAL	Alkali Density
WENDY'S, Frosty Dairy Dessert	132	3	3	24	-0.21	-0.01
WENDY'S, Homestyle Chicken Fillet Sandwich	214	14	8	22	6.99	0.32
WENDY'S, Jr. Hamburger, with cheese	256	13	11	25	5.85	0.23
WENDY'S, Jr. Hamburger, without cheese	243	13	9	28	5.33	0.19
WENDY'S, Ultimate Chicken Grill Sandwich	179	15	5	19	7.84	0.41

Grains

Food Description	Kcals	Protein	Fat	Carbs	PRAL	Alka Densi
Amaranth	374	14	7	66	7.32	0.11
Arrowroot flour	357	0	0	88	-0.49	-0.0
Barley flour or meal	345	11	2	75	6.69	0.09
Barley malt flour	361	10	2	78	8.54	0.11
Barley, hulled	354	12	2	73	2.50	0.03
Barley, pearled, cooked	123	2	0	28	0.43	0.02
Barley, pearled, raw	352	10	1	78	4.72	0.0
Buckwheat	343	13	3	71	3.43	0.05
Buckwheat flour, whole-groat	335	13	3	71	-0.52	-0.0
Buckwheat groats, roasted, cooked	92	3	1	20	0.98	0.05
Buckwheat groats, roasted, dry	346	12	3	75	4.86	0.06
Bulgur, cooked	83	3	0	19	0.59	0.03
Bulgur, dry	342	12	1	76	3.79	0.05
Corn bran, crude	224	8	1	86	3.62	0.0
Corn flour, degermed, unenriched, yellow	375	6	1	83	2.57	0.0
Corn flour, masa, enriched, white	365	9	4	76	1.87	0.0
Corn flour, masa, enriched, yellow	365	9	4	76	1.87	0.0
Corn flour, whole-grain, white	361	7	4	77	4.33	0.0
Corn flour, whole-grain, yellow	361	7	4	77	4.33	0.0
Corn, white	365	9	5	74	2.96	0.0
Corn, yellow	365	9	5	74	2.96	0.0
Cornmeal, degermed, enriched, white	369	7	2	79	3.29	0.0
Cornmeal, degermed, enriched, yellow	369	7	2	79	3.29	0.0
Cornmeal, degermed, unenriched, white	369	7	2	79	3.29	0.0
Cornmeal, degermed, unenriched, yellow	369	7	2	79	3.29	0.0
Cornmeal, self-rising, bolted, plain, enriched, white	334	8	3	73	21.52	0.2
Cornmeal, self-rising, bolted, plain, enriched, yellow	334	8	3	73	21.52	0.2
Cornmeal, self-rising, bolted, with wheat flour added, enriched, white	348	8	3	73	18.57	0.2
Cornmeal, self-rising, bolted, with wheat flour added, enriched, yellow	348	8	3	73	18.57	0.2
Cornmeal, self-rising, degermed, enriched, white	355	8	2	75	17.77	0.2
Cornmeal, self-rising, degermed, enriched, yellow	355	8	2	75	17.77	0.2
Cornmeal, whole-grain, white	362	8	4	77	3.48	0.0
Cornmeal, whole-grain, yellow	362	8	4	77	3.48	0.0
Cornstarch	381	0	0	91	0.44	0
Couscous, cooked	112	4	0	23	1.14	0.0
Couscous, dry	376	13	1	77	7.60	0.1
Hominy, canned, white	72	1	1	14	1.28	0.0
Hominy, canned, yellow	72	1	1	14	1.28	0.0

Grains

Food Description	Kcals	Protein	Fat	Carbs	PRAL	Alkali Density
Macaroni, cooked, enriched	158	6	1	31	3.50	0.11
Macaroni, cooked, unenriched	158	6	1	31	3.50	0.11
Macaroni, dry, enriched	371	13	2	75	7.04	0.09
Macaroni, dry, unenriched	371	13	2	75	7.04	0.09
Macaroni, protein-fortified, cooked, enriched, (n x 5.70)	164	20	2	68	4.01	0.06
Macaroni, protein-fortified, cooked, enriched, (n x 6.25)	164	20	2	68	4.39	0.06
Macaroni, protein-fortified, dry, enriched, (n x 5.70)	375	22	2	66	9.34	0.14
Macaroni, protein-fortified, dry, enriched, (n x 6.25)	374	22	2	66	10.28	0.16
Macaroni, vegetable, cooked, enriched	128	5	0	27	2.78	0.10
Macaroni, vegetable, dry, enriched	367	13	1	75	3.10	0.04
Macaroni, whole-wheat, cooked	124	5	1	27	4	0.15
Macaroni, whole-wheat, dry	348	15	1	75	7.96	0.11
Millet, cooked	119	4	1	24	2.93	0.12
Millet, raw	378	11	4	73	8.78	0.12
Noodles, Chinese, chow mein	527	8	31	58	5.93	0.10
Noodles, egg, cooked, enriched	138	5	2	25	3.53	0.14
Noodles, egg, cooked, enriched, with added salt	138	5	2	25	3.53	0.14
Noodles, egg, cooked, unenriched, with added salt	138	5	2	25	3.53	0.14
Noodles, egg, cooked, unenriched, without added salt	138	5	2	25	3.53	0.14
Noodles, egg, dry, enriched	384	14	4	71	8.76	0.12
Noodles, egg, dry, unenriched	384	14	4	71	8.76	0.12
Noodles, egg, spinach, cooked, enriched	132	5	2	24	2.93	0.12
Noodles, egg, spinach, dry, enriched	382	15	5	70	3.98	0.06
Noodles, Japanese, soba, cooked	99	5	0	21	2.38	0.11
Noodles, Japanese, soba, dry	336	14	1	75	8.22	0.11
Noodles, Japanese, somen, cooked	131	4	0	28	2.19	0.08
Noodles, Japanese, somen, dry	356	11	1	74	4.05	0.05
Oat bran, cooked	40	3	1	11	2.87	0.26
Oat bran, raw	246	17	7	66	16.88	0.26
Oat flour, partially debranned	404	15	9	66	11.65	0.18
Oats	389	17	7	66	13.31	0.20
Pasta, corn, cooked	126	3	1	28	2.50	0.09
Pasta, corn, dry	357	7	2	79	3.69	0.05
Pasta, fresh-refrigerated, plain, as purchased	288	11	2	55	6.42	0.12
Pasta, fresh-refrigerated, plain, cooked	131	5	1	25	3.80	0.15
Pasta, fresh-refrigerated, spinach, as purchased	289	11	2	56	3.08	0.06
Pasta, fresh-refrigerated, spinach, cooked	130	5	1	25	2.95	0.12
Pasta, homemade, made with egg, cooked	130	5	2	24	3.57	0.15
Pasta, homemade, made without egg, cooked	124	4	1	25	2.78	0.11

Grains

Food Description	Kcals	Protein	Fat	Carbs	PRAL	Alkal Density
Quinoa	374	4	2	21	-0.19	-0.01
Rice bran, crude	316	13	21	50	16.35	0.33
Rice flour, brown	363	7	3	76	6.88	0.09
Rice flour, white	366	6	1	80	3.90	0.05
Rice noodles, cooked	109	1	0	25	0.97	0.04
Rice noodles, dry	364	3	1	83	6.17	0.07
Rice, brown, long-grain, cooked	111	3	1	23	2.18	0.09
Rice, brown, long-grain, raw	370	8	3	76	7.51	0.10
Rice, brown, medium-grain, cooked	112	2	1	24	1.05	0.04
Rice, brown, medium-grain, raw	362	8	3	76	3.66	0.05
Rice, white, glutinous, cooked	97	2	0	21	0.92	0.04
Rice, white, glutinous, raw	370	7	1	82	3.60	0.04
Rice, white, long-grain, parboiled, enriched, cooked	123	3	0	26	1.80	0.07
Rice, white, long-grain, parboiled, enriched, dry	374	8	1	80	4.40	0.06
Rice, white, long-grain, parboiled, unenriched, cooked	123	3	0	26	1.80	0.07
Rice, white, long-grain, parboiled, unenriched, dry	374	8	1	80	4.40	0.06
Rice, white, long-grain, precooked or instant, enriched, dry	380	8	1	82	6.98	0.09
Rice, white, long-grain, precooked or instant, enriched, prepared	117	2	0	27	2.01	0.07
Rice, white, long-grain, regular, cooked	130	3	0	28	1.73	0.06
Rice, white, long-grain, regular, cooked, enriched, with salt	130	3	0	28	1.73	0.06
Rice, white, long-grain, regular, cooked, unenriched, with salt	130	3	0	28	1.73	0.06
Rice, white, long-grain, regular, cooked, unenriched, without salt	130	3	0	28	1.73	0.06
Rice, white, long-grain, regular, raw, enriched	365	7	1	80	4.32	0.05
Rice, white, long-grain, regular, raw, unenriched	365	7	1	80	4.32	0.05
Rice, white, medium-grain, cooked	130	2	0	29	1.54	0.05
Rice, white, medium-grain, cooked, unenriched	130	2	0	29	1.54	0.05
Rice, white, medium-grain, raw, enriched	360	7	1	80	4.40	0.06
Rice, white, medium-grain, raw, unenriched	360	7	1	80	4.40	0.06
Rice, white, short-grain, cooked	130	2	0	29	1.61	0.06
Rice, white, short-grain, cooked, unenriched	130	2	0	29	1.61	0.06
Rice, white, short-grain, raw	358	6	1	79	4.46	0.06
Rice, white, short-grain, raw, unenriched	358	6	1	79	4.46	0.06
Rice, white, with pasta, cooked	122	5	6	43	1.31	0.03
Rice, white, with pasta, dry	368	9	2	75	4.41	0.06
Rye	335	15	3	70	11.95	0.17
Rye flour, dark	324	14	3	69	7.75	0.11
Rye flour, light	367	8	1	80	4.30	0.05
Rye flour, medium	354	9	2	77	2.85	0.04

Grains

Food Description	Kcals	Protein	Fat	Carbs	PRAL	Alkali Density
Semolina, enriched	360	13	1	73	5.89	0.08
Semolina, unenriched	360	13	1	73	5.89	0.08
Spaghetti, cooked, enriched, with added salt	157	6	1	31	3.50	0.11
Spaghetti, cooked, enriched, without added salt	158	6	1	31	3.50	0.11
Spaghetti, cooked, unenriched, with added salt	157	6	1	31	3.50	0.11
Spaghetti, cooked, unenriched, without added salt	158	6	1	31	3.50	0.11
Spaghetti, dry, enriched	371	13	2	75	7.04	0.09
Spaghetti, dry, unenriched	371	13	2	75	7.04	0.09
Spaghetti, protein-fortified, cooked, enriched (N x 5.70)	164	8	0	32	4.01	0.13
Spaghetti, protein-fortified, cooked, enriched (n x 6.25)	164	8	0	32	4.39	0.14
Spaghetti, protein-fortified, dry, enriched (n x 5.70)	375	22	2	66	9.34	0.14
Spaghetti, protein-fortified, dry, enriched (n x 6.25)	374	22	2	66	10.28	0.16
Spaghetti, spinach, cooked	130	5	1	26	3.02	0.12
Spaghetti, spinach, dry	372	13	2	75	5.65	0.08
Spaghetti, whole-wheat, cooked	124	5	1	27	4	0.15
Spaghetti, whole-wheat, dry	348	15	1	75	7.96	0.11
Tapioca, pearl, dry	358	0	0	88	-0.16	0
Triticale	336	13	2	42	8.80	0.21
Triticale flour, whole-grain	338	13	2	73	4.11	0.06
Vital wheat gluten	370	75	2	14	41.85	2.99
Wheat bran, crude	216	16	4	65	3.44	0.05
Wheat flour, white (industrial), 10% protein, bleached, enriched	366	10	1	76	4.67	0.06
Wheat flour, white (industrial), 10% protein, bleached, unenriched	366	10	1	76	4.67	0.06
Wheat flour, white (industrial), 10% protein, unbleached, enriched	366	10	1	76	4.67	0.06
Wheat flour, white (industrial), 11.5% protein, bleached, enriched	363	11	1	74	5.84	0.08
Wheat flour, white (industrial), 11.5% protein, bleached, unenriched	363	11	1	74	5.84	0.08
Wheat flour, white (industrial), 11.5% protein, unbleached, enriched	363	11	1	74	5.84	0.08
Wheat flour, white (industrial), 13% protein, bleached, enriched	362	13	1	72	6.89	0.10
Wheat flour, white (industrial), 13% protein, bleached, unenriched	362	13	1	72	6.89	0.10
Wheat flour, white (industrial), 15% protein, bleached, enriched	362	15	1	70	8.51	0.12
Wheat flour, white (industrial), 15% protein, bleached, unenriched	362	15	1	70	8.51	0.12
Wheat flour, white (industrial), 9% protein, bleached, enriched	367	9	1	77	3.97	0.05
Wheat flour, white (industrial), 9% protein, bleached, unenriched	367	9	1	77	3.97	0.05
Wheat flour, white, all-purpose, enriched, bleached	364	13	1	76	6.04	0.08
Wheat flour, white, all-purpose, enriched, calcium-fortified	364	13	1	76	2.96	0.04
Wheat flour, white, all-purpose, enriched, unbleached	364	13	1	76	6.04	0.08

Grains

Food Description	Kcals	Protein	Fat	Carbs	PRAL	Alkal Density
Wheat flour, white, all-purpose, self-rising, enriched	354	10	1	74	19.36	0.26
Wheat flour, white, all-purpose, unenriched	364	13	1	76	6.04	0.08
Wheat flour, white, bread, enriched	361	12	2	73	6.51	0.09
Wheat flour, white, cake, enriched	362	12	2	73	4.36	0.06
Wheat flour, white, tortilla mix, enriched	405	10	11	67	7.19	0.11
Wheat flour, whole-grain	339	14	2	73	6.98	0.10
Wheat flours, bread, unenriched	361	12	2	73	6.51	0.09
Wheat germ, crude	360	23	10	52	17.04	0.33
Wheat, durum	339	14	2	71	12.26	0.17
Wheat, hard red spring	329	15	2	68	9.14	0.13
Wheat, hard red winter	327	13	2	71	5.55	0.08
Wheat, hard white	342	11	2	76	6.77	0.09
Wheat, soft red winter	331	10	2	74	11.34	0.15
Wheat, soft white	340	11	2	75	8.19	0.11
Wheat, sprouted	198	7	1	43	5.02	0.12
Wild rice, cooked	101	4	0	21	1.99	0.09
Wild rice, raw	357	15	1	75	9.39	0.13

Baked Goods

Food Description	Kcals	Protein	Fat	Carbs	PRAL	Alkali Density
Bagels, cinnamon-raisin	273	10	2	55	4.41	0.08
Bagels, cinnamon-raisin, toasted	294	11	2	59	3.98	0.07
Bagels, egg	278	11	2	53	6.05	0.11
Bagels, oat bran	255	11	1	53	5.93	0.11
Bagels, plain, enriched, with calcium propionate (includes onion, poppy, sesame)	257	10	2	51	4.82	0.09
Bagels, plain, enriched, without calcium propionate (includes onion, poppy, sesame)	275	11	2	53	5.58	0.11
Bagels, plain, toasted, enriched, with calcium propionate (includes onion, poppy, sesame)	288	11	2	57	5.16	0.09
Bagels, plain, unenriched, with calcium propionate (includes onion, poppy, sesame)	275	11	2	53	4.86	0.09
Bagels, plain, unenriched, without calcium propionate(includes onion, poppy, sesame)	275	11	2	53	5.58	0.11
Biscuits, mixed grain, refrigerated dough	263	6	6	47	1.14	0.02
Biscuits, plain or buttermilk, commercially baked	365	6	17	48	13.16	0.27
Biscuits, plain or buttermilk, dry mix	428	8	15	63	19.16	0.30
Biscuits, plain or buttermilk, dry mix, prepared	335	7	12	48	13.96	0.29
Biscuits, plain or buttermilk, prepared from recipe	353	7	16	45	3.43	0.08
Biscuits, plain or buttermilk, refrigerated dough, higher fat	322	7	14	43	16.14	0.38
Biscuits, plain or buttermilk, refrigerated dough, higher fat, baked	352	7	15	47	17.63	0.38
Biscuits, plain or buttermilk, refrigerated dough, lower fat	257	7	5	48	14.13	0.29
Biscuits, plain or buttermilk, refrigerated dough, lower fat, baked	300	8	5	55	16.45	0.30
Bread crumbs, dry, grated, plain	395	13	5	72	5.03	0.07
Bread crumbs, dry, grated, seasoned	383	14	5	68	5.06	0.07
Bread sticks, plain	412	12	9	68	6.63	0.10
Bread stuffing, bread, dry mix	386	11	3	76	3.14	0.04
Bread stuffing, bread, dry mix, prepared	177	3	9	22	0.84	0.04
Bread stuffing, cornbread, dry mix	389	10	4	77	2.63	0.03
Bread stuffing, cornbread, dry mix, prepared	179	3	9	22	0.70	0.03
Bread, banana, prepared from recipe, made with margarine	326	4	11	55	0.80	0.01
Bread, Boston brown, canned	195	2	1	19	-2.53	-0.13
Bread, cornbread, dry mix, enriched (includes corn muffin mix)	418	7	12	69	17.78	0.26
Bread, cornbread, dry mix, prepared	314	7	10	48	13.28	0.28
Bread, cornbread, dry mix, unenriched (includes corn muffin mix)	418	7	12	68	17.78	0.26
Bread, cornbread, prepared from recipe, made with low fat (2%) milk	266	7	7	44	2.56	0.06
Bread, cracked-wheat	260	9	4	50	4.29	0.09
Bread, egg	283	9	6	48	4.45	0.09
Bread, egg, toasted	315	11	7	53	4.95	0.09
Bread, French or Vienna (includes sourdough)	289	12	2	56	5.98	0.11

Baked Goods

Food Description	Kcals	Protein	Fat	Carbs	PRAL	Alkali Density
Bread, French or Vienna, toasted (includes sourdough)	319	13	2	62	6.67	0.11
Bread, Irish soda, prepared from recipe	290	7	5	56	0.21	0
Bread, Italian	271	9	4	50	4.09	0.08
Bread, oat bran	236	10	4	40	5.47	0.14
Bread, oat bran, toasted	259	11	5	44	5.48	0.12
Bread, oatmeal	269	8	4	48	3.97	0.08
Bread, oatmeal, toasted	292	9	5	53	4.34	0.08
Bread, pita, white, enriched	275	5	1	33	3.73	0.11
Bread, pita, white, unenriched	275	5	1	33	3.73	0.11
Bread, pita, whole-wheat	266	10	3	55	5.90	0.11
Bread, protein (includes gluten)	245	12	2	44	2.71	0.06
Bread, protein, toasted (includes gluten)	270	13	2	48	2.97	0.06
Bread, pumpernickel	250	9	3	47	4.19	0.09
Bread, pumpernickel, toasted	275	9	3	52	4.56	0.09
Bread, raisin, enriched	274	8	4	52	1.60	0.03
Bread, raisin, toasted, enriched	297	9	5	57	1.75	0.03
Bread, raisin, unenriched	274	8	4	52	1.60	0.03
Bread, reduced-calorie, oat bran	201	8	3	41	4.75	0.12
Bread, reduced-calorie, oat bran, toasted	239	9	4	49	5.10	0.10
Bread, reduced-calorie, oatmeal	210	8	4	43	2.70	0.06
Bread, reduced-calorie, rye	203	9	3	40	3.72	0.09
Bread, reduced-calorie, wheat	198	9	2	44	3.61	0.08
Bread, reduced-calorie, white	207	9	3	44	5.32	0.12
Bread, rice bran	243	9	5	44	3.45	0.08
Bread, rice bran, toasted	264	10	5	47	3.78	0.08
Bread, rye	258	8	3	48	3.31	0.07
Bread, rye, toasted	284	9	4	53	3.71	0.07
Bread, wheat	266	11	4	48	4.12	0.09
Bread, wheat bran	248	9	3	48	3.32	0.07
Bread, wheat germ	261	10	3	48	1.96	0.04
Bread, wheat germ, toasted	293	11	3	54	3.44	0.06
Bread, wheat, toasted	313	13	4	56	4.94	0.09
Bread, white, commercially prepared (includes soft bread crumbs)	266	8	3	51	2.74	0.05
Bread, white, commercially prepared, low sodium no salt	267	8	4	50	2.96	0.06
Bread, white, commercially prepared, toasted	293	9	4	54	3.24	0.06
Bread, white, commercially prepared, toasted, low sodium no salt	293	9	4	54	3.24	0.06
Bread, white, prepared from recipe, made with low fat (2%) milk	285	8	6	50	3.82	0.08

Baked Goods

Food Description	Kcals	Protein	Fat	Carbs	PRAL	Alkali Density
Bread, white, prepared from recipe, made with nonfat dry milk	274	8	3	54	4.13	0.08
Bread, whole-wheat, commercially prepared	247	13	3	41	5.08	0.12
Bread, whole-wheat, commercially prepared, toasted	306	16	4	51	8.07	0.16
Bread, whole-wheat, prepared from recipe	278	8	5	51	1.90	0.04
Bread, whole-wheat, prepared from recipe, toasted	305	9	6	56	2.06	0.04
Breakfast tart, low fat	372	4	6	77	2.29	0.03
Cake, angelfood, commercially prepared	258	6	1	58	10.79	0.19
Cake, angelfood, dry mix	373	9	0	85	10.83	0.13
Cake, angelfood, dry mix, prepared	257	6	0	59	7.43	0.13
Cake, Boston cream pie, commercially prepared	252	2	8	43	1.71	0.04
Cake, carrot, dry mix, pudding-type	415	5	10	79	5.64	0.07
Cake, cherry fudge with chocolate frosting	264	2	13	38	0.45	0.01
Cake, chocolate, commercially prepared with chocolate frosting	367	4	16	55	0.88	0.02
Cake, chocolate, dry mix, pudding-type	396	5	9	79	2.96	0.04
Cake, chocolate, dry mix, regular	428	6	16	73	2.77	0.04
Cake, chocolate, prepared from recipe without frosting	358	5	15	53	1.96	0.04
Cake, fruitcake, commercially prepared	324	3	9	62	-0.71	-0.01
Cake, German chocolate, dry mix, pudding-type	401	4	9	80	7.87	0.10
Cake, gingerbread, dry mix	437	4	14	75	1.58	0.02
Cake, gingerbread, prepared from recipe	356	4	16	49	-8.05	-0.16
Cake, marble, dry mix, pudding-type	416	3	12	79	7.80	0.10
Cake, pineapple upside-down, prepared from recipe	319	4	12	50	0.49	0.01
Cake, pound, commercially prepared, butter	388	5	20	49	4.52	0.09
Cake, pound, commercially prepared, fat-free	283	5	1	61	4.91	0.08
Cake, pound, commercially prepared, other than all butter, enriched	389	5	18	53	4.11	0.08
Cake, pound, commercially prepared, other than all butter, unenriched	389	5	18	53	4.11	0.08
Cake, shortcake, biscuit-type, prepared from recipe	346	6	14	48	2.97	0.06
Cake, snack cakes, crème-filled, chocolate with frosting	399	4	16	60	-1.14	-0.02
Cake, snack cakes, crème-filled, sponge	364	3	11	64	5.81	0.09
Cake, snack cakes, cupcakes, chocolate, with frosting, low-fat	305	4	4	67	3.05	0.05
Cake, sponge, commercially prepared	289	5	3	61	4.44	0.07
Cake, sponge, prepared from recipe	297	7	4	58	3.53	0.06
Cake, white, dry mix, pudding-type, enriched	423	4	9	81	9.41	0.12
Cake, white, dry mix, pudding-type, unenriched	423	4	9	81	9.41	0.12
Cake, white, dry mix, regular	426	5	11	78	9.43	0.12
Cake, white, dry mix, special dietary (includes lemon-flavored)	397	3	8	80	8.69	0.11

Baked Goods

Food Description	Kcals	Protein	Fat	Carbs	PRAL	Alkali Density
Cake, white, prepared from recipe with coconut frosting	356	4	10	63	1.18	0.02
Cake, white, prepared from recipe without frosting	357	5	12	57	2.09	0.04
Cake, yellow, commercially prepared, with chocolate frosting	379	4	17	55	2.82	0.05
Cake, yellow, commercially prepared, with vanilla frosting	373	4	15	59	4.93	0.08
Cake, yellow, dry mix, light	404	5	5	84	10.65	0.13
Cake, yellow, dry mix, pudding-type	423	4	10	80	8.26	0.10
Cake, yellow, dry mix, regular, enriched	432	4	12	78	9.88	0.13
Cake, yellow, dry mix, regular, unenriched	432	4	12	78	9.88	0.13
Cake, yellow, prepared from recipe without frosting	361	5	15	53	2.80	0.05
Cheesecake commercially prepared	321	5	22	26	3.29	0.13
Cheesecake prepared from mix, no-bake type	274	5	13	36	4.19	0.12
Coffeecake, cheese	339	7	15	44	-0.05	0
Coffeecake, cinnamon with crumb topping, commercially prepared, enriched	418	7	23	47	3.47	0.07
Coffeecake, cinnamon with crumb topping, commercially prepared, unenriched	418	7	23	47	3.47	0.07
Coffeecake, cinnamon with crumb topping, dry mix	436	5	12	78	7.57	0.10
Coffeecake, cinnamon with crumb topping, dry mix, prepared	318	5	10	53	6.06	0.11
Coffeecake, crème-filled with chocolate frosting	331	5	11	54	2.70	0.05
Coffeecake, fruit	311	5	10	51	3.99	0.08
Cookies, animal crackers (includes arrowroot, tea biscuits)	446	7	14	76	4.47	0.06
Cookies, brownies, commercially prepared	405	5	16	64	1.77	0.03
Cookies, brownies, dry mix, regular	434	4	15	77	-0.89	-0.01
Cookies, brownies, dry mix, special dietary	426	3	13	80	-3.76	-0.05
Cookies, brownies, dry mix, special dietary, prepared	384	4	11	71	-3.12	-0.04
Cookies, brownies, prepared from recipe	466	6	29	50	2.10	0.04
Cookies, butter, commercially prepared, enriched	467	6	19	69	3.74	0.05
Cookies, butter, commercially prepared, unenriched	467	6	19	69	3.74	0.05
Cookies, chocolate chip, commercially prepared, regular, higher fat, enriched	489	5	25	64	2.17	0.03
Cookies, chocolate chip, commercially prepared, regular, higher fat, unenriched	481	5	23	67	2.67	0.04
Cookies, chocolate chip, commercially prepared, regular, lower fat	453	6	15	73	2.39	0.03
Cookies, chocolate chip, commercially prepared, soft-type	458	4	24	59	0.50	0.01
Cookies, chocolate chip, commercially prepared, special dietary	450	4	17	73	0.62	0.01
Cookies, chocolate chip, dry mix	497	5	25	66	-0.64	-0.01
Cookies, chocolate chip, prepared from recipe, made with butter	488	6	28	58	-0.07	0
Cookies, chocolate chip, prepared from recipe, made with margarine	488	6	28	58	-0.14	0

Baked Goods

Food Description	Kcals	Protein	Fat	Carbs	PRAL	Alkali Density
Cookies, chocolate chip, refrigerated dough	443	4	20	61	-0.02	0
Cookies, chocolate chip, refrigerated dough, baked	492	5	23	68	-0.05	0
Cookies, chocolate sandwich, with crème filling, regular	466	5	19	72	0.56	0.01
Cookies, chocolate sandwich, with crème filling, regular, chocolate-coated	481	4	26	69	-1.41	-0.02
Cookies, chocolate sandwich, with crème filling, special dietary	461	5	22	68	1.46	0.02
Cookies, chocolate sandwich, with extra crème filling	497	4	25	69	0.65	0.01
Cookies, chocolate wafers	433	7	14	72	1.92	0.03
Cookies, coconut macaroons, prepared from recipe	404	4	13	72	-0.55	-0.01
Cookies, fig bars	348	4	7	71	-1.77	-0.02
Cookies, fortune	378	4	3	84	2.15	0.03
Cookies, fudge, cake-type (includes trolley cakes)	349	5	4	78	1.34	0.02
Cookies, gingersnaps	416	6	10	77	-3.72	-0.05
Cookies, graham crackers, chocolate-coated	484	6	23	67	1.14	0.02
Cookies, graham crackers, plain or honey (includes cinnamon)	423	7	10	77	3.30	0.04
Cookies, ladyfingers, with lemon juice and rind	365	11	9	60	8.29	0.14
Cookies, ladyfingers, without lemon juice and rind	365	11	9	60	8.29	0.14
Cookies, marshmallow, chocolate-coated (includes marshmallow pies)	421	4	17	68	0.19	0
Cookies, molasses	430	6	13	74	-3.32	-0.04
Cookies, oatmeal, commercially prepared, fat-free	326	6	1	79	0.89	0.01
Cookies, oatmeal, commercially prepared, regular	450	6	18	69	3.82	0.06
Cookies, oatmeal, commercially prepared, soft-type	409	6	15	66	5.93	0.09
Cookies, oatmeal, commercially prepared, special dietary	449	5	18	70	2.04	0.03
Cookies, oatmeal, dry mix	462	6	19	67	3.80	0.06
Cookies, oatmeal, prepared from recipe, with raisins	435	6	16	68	1.73	0.03
Cookies, oatmeal, prepared from recipe, without raisins	447	7	18	66	3.20	0.05
Cookies, oatmeal, refrigerated dough	424	5	19	59	2.27	0.04
Cookies, oatmeal, refrigerated dough, baked	471	6	21	66	2.52	0.04
Cookies, peanut butter sandwich, regular	478	9	21	66	5.27	0.08
Cookies, peanut butter sandwich, special dietary	535	10	34	51	2.53	0.05
Cookies, peanut butter, commercially prepared, regular	477	10	24	59	2.75	0.05
Cookies, peanut butter, commercially prepared, soft-type	457	5	24	58	2.58	0.04
Cookies, peanut butter, prepared from recipe	475	9	24	59	2.33	0.04
Cookies, peanut butter, refrigerated dough	458	8	25	52	4.19	0.08
Cookies, peanut butter, refrigerated dough, baked	503	9	27	57	4.62	0.08

Baked Goods

Food Description	Kcals	Protein	Fat	Carbs	PRAL	Alkali Density
Cookies, raisin, soft-type	401	4	14	68	0.99	0.01
Cookies, shortbread, commercially prepared, pecan	542	5	32	58	3.15	0.05
Cookies, shortbread, commercially prepared, plain	502	6	24	65	3.98	0.06
Cookies, sugar wafers with crème filling, regular	511	4	24	70	2.32	0.03
Cookies, sugar wafers with crème filling, special dietary	502	3	26	66	0.65	0.01
Cookies, sugar, commercially prepared, regular (includes vanilla)	478	5	21	68	3.55	0.05
Cookies, sugar, commercially prepared, special dietary	431	4	13	77	1.96	0.03
Cookies, sugar, prepared from recipe, made with margarine	472	6	23	60	3.34	0.06
Cookies, sugar, refrigerated dough	436	4	21	59	3.98	0.07
Cookies, sugar, refrigerated dough, baked	484	5	23	66	4.42	0.07
Cookies, vanilla sandwich with crème filling	483	5	20	72	2.35	0.03
Cookies, vanilla wafers, higher fat	473	4	19	71	1.59	0.02
Cookies, vanilla wafers, lower fat	441	5	15	74	3.27	0.04
Cracker meal	383	9	2	81	5.06	0.06
Crackers, cheese, low sodium	503	10	25	58	7.89	0.14
Crackers, cheese, regular	503	10	25	58	7.07	0.12
Crackers, cheese, sandwich-type with cheese filling	490	9	24	59	6.94	0.12
Crackers, cheese, sandwich-type with peanut butter filling	496	12	25	57	9.31	0.16
Crackers, crispbread, rye	366	8	1	82	4.69	0.06
Crackers, matzo, egg	391	12	2	79	7.20	0.09
Crackers, matzo, egg and onion	391	10	4	77	5.20	0.07
Crackers, matzo, plain	395	10	1	84	5.02	0.06
Crackers, matzo, whole-wheat	351	13	1	79	7.28	0.09
Crackers, melba toast, plain	390	12	3	77	6.19	0.08
Crackers, melba toast, plain, without salt	390	12	3	77	6.19	0.08
Crackers, melba toast, rye (includes pumpernickel)	389	12	3	77	6.37	0.08
Crackers, melba toast, wheat	374	13	2	76	7.30	0.10
Crackers, milk	455	8	16	70	9.73	0.14
Crackers, rusk toast	407	13	7	72	5.84	0.08
Crackers, rye, sandwich-type with cheese filling	481	9	22	61	6.02	0.10
Crackers, rye, wafers, plain	334	10	1	80	3	0.04
Crackers, rye, wafers, seasoned	381	9	9	74	2.90	0.04
Crackers, saltines (includes oyster, soda, soup)	428	9	11	71	3.56	0.05
Crackers, saltines, fat-free, low-sodium	393	11	2	82	5.94	0.07
Crackers, saltines, low salt (includes oyster, soda, soup)	434	9	12	71	-9.06	-0.13
Crackers, saltines, unsalted tops (includes oyster, soda, soup)	434	9	12	71	3.45	0.05

Baked Goods

Food Description	Kcals	Protein	Fat	Carbs	PRAL	Alkali Density
Crackers, standard snack-type, regular	502	7	25	61	7	0.11
Crackers, standard snack-type, regular, low salt	502	7	25	61	2.34	0.04
Crackers, standard snack-type, sandwich, with cheese filling	477	9	21	62	6.29	0.10
Crackers, standard snack-type, sandwich, with peanut butter filling	494	11	25	58	8.76	0.15
Crackers, wheat, low salt	473	9	21	65	5.84	0.09
Crackers, wheat, regular	473	9	21	65	6.26	0.10
Crackers, wheat, sandwich, with cheese filling	497	10	25	58	8.45	0.15
Crackers, wheat, sandwich, with peanut butter filling	495	13	27	54	10.01	0.19
Crackers, whole-wheat	443	9	17	69	5.76	0.08
Crackers, whole-wheat, low salt	443	9	17	69	5.76	0.08
Cream puffs, prepared from recipe, shell (includes eclair)	362	9	26	23	5.99	0.26
Cream puffs, prepared from recipe, shell, with custard filling	258	7	15	23	3.73	0.16
Croissants, apple	254	7	9	37	3.15	0.09
Croissants, butter	406	8	21	46	4.52	0.10
Croissants, cheese	414	9	21	47	5.23	0.11
Croutons, plain	407	12	7	73	5.68	0.08
Croutons, seasoned	465	11	18	63	4.33	0.07
Danish pastry, cheese	374	8	22	37	5.01	0.14
Danish pastry, cinnamon, enriched	403	7	22	45	3.34	0.07
Danish pastry, cinnamon, unenriched	403	7	22	45	3.34	0.07
Danish pastry, fruit, enriched (includes apple, cinnamon, raisin, lemon, raspberry, strawberry)	371	5	18	48	3.20	0.07
Danish pastry, fruit, unenriched (includes apple, cinnamon, raisin, strawberry)	371	5	18	48	3.20	0.07
Danish pastry, lemon, unenriched	371	5	18	48	3.20	0.07
Danish pastry, nut (includes almond, raisin nut, cinnamon nut)	430	7	25	46	3.50	0.08
Danish pastry, raspberry, unenriched	371	5	18	48	3.20	0.07
Doughnuts, cake-type, chocolate, sugared or glazed	417	5	20	57	2.32	0.04
Doughnuts, cake-type, plain (includes unsugared, old-fashioned)	418	6	24	46	9.41	0.20
Doughnuts, cake-type, plain, chocolate-coated or frosted	452	5	25	51	4.87	0.10
Doughnuts, cake-type, plain, sugared or glazed	426	5	23	51	3.51	0.07
Doughnuts, cake-type, wheat, sugared or glazed	360	6	19	43	2.61	0.06
Doughnuts, French crullers, glazed	412	3	18	60	3.78	0.06
Doughnuts, yeast-leavened, glazed, enriched (includes honey buns)	399	6	19	51	4.98	0.10
Doughnuts, yeast-leavened, glazed, unenriched (includes honey buns)	403	6	23	44	3.17	0.07
Doughnuts, yeast-leavened, with crème filling	361	6	24	30	3.42	0.11
Doughnuts, yeast-leavened, with jelly filling	340	6	19	39	3.53	0.09

Baked Goods

Food Description	Kcals	Protein	Fat	Carbs	PRAL	Alkali Density
Eclairs, custard-filled with chocolate glaze, prepared from recipe	262	6	16	24	3.42	0.14
English muffins, mixed-grain (includes granola)	235	9	2	46	0.56	0.01
English muffins, mixed-grain, toasted (includes granola)	255	10	2	50	3.27	0.07
English muffins, plain, enriched, with ca prop (includes sourdough)	227	9	2	44	2.71	0.06
English muffins, plain, enriched, without calcium propionate(includes sourdough)	235	8	2	46	4.72	0.10
English muffins, plain, toasted, enriched, with calcium propionate (includes sourdough)	270	10	2	53	3.01	0.06
English muffins, plain, unenriched, with calcium propionate (includes sourdough)	235	8	2	46	3.13	0.07
English muffins, plain, unenriched, without calcium propionate (includes sourdough)	235	8	2	46	4.72	0.10
English muffins, raisin-cinnamon (includes apple-cinnamon)	240	8	2	49	1.53	0.03
English muffins, raisin-cinnamon, toasted (includes apple-cinnamon)	276	9	2	55	1.73	0.03
English muffins, wheat	223	9	2	45	1.04	0.02
English muffins, wheat, toasted	243	9	2	49	1.38	0.03
English muffins, whole-wheat	203	9	2	40	5.04	0.13
English muffins, whole-wheat, toasted	221	10	2	44	5.52	0.13
French toast, frozen, ready-to-heat	213	7	6	32	4.12	0.13
French toast, prepared from recipe, made with low fat (2%) milk	229	8	11	25	3.54	0.14
Hush puppies, prepared from recipe	337	8	13	46	3.50	0.08
Ice cream cones, cake or wafer-type	417	8	7	79	4.20	0.05
Ice cream cones, sugar, rolled-type	402	8	4	84	3.25	0.04
KELLOGG, KELLOG'S NUTRI-GRAIN CEREAL BARS, Mixed Berry	370	4	8	73	0.60	0.01
KELLOGG'S Eggo Golden Oat Waffles	198	7	3	38	9.28	0.24
KELLOGG'S Eggo Lowfat Blueberry Nutri-Grain Waffles	208	6	3	43	2.14	0.05
KELLOGG'S Eggo Lowfat Homestyle Waffles	236	7	4	44	0.93	0.02
KELLOGG'S Eggo Lowfat Nutri-Grain Waffles	203	6	3	40	2.31	0.06
Leavening agents, baking powder, double-acting, sodium aluminum sulfate	53	0	0	28	3.55	0.13
Leavening agents, baking powder, double-acting, straight phosphate	51	0	0	24	270.16	11.26
Leavening agents, baking powder, low-sodium	97	0	0	47	-14.96	-0.32
Leavening agents, baking soda	0	0	0	0	0	
Leavening agents, cream of tartar	258	0	0	61	-346.47	-5.68
Leavening agents, yeast, baker's, active dry	295	38	5	38	21.11	0.56
Leavening agents, yeast, baker's, compressed	105	8	2	18	2.64	0.15
Muffins, blueberry, commercially prepared (Includes mini-muffins)	393	5	19	50	4.48	0.09
Muffins, blueberry, dry mix	366	5	10	63	8.11	0.13
Muffins, blueberry, prepared from recipe, made with low fat (2%) milk	285	6	11	41	3.09	0.08
Muffins, blueberry, toaster-type	313	5	9	53	2.21	0.04

Baked Goods

Food Description	Kcals	Protein	Fat	Carbs	PRAL	Alkali Density
Muffins, blueberry, toaster-type, toasted	333	5	10	57	7.08	0.12
Muffins, corn, commercially prepared	305	6	8	51	10.15	0.20
Muffins, corn, dry mix, prepared	321	7	10	49	13.56	0.28
Muffins, corn, prepared from recipe, made with low fat (2%) milk	316	7	12	44	3.01	0.07
Muffins, corn, toaster-type	346	5	11	58	5.64	0.10
Muffins, oat bran	270	7	7	48	1.79	0.04
Muffins, plain, prepared from recipe, made with low fat (2%) milk	296	7	11	41	3.45	0.08
Muffins, wheat bran, dry mix	396	7	12	73	14.30	0.20
Muffins, wheat bran, toaster-type with raisins	295	5	9	52	5.10	0.10
Muffins, wheat bran, toaster-type with raisins, toasted	313	5	9	56	8.43	0.15
Pancakes plain, frozen, ready-to-heat (includes buttermilk)	225	5	5	41	9.56	0.23
Pancakes, blueberry, prepared from recipe	222	6	9	29	2.58	0.09
Pancakes, buckwheat, dry mix, incomplete	340	11	3	71	21.35	0.30
Pancakes, buttermilk, prepared from recipe	227	7	9	29	2.99	0.10
Pancakes, plain, dry mix, complete (includes buttermilk)	376	10	5	71	17.70	0.25
Pancakes, plain, dry mix, complete, prepared	194	5	3	37	9.07	0.25
Pancakes, plain, dry mix, incomplete (includes buttermilk)	355	10	2	74	18.83	0.25
Pancakes, plain, dry mix, incomplete, prepared	218	8	8	29	7.85	0.27
Pancakes, plain, frozen, ready-to-heat, microwave (includes buttermilk)	239	6	5	43	11.91	0.28
Pancakes, plain, prepared from recipe	227	6	10	28	2.98	0.11
Pancakes, special dietary, dry mix	349	9	1	74	9.70	0.13
Pancakes, whole-wheat, dry mix, incomplete	344	13	1	71	17.32	0.24
Pancakes, whole-wheat, dry mix, incomplete, prepared	208	8	6	29	7.66	0.26
Phyllo dough	299	7	6	53	4.16	0.08
Pie crust, cookie-type, prepared from recipe, chocolate wafer, chilled	506	5	31	54	1.42	0.03
Pie crust, cookie-type, prepared from recipe, graham cracker, baked	494	4	25	65	1.87	0.03
Pie crust, cookie-type, prepared from recipe, graham cracker, chilled	484	4	24	64	1.84	0.03
Pie crust, cookie-type, prepared from recipe, vanilla wafer, chilled	531	4	36	50	2.23	0.04
Pie crust, standard-type, dry mix	518	7	31	52	4.03	0.08
Pie crust, standard-type, dry mix, prepared, baked	501	7	30	50	3.91	0.08
Pie crust, standard-type, frozen, ready-to-bake, baked	514	4	33	50	1.28	0.03
Pie crust, standard-type, frozen, ready-to-bake, enriched	457	4	29	44	1.16	0.03
Pie crust, standard-type, frozen, ready-to-bake, unenriched	457	4	29	44	1.16	0.03
Pie crust, standard-type, prepared from recipe, baked	527	6	35	47	3.71	0.08

Baked Goods

Food Description	Kcals	Protein	Fat	Carbs	PRAL	Alkali Density
Pie crust, standard-type, prepared from recipe, unbaked	469	6	31	42	3.34	0.08
Pie, apple, commercially prepared, enriched flour	237	2	11	34	0.12	0
Pie, apple, commercially prepared, unenriched flour	237	2	11	34	0.12	0
Pie, apple, prepared from recipe	265	2	13	37	0.28	0.01
Pie, banana cream, prepared from mix, no-bake type	251	3	13	32	4.21	0.13
Pie, banana cream, prepared from recipe	269	4	14	33	0.70	0.02
Pie, blueberry, commercially prepared	232	2	10	35	0.44	0.01
Pie, blueberry, prepared from recipe	245	3	12	33	1.08	0.03
Pie, cherry, commercially prepared	260	2	11	40	-0.01	0
Pie, cherry, prepared from recipe	270	3	12	38	0.50	0.01
Pie, chocolate crème, commercially prepared	304	3	19	34	0.10	0
Pie, chocolate mousse, prepared from mix, no-bake type	260	4	15	30	2.44	0.08
Pie, coconut cream, prepared from mix, no-bake type	276	3	18	28	3.28	0.12
Pie, coconut crème, commercially prepared	298	2	17	38	1.91	0.05
Pie, coconut custard, commercially prepared	260	6	13	30	2.20	0.07
Pie, egg custard, commercially prepared	210	5	12	21	3.28	0.16
Pie, fried pies, cherry	316	3	16	43	1.15	0.03
Pie, fried pies, fruit	316	3	16	43	1.15	0.03
Pie, fried pies, lemon	316	3	16	43	1.15	0.03
Pie, lemon meringue, commercially prepared	268	1	9	47	1.63	0.03
Pie, lemon meringue, prepared from recipe	285	4	13	39	1.73	0.04
Pie, mince, prepared from recipe	289	3	11	48	-2.08	-0.04
Pie, peach	223	2	10	33	-1.14	-0.03
Pie, pecan, commercially prepared	400	4	18	57	2.56	0.04
Pie, pecan, prepared from recipe	412	5	22	52	1.99	0.04
Pie, pumpkin, commercially prepared	210	4	9	27	0.13	0
Pie, pumpkin, prepared from recipe	204	5	9	26	0.20	0.01
Pie, vanilla cream, prepared from recipe	278	5	14	33	2.04	0.06
Popovers, dry mix, enriched	371	10	4	71	5.63	0.08
Popovers, dry mix, unenriched	371	10	4	71	5.63	0.08
Puff pastry, frozen, ready-to-bake	551	7	38	45	3.97	0.09
Puff pastry, frozen, ready-to-bake, baked	558	7	38	46	3.99	0.09
Rolls, dinner, egg	307	9	6	52	4.79	0.09
Rolls, dinner, oat bran	236	9	5	40	4.40	0.11
Rolls, dinner, plain, commercially prepared (includes brown-and-serve)	310	9	6	52	3.92	0.08
Rolls, dinner, plain, prepared from recipe, made with low fat (2%) milk	316	8	7	53	4.36	0.08
Rolls, dinner, rye	286	10	3	53	5.35	0.10

Baked Goods

Food Description	Kcals	Protein	Fat	Carbs	PRAL	Alkali Density
Rolls, dinner, wheat	273	9	6	46	2.42	0.05
Rolls, dinner, whole-wheat	266	9	5	51	3.25	0.06
Rolls, French	277	9	4	50	3.22	0.06
Rolls, hamburger or hotdog, mixed-grain	263	10	6	45	3.47	0.08
Rolls, hamburger or hotdog, plain	279	9	4	49	2.63	0.05
Rolls, hamburger or hotdog, reduced-calorie	196	8	2	42	4.25	0.10
Rolls, hard (includes kaiser)	293	10	4	53	4.34	0.08
Rolls, pumpernickel	277	11	3	53	4.97	0.09
Strudel, apple	274	3	11	41	-0.72	-0.02
Sweet rolls, cheese	360	7	18	44	2.20	0.05
Sweet rolls, cinnamon, commercially prepared with raisins	372	6	16	51	2.14	0.04
Sweet rolls, cinnamon, refrigerated dough with frosting	333	5	12	52	12.42	0.24
Sweet rolls, cinnamon, refrigerated dough with frosting, baked	362	5	13	56	13.44	0.24
Taco shells, baked	467	7	21	63	3.62	0.06
Taco shells, baked, without added salt	468	7	23	62	4.13	0.07
Toaster pastries, brown-sugar-cinnamon	412	5	14	68	3.96	0.06
Toaster pastries, fruit (includes apple, blueberry, cherry, strawberry)	391	5	11	69	2.88	0.04
Toaster pastries, fruit, toasted (include apple, blueberry, cherry, strawberry)	409	5	11	73	2.95	0.04
Tortillas, ready-to-bake or -fry, corn	218	6	3	45	7.58	0.17
Tortillas, ready-to-bake or -fry, corn, without added salt	222	6	3	47	7.21	0.15
Tortillas, ready-to-bake or -fry, flour	312	8	8	51	3.14	0.06
Tortillas, ready-to-bake or -fry, flour, without added calcium	325	9	7	56	4.91	0.09
USDA Commodity, Bakery , Flour Mix Low-fat	361	9	5	71	21.82	0.31
USDA Commodity, Bakery, Flour Mix	400	8	13	65	21.90	0.34
Waffle, buttermilk, frozen, ready-to-heat, microwaved	289	7	9	45	14.10	0.31
Waffle, buttermilk, frozen, ready-to-heat, toasted	309	7	9	49	12.70	0.26
Waffle, plain, frozen, ready-to-heat, microwave	298	7	10	46	12.13	0.26
Waffles, buttermilk, frozen, ready-to-heat	273	7	9	42	10.81	0.26
Waffles, plain, frozen, ready -to-heat, toasted	312	25	14	0	11.75	
Waffles, plain, frozen, ready-to-heat	285	6	10	43	9.30	0.22
Waffles, plain, prepared from recipe	291	8	14	33	3.75	0.11
Wonton wrappers (includes egg roll wrappers)	291	10	1	58	4.94	0.09

Lamb, Veal, and Game Products

Food Description	Kcals	Protein	Fat	Carbs	PRAL	Acid Density
Game meat, bison, ground, raw	223	19	16	0	8.76	0.46
Game meat, bison, top sirloin, separable lean only, 1" steak, cooked, broiled	171	28	6	0	14.21	0.51
Game meat, antelope, cooked, roasted	150	100	9	0	13.60	0.14
Game meat, antelope, raw	114	22	2	0	9.76	0.44
Game meat, bear, cooked, simmered	259	32	13	0	15.99	0.50
Game meat, beaver, cooked, roasted	212	35	7	0	18.37	0.52
Game meat, beaver, raw	146	24	5	0	12.40	0.52
Game meat, bison, chuck, shoulder clod, separable lean only, 3-5 lb roast, raw	119	21	3	0	10.12	0.48
Game meat, bison, chuck, shoulder clod, separable lean only, 3-5 lb roast, cooked, braised	193	34	5	0	17.99	0.53
Game meat, bison, ground, cooked, pan-broiled	238	24	15	0	11.33	0.47
Game meat, bison, ribeye, separable lean only, 1" steak, cooked, broiled	177	29	6	0	14.67	0.51
Game meat, bison, ribeye, separable lean only, trimmed to 0" fat, raw	116	22	2	0	10.22	0.46
Game meat, bison, separable lean only, cooked, roasted	143	28	2	0	13.30	0.48
Game meat, bison, separable lean only, raw	109	22	2	0	9.58	0.44
Game meat, bison, shoulder clod, separable lean only, trimmed to 0" fat, raw	109	21	2	0	9.89	0.47
Game meat, bison, top round, separable lean only, 1" steak, cooked, broiled	174	30	5	0	15.48	0.52
Game meat, bison, top round, separable lean only, 1" steak, raw	122	23	2	0	11.23	0.49
Game meat, bison, top sirloin, separable lean only, trimmed to 0" fat, raw	113	21	2	0	10.27	0.49
Game meat, boar, wild, cooked, roasted	160	28	4	0	9.59	0.34
Game meat, buffalo, water, cooked, roasted	131	27	2	0	13.66	0.51
Game meat, buffalo, water, raw	99	20	1	0	10.05	0.50
Game meat, caribou, cooked, roasted	167	30	4	0	15.71	0.52
Game meat, caribou, raw	127	23	3	0	11.69	0.51
Game meat, deer, cooked, roasted	158	30	3	0	15.41	0.51
Game meat, deer, ground, cooked, pan-broiled	187	26	8	0	12.94	0.50
Game meat, deer, ground, raw	157	22	7	0	10.49	0.48
Game meat, deer, loin, separable lean only, 1" steak, cooked, broiled	150	30	2	0	15.83	0.53
Game meat, deer, raw	120	23	2	0	11.38	0.49
Game meat, deer, shoulder clod, separable lean only, 3-5 lb roast, cooked, braised	191	36	4	0	20.05	0.56
Game meat, deer, tenderloin, separable lean only, 0.5-1 lb roast, cooked, broiled	149	30	2	0	15.67	0.52
Game meat, deer, top round, separable lean only, 1" steak, cooked, broiled	152	31	2	0	16.73	0.54
Game meat, elk, cooked, roasted	146	30	2	0	13.87	0.46
Game meat, elk, ground, cooked, pan-broiled	193	27	9	0	13.04	0.48
Game meat, elk, ground, raw	172	22	9	0	10.38	0.47
Game meat, elk, loin, separable lean only, cooked, broiled	167	31	4	0	15.38	0.50

Lamb, Veal, and Game Products

Food Description	Kcals	Protein	Fat	Carbs	PRAL	Acid Density
Game meat, elk, raw	111	23	1	0	10	0.43
Game meat, elk, round, separable lean only, cooked, broiled	156	31	3	0	15.97	0.52
Game meat, elk, tenderloin, separable lean only, cooked, broiled	162	31	3	0	16.56	0.53
Game meat, goat, cooked, roasted	143	27	3	0	11.99	0.44
Game meat, horse, cooked, roasted	175	28	6	0	14.21	0.51
Game meat, horse, raw	133	21	5	0	10.39	0.49
Game meat, moose, cooked, roasted	134	29	1	0	13.13	0.45
Game meat, moose, raw	102	22	1	0	9.42	0.43
Game meat, muskrat, cooked, roasted	234	30	12	0	16.90	0.56
Game meat, muskrat, raw	162	21	8	0	11.61	0.55
Game meat, opossum, cooked, roasted	221	30	10	0	14.78	0.49
Game meat, rabbit, domesticated, composite of cuts, cooked, roasted	197	29	8	0	15.13	0.52
Game meat, rabbit, domesticated, composite of cuts, cooked, stewed	206	30	8	0	16.16	0.54
Game meat, rabbit, domesticated, composite of cuts, raw	136	20	6	0	10.11	0.51
Game meat, rabbit, wild, cooked, stewed	173	33	4	0	16.81	0.51
Game meat, rabbit, wild, raw	114	22	2	0	10.19	0.46
Game meat, raccoon, cooked, roasted	255	29	15	0	14.64	0.50
Game meat, squirrel, cooked, roasted	173	31	5	0	14.72	0.47
Game meat, squirrel, raw	120	21	3	0	9.73	0.46
Lamb, Australian, imported, fresh, composite of trimmed retail cuts, separable lean and fat, trimmed to 1/8" fat, raw	229	18	17	0	8.30	0.46
Lamb, Australian, imported, fresh, composite of trimmed retail cuts, separable lean only, trimmed to 1/8" fat, raw	142	20	6	0	9.43	0.47
Lamb, Australian, imported, fresh, composite of trimmed retail cuts, separable lean and fat, trimmed to 1/8" fat, cooked	256	25	17	0	12.11	0.48
Lamb, Australian, imported, fresh, composite of trimmed retail cuts, separable lean only, trimmed to 1/8" fat, cooked	201	27	10	0	13.23	0.49
Lamb, Australian, imported, fresh, foreshank, separable lean and fat, trimmed to 1/8" fat, raw	195	19	13	0	8.76	0.46
Lamb, Australian, imported, fresh, foreshank, separable lean and fat, trimmed to 1/8" fat, cooked, braised	236	25	14	0	12.44	0.50
Lamb, Australian, imported, fresh, foreshank, separable lean only, trimmed to 1/8" fat, raw	123	21	4	0	9.67	0.46
Lamb, Australian, imported, fresh, foreshank, separable lean only, trimmed to 1/8" fat, cooked, braised	165	27	5	0	13.91	0.52
Lamb, Australian, imported, fresh, leg, center slice, bone-in, separable lean only, trimmed to 1/8" fat, raw	143	21	6	0	10.08	0.48
Lamb, Australian, imported, fresh, leg, center slice, bone-in, separable lean and fat, trimmed to 1/8" fat, raw	195	19	13	0	9.35	0.49

Lamb, Veal, and Game Products

Food Description	Kcals	Protein	Fat	Carbs	PRAL	Acid Density
Lamb, Australian, imported, fresh, leg, center slice, bone-in, separable lean and fat, trimmed to 1/8" fat, cooked, broiled	215	26	12	0	12.93	0.50
Lamb, Australian, imported, fresh, leg, center slice, bone-in, separable lean only, trimmed to 1/8" fat, cooked, broiled	183	27	8	0	13.59	0.50
Lamb, Australian, imported, fresh, leg, shank half, separable lean and fat, trimmed to 1/8" fat, raw	201	19	13	0	8.66	0.46
Lamb, Australian, imported, fresh, leg, shank half, separable lean only, trimmed to 1/8" fat, raw	133	20	5	0	9.51	0.48
Lamb, Australian, imported, fresh, leg, shank half, separable lean only, trimmed to 1/8" fat, cooked, roasted	182	27	7	0	13.53	0.50
Lamb, Australian, imported, fresh, leg, shank half, separable lean and fat, trimmed to 1/8" fat, cooked, roasted	231	25	14	0	12.58	0.50
Lamb, Australian, imported, fresh, leg, sirloin chops, boneless, separable lean and fat, trimmed to 1/8" fat, raw	208	18	14	0	8.90	0.49
Lamb, Australian, imported, fresh, leg, sirloin chops, boneless, separable lean only, trimmed to 1/8" fat, raw	132	20	5	0	9.98	0.50
Lamb, Australian, imported, fresh, leg, sirloin chops, boneless, separable lean and fat, trimmed to 1/8" fat, cooked, broiled	235	26	14	0	13.01	0.50
Lamb, Australian, imported, fresh, leg, sirloin chops, boneless, separable lean only, trimmed to 1/8" fat, cooked, broiled	188	28	8	0	14.02	0.50
Lamb, Australian, imported, fresh, leg, sirloin half, boneless, separable lean and fat, trimmed to 1/8" fat, raw	254	17	20	0	8.09	0.48
Lamb, Australian, imported, fresh, leg, sirloin half, boneless, separable lean only, trimmed to 1/8" fat, raw	138	20	6	0	9.63	0.48
Lamb, Australian, imported, fresh, leg, sirloin half, boneless, separable lean only, trimmed to 1/8" fat, cooked, roasted	215	28	11	0	14.01	0.50
Lamb, Australian, imported, fresh, leg, sirloin half, boneless, separable lean and fat, trimmed to 1/8" fat, cooked, roasted	281	25	19	0	12.52	0.50
Lamb, Australian, imported, fresh, leg, whole (shank and sirloin), separable lean only, trimmed to 1/8" fat, raw	135	20	5	0	9.51	0.48
Lamb, Australian, imported, fresh, leg, whole (shank and sirloin), separable lean and fat, trimmed to 1/8" fat, cooked, roasted	244	25	15	0	12.57	0.50
Lamb, Australian, imported, fresh, leg, whole (shank and sirloin), separable lean only, trimmed to 1/8" fat, cooked, roasted	190	27	8	0	13.68	0.51
Lamb, Australian, imported, fresh, leg, whole (shank and sirloin), separable lean and fat, trimmed to 1/8" fat, raw	215	16	13	0	8.49	0.53
Lamb, Australian, imported, fresh, loin, separable lean and fat, trimmed to 1/8" fat, raw	203	19	13	0	9.20	0.48
Lamb, Australian, imported, fresh, loin, separable lean and fat, trimmed to 1/8" fat, cooked, broiled	219	25	12	0	12.53	0.50
Lamb, Australian, imported, fresh, loin, separable lean only, trimmed to 1/8" fat, raw	146	21	6	0	9.96	0.47

Lamb, Veal, and Game Products

Food Description	Kcals	Protein	Fat	Carbs	PRAL	Acid Density
Lamb, Australian, imported, fresh, loin, separable lean only, trimmed to 1/8" fat, cooked, broiled	192	27	9	0	13.05	0.48
Lamb, Australian, imported, fresh, rib, separable lean and fat, trimmed to 1/8" fat, raw	289	16	24	0	7.86	0.49
Lamb, Australian, imported, fresh, rib, separable lean and fat, trimmed to 1/8" fat, cooked, roasted	277	22	20	0	10.94	0.50
Lamb, Australian, imported, fresh, rib, separable lean only, trimmed to 1/8" fat, raw	160	20	8	0	9.63	0.48
Lamb, Australian, imported, fresh, rib, separable lean only, trimmed to 1/8" fat, cooked, roasted	210	25	12	0	12.14	0.49
Lamb, Australian, imported, fresh, separable fat, cooked	639	9	66	0	4.41	0.49
Lamb, Australian, imported, fresh, separable fat, raw	648	6	69	0	2.91	0.49
Lamb, Australian, imported, fresh, shoulder, blade, separable lean only, trimmed to 1/8" fat, cooked, broiled	231	24	14	0	11.10	0.46
Lamb, Australian, imported, fresh, shoulder, arm, separable lean only, trimmed to 1/8" fat, raw	137	20	6	0	9.29	0.46
Lamb, Australian, imported, fresh, shoulder, arm, separable lean and fat, trimmed to 1/8" fat, raw	243	17	19	0	7.97	0.47
Lamb, Australian, imported, fresh, shoulder, arm, separable lean and fat, trimmed to 1/8" fat, cooked, braised	311	30	20	0	15.41	0.51
Lamb, Australian, imported, fresh, shoulder, arm, separable lean only, trimmed to 1/8" fat, cooked, braised	238	34	10	0	17.89	0.53
Lamb, Australian, imported, fresh, shoulder, blade, separable lean only, trimmed to 1/8" fat, raw	164	19	9	0	8.62	0.45
Lamb, Australian, imported, fresh, shoulder, blade, separable lean and fat, trimmed to 1/8" fat, cooked, broiled	291	22	22	0	10.10	0.46
Lamb, Australian, imported, fresh, shoulder, blade, separable lean and fat, trimmed to 1/8" fat, raw	262	16	21	0	7.47	0.47
Lamb, Australian, imported, fresh, shoulder, whole (arm and blade), separable lean and fat, trimmed to 1/8" fat, raw	256	19	8	0	7.63	0.40
Lamb, Australian, imported, fresh, shoulder, whole (arm and blade), separable lean and fat, trimmed to 1/8" fat, cooked	296	26	13	0	11.36	0.44
Lamb, Australian, imported, fresh, shoulder, whole (arm and blade), separable lean only, trimmed to 1/8" fat, raw	155	19	8	0	8.86	0.47
Lamb, Australian, imported, fresh, shoulder, whole (arm and blade), separable lean only, trimmed to 1/8" fat, cooked	233	26	13	0	12.63	0.49
Lamb, domestic, composite of trimmed retail cuts, separable fat, trimmed to 1/4" fat, choice, cooked	586	12	59	0	5.46	0.46
Lamb, domestic, composite of trimmed retail cuts, separable fat, trimmed to 1/4" fat, choice, raw	665	7	71	0	3.75	0.54
Lamb, domestic, composite of trimmed retail cuts, separable lean and fat, trimmed to 1/4" fat, choice, cooked	294	25	21	0	11.64	0.47

Lamb, Veal, and Game Products

Food Description	Kcals	Protein	Fat	Carbs	PRAL	Acid Density
Lamb, domestic, composite of trimmed retail cuts, separable lean and fat, trimmed to 1/8" fat, choice, cooked	271	26	18	0	12.13	0.47
Lamb, domestic, composite of trimmed retail cuts, separable lean only, trimmed to 1/4" fat, choice, cooked	206	28	10	0	13.50	0.48
Lamb, domestic, composite of trimmed retail cuts, separable lean and fat, trimmed to 1/8" fat, choice, raw	243	18	19	0	8.99	0.50
Lamb, domestic, composite of trimmed retail cuts, separable lean and fat, trimmed to 1/4" fat, choice, raw	267	17	22	0	8.63	0.51
Lamb, domestic, composite of trimmed retail cuts, separable lean only, trimmed to 1/4" fat, choice, raw	134	20	5	0	10.24	0.51
Lamb, domestic, cubed for stew or kabob (leg and shoulder), separable lean only, trimmed to 1/4" fat, cooked, broiled	186	28	7	0	14.03	0.50
Lamb, domestic, cubed for stew or kabob (leg and shoulder), separable lean only, trimmed to 1/4" fat, raw	134	20	5	0	10.13	0.51
Lamb, domestic, cubed for stew or kabob (leg and shoulder), separable lean only, trimmed to 1/4" fat, cooked, braised	223	34	9	0	17.71	0.52
Lamb, domestic, foreshank, separable lean and fat, trimmed to 1/4" fat, choice, cooked, braised	243	28	13	0	13.81	0.49
Lamb, domestic, foreshank, separable lean and fat, trimmed to 1/4" fat, choice, raw	201	19	13	0	10.34	0.54
Lamb, domestic, foreshank, separable lean and fat, trimmed to 1/8" fat, cooked, braised	243	28	13	0	13.81	0.49
Lamb, domestic, foreshank, separable lean and fat, trimmed to 1/8" fat, choice, raw	201	19	13	0	10.34	0.54
Lamb, domestic, foreshank, separable lean only, trimmed to 1/4" fat, choice, cooked, braised	187	31	6	0	15.20	0.49
Lamb, domestic, foreshank, separable lean only, trimmed to 1/4" fat, choice, raw	120	21	3	0	11.50	0.55
Lamb, domestic, leg, shank half, separable lean and fat, trimmed to 1/8" fat, choice, cooked, roasted	217	27	11	0	12.82	0.47
Lamb, domestic, leg, shank half, separable lean and fat, trimmed to 1/4" fat, choice, cooked, roasted	225	26	12	0	12.64	0.49
Lamb, domestic, leg, shank half, separable lean and fat, trimmed to 1/4" fat, choice, raw	201	19	13	0	9.48	0.50
Lamb, domestic, leg, shank half, separable lean and fat, trimmed to 1/8" fat, choice, raw	185	19	11	0	9.69	0.51
Lamb, domestic, leg, shank half, separable lean only, trimmed to 1/4" fat, choice, cooked, roasted	180	28	7	0	13.53	0.48
Lamb, domestic, leg, shank half, separable lean only, trimmed to 1/4" fat, choice, raw	125	21	4	0	10.40	0.50
Lamb, domestic, leg, sirloin half, separable lean and fat, trimmed to 1/4" fat, choice, cooked, roasted	292	25	21	0	11.80	0.47
Lamb, domestic, leg, sirloin half, separable lean and fat, trimmed to 1/8" fat, choice, cooked, roasted	284	25	20	0	11.94	0.48
Lamb, domestic, leg, sirloin half, separable lean and fat, trimmed to 1/4" fat, choice, raw	272	17	22	0	8.63	0.51
Lamb, domestic, leg, sirloin half, separable lean and fat, trimmed to 1/8" fat, choice, raw	261	17	21	0	8.72	0.51
Lamb, domestic, leg, sirloin half, separable lean only, trimmed to 1/4" fat, choice, cooked, roasted	204	28	9	0	13.65	0.49

Lamb, Veal, and Game Products

Food Description	Kcals	Protein	Fat	Carbs	PRAL	Acid Density
Lamb, domestic, leg, sirloin half, separable lean only, trimmed to 1/4" fat, choice, raw	134	21	5	0	10.30	0.49
Lamb, domestic, leg, whole (shank and sirloin), separable lean and fat, trimmed to 1/4" fat, choice, cooked, roasted	258	26	16	0	12.24	0.47
Lamb, domestic, leg, whole (shank and sirloin), separable lean and fat, trimmed to 1/8" fat, choice, cooked, roasted	242	26	14	0	12.56	0.48
Lamb, domestic, leg, whole (shank and sirloin), separable lean and fat, trimmed to 1/4" fat, choice, raw	230	18	17	0	9.12	0.51
Lamb, domestic, leg, whole (shank and sirloin), separable lean and fat, trimmed to 1/8" fat, choice, raw	209	18	14	0	9.37	0.52
Lamb, domestic, leg, whole (shank and sirloin), separable lean only, trimmed to 1/4" fat, choice, cooked, roasted	191	28	8	0	13.61	0.49
Lamb, domestic, leg, whole (shank and sirloin), separable lean only, trimmed to 1/4" fat, choice, raw	128	21	5	0	10.36	0.49
Lamb, domestic, loin, separable lean and fat, trimmed to 1/4" fat, choice, cooked, broiled	316	25	23	0	11.83	0.47
Lamb, domestic, loin, separable lean and fat, trimmed to 1/4" fat, choice, cooked, roasted	309	23	24	0	11.71	0.51
Lamb, domestic, loin, separable lean and fat, trimmed to 1/4" fat, choice, raw	310	16	27	0	8.38	0.52
Lamb, domestic, loin, separable lean and fat, trimmed to 1/8" fat, choice, cooked, broiled	297	26	21	0	12.24	0.47
Lamb, domestic, loin, separable lean and fat, trimmed to 1/8" fat, choice, raw	279	17	23	0	8.80	0.52
Lamb, domestic, loin, separable lean and fat, trimmed to 1/8" fat, choice, cooked, roasted	290	23	21	0	12.13	0.53
Lamb, domestic, loin, separable lean only, trimmed to 1/4" fat, choice, cooked, broiled	216	30	10	0	14.18	0.47
Lamb, domestic, loin, separable lean only, trimmed to 1/4" fat, choice, raw	143	21	6	0	10.60	0.50
Lamb, domestic, loin, separable lean only, trimmed to 1/4" fat, choice, cooked, roasted	202	27	10	0	14.12	0.52
Lamb, domestic, rib, separable lean and fat, trimmed to 1/4" fat, choice, cooked, roasted	359	21	30	0	9.99	0.48
Lamb, domestic, rib, separable lean and fat, trimmed to 1/4" fat, choice, cooked, broiled	361	22	30	0	10.91	0.50
Lamb, domestic, rib, separable lean and fat, trimmed to 1/4" fat, choice, raw	372	15	34	0	7.53	0.50
Lamb, domestic, rib, separable lean and fat, trimmed to 1/8" fat, choice, cooked, roasted	341	22	28	0	10.35	0.47
Lamb, domestic, rib, separable lean and fat, trimmed to 1/8" fat, choice, cooked, broiled	340	23	27	0	11.43	0.50
Lamb, domestic, rib, separable lean and fat, trimmed to 1/8" fat, choice, raw	342	15	31	0	7.90	0.53
Lamb, domestic, rib, separable lean only, trimmed to 1/4" fat, choice, cooked, roasted	232	26	13	0	12.54	0.48
Lamb, domestic, rib, separable lean only, trimmed to 1/4" fat, choice, cooked, broiled	235	28	13	0	13.93	0.50
Lamb, domestic, rib, separable lean only, trimmed to 1/4" fat, choice, raw	169	20	9	0	10.11	0.51
Lamb, domestic, shoulder, arm, separable lean and fat, trimmed to 1/8" fat, cooked, broiled	269	25	18	0	12.07	0.48
Lamb, domestic, shoulder, arm, separable lean and fat, trimmed to 1/4" fat, choice, raw	260	17	21	0	8.38	0.49

Lamb, Veal, and Game Products

Food Description	Kcals	Protein	Fat	Carbs	PRAL	Acid Density
Lamb, domestic, shoulder, arm, separable lean and fat, trimmed to 1/4" fat, choice, cooked, broiled	281	24	20	0	11.86	0.49
Lamb, domestic, shoulder, arm, separable lean and fat, trimmed to 1/8" fat, choice, cooked, braised	337	31	23	0	15.47	0.50
Lamb, domestic, shoulder, arm, separable lean and fat, trimmed to 1/4" fat, choice, cooked, roasted	279	23	20	0	11.54	0.50
Lamb, domestic, shoulder, arm, separable lean and fat, trimmed to 1/8" fat, choice, raw	244	17	19	0	8.53	0.50
Lamb, domestic, shoulder, arm, separable lean and fat, trimmed to 1/4" fat, choice, cooked, braised	346	30	24	0	15.08	0.50
Lamb, domestic, shoulder, arm, separable lean and fat, trimmed to 1/8" fat, choice, roasted	267	23	19	0	11.76	0.51
Lamb, domestic, shoulder, arm, separable lean only, trimmed to 1/4" fat, choice, cooked, broiled	200	28	9	0	13.54	0.48
Lamb, domestic, shoulder, arm, separable lean only, trimmed to 1/4" fat, choice, raw	132	20	5	0	9.84	0.49
Lamb, domestic, shoulder, arm, separable lean only, trimmed to 1/4" fat, choice, cooked, braised	279	36	14	0	17.80	0.49
Lamb, domestic, shoulder, arm, separable lean only, trimmed to 1/4" fat, choice, cooked, roasted	192	25	9	0	13.24	0.53
Lamb, domestic, shoulder, blade, separable lean and fat, trimmed to 1/8" fat, choice, cooked, broiled	267	59	46	0	10.84	0.18
Lamb, domestic, shoulder, blade, separable lean and fat, trimmed to 1/4" fat, choice, cooked, broiled	278	23	20	0	10.64	0.46
Lamb, domestic, shoulder, blade, separable lean and fat, trimmed to 1/4" fat, choice, raw	259	17	21	0	8.49	0.50
Lamb, domestic, shoulder, blade, separable lean and fat, trimmed to 1/4" fat, choice, cooked, braised	345	29	25	0	14.73	0.51
Lamb, domestic, shoulder, blade, separable lean and fat, trimmed to 1/8" fat, choice, raw	244	17	19	0	8.68	0.51
Lamb, domestic, shoulder, blade, separable lean and fat, trimmed to 1/8" fat, choice, cooked, roasted	270	23	19	0	11.85	0.52
Lamb, domestic, shoulder, blade, separable lean and fat, trimmed to 1/8" fat, choice, cooked, braised	339	29	24	0	14.99	0.52
Lamb, domestic, shoulder, blade, separable lean and fat, trimmed to 1/4" fat, choice, cooked, roasted	281	22	21	0	11.66	0.53
Lamb, domestic, shoulder, blade, separable lean only, trimmed to 1/4" fat, choice, cooked, broiled	211	25	11	0	11.76	0.47
Lamb, domestic, shoulder, blade, separable lean only, trimmed to 1/4" fat, choice, raw	151	19	8	0	9.76	0.51
Lamb, domestic, shoulder, blade, separable lean only, trimmed to 1/4" fat, choice, cooked, roasted	209	25	12	0	13.08	0.52
Lamb, domestic, shoulder, blade, separable lean only, trimmed to 1/4" fat, choice, cooked, braised	288	32	17	0	16.95	0.53
Lamb, domestic, shoulder, whole (arm and blade), separable lean and fat, trimmed to 1/8" fat, choice, raw	244	20	7	0	8.66	0.43
Lamb, domestic, shoulder, whole (arm and blade), separable lean and fat, trimmed to 1/8" fat, choice, cooked, broiled	268	24	18	0	11.13	0.46

Lamb, Veal, and Game Products

Food Description	Kcals	Protein	Fat	Carbs	PRAL	Acid Density
Lamb, domestic, shoulder, whole (arm and blade), separable lean and fat, trimmed to 1/8" fat, choice, cooked, roasted	269	25	11	0	11.83	0.47
Lamb, domestic, shoulder, whole (arm and blade), separable lean and fat, trimmed to 1/4" fat, choice, raw	264	17	21	0	8.38	0.49
Lamb, domestic, shoulder, whole (arm and blade), separable lean and fat, trimmed to 1/4" fat, choice, cooked, broiled	278	24	19	0	12.02	0.50
Lamb, domestic, shoulder, whole (arm and blade), separable lean and fat, trimmed to 1/4" fat, choice, cooked, roasted	276	23	20	0	11.70	0.51
Lamb, domestic, shoulder, whole (arm and blade), separable lean and fat, trimmed to 1/4" fat, choice, cooked, braised	344	29	25	0	14.77	0.51
Lamb, domestic, shoulder, whole (arm and blade), separable lean and fat, trimmed to 1/8" fat, choice, cooked, braised	338	29	24	0	15.09	0.52
Lamb, domestic, shoulder, whole (arm and blade), separable lean only, trimmed to 1/4" fat, choice, raw	144	20	7	0	9.81	0.49
Lamb, domestic, shoulder, whole (arm and blade), separable lean only, trimmed to 1/4" fat, choice, cooked, broiled	210	27	11	0	13.48	0.50
Lamb, domestic, shoulder, whole (arm and blade), separable lean only, trimmed to 1/4" fat, choice, cooked, braised	283	33	16	0	17.10	0.52
Lamb, domestic, shoulder, whole (arm and blade), separable lean only, trimmed to 1/4" fat, choice, cooked, roasted	204	25	11	0	13.15	0.53
Lamb, ground, cooked, broiled	283	25	20	0	11.53	0.46
Lamb, ground, raw	282	17	23	0	8.50	0.50
Lamb, New Zealand, imported, frozen, composite of trimmed retail cuts, separable lean only, cooked	206	30	9	0	18.91	0.63
Lamb, New Zealand, imported, frozen, composite of trimmed retail cuts, separable lean only, raw	128	21	4	0	13.45	0.64
Lamb, New Zealand, imported, frozen, composite of trimmed retail cuts, separable lean and fat, trimmed to 1/8" fat, cooked	270	25	18	0	16.11	0.64
Lamb, New Zealand, imported, frozen, composite of trimmed retail cuts, separable lean and fat, raw	277	17	23	0	11	0.65
Lamb, new Zealand, imported, frozen, composite of trimmed retail cuts, separable lean and fat, trimmed to 1/8" fat, raw	232	18	17	0	11.77	0.65
Lamb, New Zealand, imported, frozen, composite of trimmed retail cuts, separable lean and fat, cooked	305	24	22	0	15.87	0.66
Lamb, New Zealand, imported, frozen, composite of trimmed retail cuts, separable fat, raw	640	7	68	0	5.04	0.72
Lamb, New Zealand, imported, frozen, composite of trimmed retail cuts, separable fat, cooked	586	10	60	0	7.29	0.73
Lamb, New Zealand, imported, frozen, foreshank, separable lean and fat, cooked, braised	258	27	16	0	16.64	0.62

Lamb, Veal, and Game Products

Food Description	Kcals	Protein	Fat	Carbs	PRAL	Acid Density
Lamb, new Zealand, imported, frozen, foreshank, separable lean and fat, trimmed to 1/8" fat, cooked, braised	258	27	16	0	16.64	0.62
Lamb, New Zealand, imported, frozen, foreshank, separable lean and fat, raw	223	18	16	0	11.85	0.66
Lamb, new Zealand, imported, frozen, foreshank, separable lean and fat, trimmed to 1/8" fat, raw	223	18	16	0	11.85	0.66
Lamb, New Zealand, imported, frozen, foreshank, separable lean only, cooked, braised	186	31	6	0	18.70	0.60
Lamb, New Zealand, imported, frozen, foreshank, separable lean only, raw	118	21	3	0	13.54	0.64
Lamb, New Zealand, imported, frozen, leg, whole (shank and sirloin), separable lean only, cooked, roasted	181	28	7	0	17.74	0.63
Lamb, New Zealand, imported, frozen, leg, whole (shank and sirloin), separable lean and fat, cooked, roasted	246	25	16	0	16.06	0.64
Lamb, New Zealand, imported, frozen, leg, whole (shank and sirloin), separable lean only, raw	123	21	4	0	13.54	0.64
Lamb, new Zealand, imported, frozen, leg, whole (shank and sirloin), separable lean and fat, trimmed to 1/8" fat, raw	201	19	13	0	12.26	0.65
Lamb, new Zealand, imported, frozen, leg, whole (shank and sirloin), separable lean and fat, trimmed to 1/8" fat, cooked, roasted	234	25	14	0	16.38	0.66
Lamb, New Zealand, imported, frozen, leg, whole (shank and sirloin), separable lean and fat, raw	216	18	15	0	12.04	0.67
Lamb, new Zealand, imported, frozen, loin, separable lean and fat, trimmed to 1/8" fat, cooked, broiled	296	24	21	0	15.57	0.65
Lamb, New Zealand, imported, frozen, loin, separable lean and fat, cooked, broiled	315	23	24	0	15.04	0.65
Lamb, new Zealand, imported, frozen, loin, separable lean and fat, trimmed to 1/8" fat, raw	273	17	22	0	11.40	0.67
Lamb, New Zealand, imported, frozen, loin, separable lean and fat, raw	303	16	26	0	10.88	0.68
Lamb, New Zealand, imported, frozen, loin, separable lean only, cooked, broiled	199	29	8	0	18.42	0.64
Lamb, New Zealand, imported, frozen, loin, separable lean only, raw	130	21	4	0	13.89	0.66
Lamb, new Zealand, imported, frozen, rib, separable lean and fat, trimmed to 1/8" fat, cooked, roasted	317	20	26	0	12.82	0.64
Lamb, new Zealand, imported, frozen, rib, separable lean and fat, trimmed to 1/8" fat, raw	311	16	27	0	10.38	0.65
Lamb, New Zealand, imported, frozen, rib, separable lean and fat, cooked, roasted	340	19	29	0	12.37	0.65
Lamb, New Zealand, imported, frozen, rib, separable lean and fat, raw	346	15	31	0	9.79	0.65
Lamb, New Zealand, imported, frozen, rib, separable lean only, cooked, roasted	196	24	10	0	15.36	0.64
Lamb, New Zealand, imported, frozen, rib, separable lean only, raw	142	20	6	0	13.09	0.65
Lamb, New Zealand, imported, frozen, shoulder, whole (arm and blade), separable lean only, cooked, braised	285	34	15	0	20.28	0.60
Lamb, New Zealand, imported, frozen, shoulder, whole (arm and blade), separable lean and fat, cooked, braised	357	28	26	0	17.16	0.61

Lamb, Veal, and Game Products

Food Description	Kcals	Protein	Fat	Carbs	PRAL	Acid Density
Lamb, new Zealand, imported, frozen, shoulder, whole (arm and blade), separable lean and fat, trimmed to 1/8" fat, cooked, braised	342	29	24	0	17.83	0.61
Lamb, New Zealand, imported, frozen, shoulder, whole (arm and blade), separable lean and fat, raw	272	17	22	0	10.82	0.64
Lamb, New Zealand, imported, frozen, shoulder, whole (arm and blade), separable lean only, raw	135	20	5	0	12.97	0.65
Lamb, new Zealand, imported, frozen, shoulder, whole (arm and blade), separable lean and fat, trimmed to 1/8" fat, raw	251	17	20	0	11.15	0.66
Lamb, variety meats and by-products, brain, cooked, braised	145	13	10	0	13.79	1.06
Lamb, variety meats and by-products, brain, cooked, pan-fried	273	17	22	0	18.26	1.07
Lamb, variety meats and by-products, brain, raw	122	10	9	0	8.44	0.84
Lamb, variety meats and by-products, heart, cooked, braised	185	25	8	2	16.87	0.67
Lamb, variety meats and by-products, heart, raw	122	16	6	0	7.38	0.46
Lamb, variety meats and by-products, kidneys, cooked, braised	137	24	4	1	17.82	0.74
Lamb, variety meats and by-products, kidneys, raw	97	16	3	1	10.38	0.65
Lamb, variety meats and by-products, liver, cooked, braised	220	31	9	3	25.20	0.81
Lamb, variety meats and by-products, liver, cooked, pan-fried	238	25	13	4	20.20	0.81
Lamb, variety meats and by-products, liver, raw	139	20	5	2	16.29	0.81
Lamb, variety meats and by-products, lungs, cooked, braised	113	20	3	0	13.58	0.68
Lamb, variety meats and by-products, lungs, raw	95	17	3	0	10.79	0.63
Lamb, variety meats and by-products, mechanically separated, raw	276	15	24	0	11.18	0.75
Lamb, variety meats and by-products, pancreas, cooked, braised	234	23	15	0	20.37	0.89
Lamb, variety meats and by-products, pancreas, raw	152	15	10	0	12.60	0.84
Lamb, variety meats and by-products, spleen, cooked, braised	156	26	5	0	19.65	0.76
Lamb, variety meats and by-products, spleen, raw	101	17	3	0	10.60	0.62
Lamb, variety meats and by-products, tongue, cooked, braised	275	22	20	0	11.66	0.53
Lamb, variety meats and by-products, tongue, raw	222	16	17	0	8.44	0.53
Veal, breast, plate half, boneless, separable lean and fat, cooked, braised	282	26	19	0	13.40	0.52
Veal, breast, point half, boneless, separable lean and fat, cooked, braised	248	28	14	0	14.62	0.52
Veal, breast, separable fat, cooked	521	9	53	0	4.24	0.47
Veal, breast, whole, boneless, separable lean and fat, cooked, braised	266	27	17	0	13.93	0.52
Veal, breast, whole, boneless, separable lean and fat, raw	208	17	15	0	8.35	0.49
Veal, breast, whole, boneless, separable lean only, cooked, braised	218	30	10	0	15.79	0.53
Veal, composite of trimmed retail cuts, separable fat, cooked	642	9	67	0	4.96	0.55

Lamb, Veal, and Game Products

Food Description	Kcals	Protein	Fat	Carbs	PRAL	Acid Density
Veal, composite of trimmed retail cuts, separable fat, raw	638	6	68	0	3.18	0.53
Veal, composite of trimmed retail cuts, separable lean and fat, cooked	231	30	11	0	15.80	0.53
Veal, composite of trimmed retail cuts, separable lean and fat, raw	144	19	7	0	9.55	0.50
Veal, composite of trimmed retail cuts, separable lean only, cooked	196	32	7	0	16.74	0.52
Veal, composite of trimmed retail cuts, separable lean only, raw	112	20	3	0	9.97	0.50
Veal, cubed for stew (leg and shoulder), separable lean only, cooked, braised	188	35	4	0	17.67	0.50
Veal, cubed for stew (leg and shoulder), separable lean only, raw	109	20	3	0	9.99	0.50
Veal, ground, cooked, broiled	172	24	8	0	12.05	0.50
Veal, ground, raw	144	19	7	0	9.55	0.50
Veal, leg (top round), separable lean and fat, cooked, braised	211	36	6	0	18.03	0.50
Veal, leg (top round), separable lean and fat, cooked, pan-fried, breaded	228	27	0	10	13.51	0.50
Veal, leg (top round), separable lean and fat, cooked, pan-fried, not breaded	211	32	8	0	16.07	0.50
Veal, leg (top round), separable lean and fat, cooked, roasted	160	28	5	0	13.25	0.47
Veal, leg (top round), separable lean and fat, raw	117	21	3	0	9.97	0.47
Veal, leg (top round), separable lean only, cooked, braised	203	37	5	0	18.28	0.49
Veal, leg (top round), separable lean only, cooked, pan-fried, breaded	216	28	6	10	14.08	0.50
Veal, leg (top round), separable lean only, cooked, pan-fried, not breaded	183	33	5	0	16.77	0.51
Veal, leg (top round), separable lean only, cooked, roasted	150	28	3	0	13.42	0.48
Veal, leg (top round), separable lean only, raw	107	21	2	0	10.09	0.48
Veal, loin, separable lean and fat, cooked, braised	284	30	17	0	16.06	0.54
Veal, loin, separable lean and fat, cooked, roasted	217	25	12	0	12.27	0.49
Veal, loin, separable lean and fat, raw	163	19	9	0	9.42	0.50
Veal, loin, separable lean only, cooked, braised	226	34	9	0	17.86	0.53
Veal, loin, separable lean only, cooked, roasted	175	26	7	0	13.02	0.50
Veal, loin, separable lean only, raw	116	20	3	0	10.01	0.50
Veal, rib, separable lean and fat, cooked, braised	251	32	13	0	16.29	0.51
Veal, rib, separable lean and fat, cooked, roasted	228	24	14	0	12.11	0.50
Veal, rib, separable lean and fat, raw	162	19	9	0	9.21	0.48
Veal, rib, separable lean only, cooked, braised	218	34	8	0	17.27	0.51
Veal, rib, separable lean only, cooked, roasted	177	26	7	0	12.97	0.50
Veal, rib, separable lean only, raw	120	20	4	0	9.75	0.49
Veal, shank (fore and hind), separable lean and fat, cooked, braised	191	32	6	0	16.29	0.51
Veal, shank (fore and hind), separable lean and fat, raw	113	18	3	0	9.05	0.50
Veal, shank (fore and hind), separable lean only, cooked, braised	177	32	4	0	16.64	0.52

Lamb, Veal, and Game Products

Food Description	Kcals	Protein	Fat	Carbs	PRAL	Acid Density
Veal, shank (fore and hind), separable lean only, raw	108	19	3	0	9.10	0.48
Veal, shoulder, arm, separable lean and fat, cooked, braised	236	34	10	0	18.09	0.53
Veal, shoulder, arm, separable lean and fat, cooked, roasted	183	25	8	0	12.33	0.49
Veal, shoulder, arm, separable lean and fat, raw	132	19	5	0	9.38	0.49
Veal, shoulder, arm, separable lean only, cooked, braised	201	36	5	0	19.26	0.54
Veal, shoulder, arm, separable lean only, cooked, roasted	164	26	6	0	12.63	0.49
Veal, shoulder, arm, separable lean only, raw	105	20	2	0	9.69	0.48
Veal, shoulder, blade, separable lean and fat, cooked, braised	225	31	10	0	16.93	0.55
Veal, shoulder, blade, separable lean and fat, cooked, roasted	186	25	9	0	12.75	0.51
Veal, shoulder, blade, separable lean and fat, raw	129	19	5	0	9.85	0.52
Veal, shoulder, blade, separable lean only, cooked, braised	198	33	6	0	17.67	0.54
Veal, shoulder, blade, separable lean only, cooked, roasted	171	26	7	0	13.02	0.50
Veal, shoulder, blade, separable lean only, raw	113	20	3	0	10.08	0.50
Veal, shoulder, whole (arm and blade), separable lean and fat, cooked, roasted	184	25	8	0	12.59	0.50
Veal, shoulder, whole (arm and blade), separable lean and fat, cooked, braised	228	32	10	0	17.31	0.54
Veal, shoulder, whole (arm and blade), separable lean and fat, raw	130	19	5	0	9.72	0.51
Veal, shoulder, whole (arm and blade), separable lean only, cooked, roasted	170	26	7	0	12.84	0.49
Veal, shoulder, whole (arm and blade), separable lean only, cooked, braised	199	34	6	0	18.21	0.54
Veal, shoulder, whole (arm and blade), separable lean only, raw	112	20	3	0	9.95	0.50
Veal, sirloin, separable lean and fat, cooked, braised	252	31	13	0	16.64	0.54
Veal, sirloin, separable lean and fat, cooked, roasted	202	25	10	0	12.35	0.49
Veal, sirloin, separable lean and fat, raw	152	19	8	0	9.40	0.49
Veal, sirloin, separable lean only, cooked, braised	204	34	7	0	18.10	0.53
Veal, sirloin, separable lean only, cooked, roasted	168	26	6	0	12.89	0.50
Veal, sirloin, separable lean only, raw	110	20	3	0	9.91	0.50
Veal, variety meats and by-products, brain, cooked, braised	136	11	10	0	14.75	1.34
Veal, variety meats and by-products, brain, cooked, pan-fried	213	14	17	0	12.64	0.90
Veal, variety meats and by-products, brain, raw	118	10	8	0	8.08	0.81
Veal, variety meats and by-products, heart, cooked, braised	186	29	7	0	18.76	0.65
Veal, variety meats and by-products, heart, raw	110	17	4	0	10.21	0.60
Veal, variety meats and by-products, kidneys, cooked, braised	163	26	6	0	22.32	0.86
Veal, variety meats and by-products, kidneys, raw	99	16	3	1	10.36	0.65
Veal, variety meats and by-products, liver, cooked, braised	192	28	6	4	23.43	0.84

Lamb, Veal, and Game Products

Food Description	Kcals	Protein	Fat	Carbs	PRAL	Acid Density
Veal, variety meats and by-products, liver, cooked, pan-fried	193	27	7	4	23.18	0.86
Veal, variety meats and by-products, liver, raw	140	20	5	3	16.73	0.84
Veal, variety meats and by-products, lungs, cooked, braised	104	19	3	0	14.48	0.76
Veal, variety meats and by-products, lungs, raw	90	16	2	0	12.48	0.78
Veal, variety meats and by-products, pancreas, cooked, braised	256	29	15	0	26.50	0.91
Veal, variety meats and by-products, pancreas, raw	182	15	13	0	12.97	0.86
Veal, variety meats and by-products, spleen, cooked, braised	129	24	3	0	18.37	0.77
Veal, variety meats and by-products, spleen, raw	98	18	2	0	13.38	0.74
Veal, variety meats and by-products, thymus, cooked, braised	125	23	3	0	24.49	1.06
Veal, variety meats and by-products, thymus, raw	101	17	3	0	17.26	1.02
Veal, variety meats and by-products, tongue, cooked, braised	202	26	10	0	14.82	0.57
Veal, variety meats and by-products, tongue, raw	131	17	5	2	8.07	0.47

Legumes and Legume Products

Food Description	Kcals	Protein	Fat	Carbs	PRAL	Alkali Density
Bacon bits, meatless	476	32	26	29	16.88	0.58
Bacon, meatless	310	11	30	6	3.46	0.58
Baked beans, canned, no salt added	105	5	0	20	-1.49	-0.07
Bean beverage	34	3	0	6	-3.77	-0.63
Beans, adzuki, mature seed, cooked, boiled, with salt	128	8	0	25	-2.98	-0.12
Beans, adzuki, mature seeds, canned, sweetened	237	4	0	55	1	0.02
Beans, adzuki, mature seeds, cooked, boiled, without salt	128	8	0	25	-2.98	-0.12
Beans, adzuki, mature seeds, raw	329	20	1	63	-6.66	-0.11
Beans, adzuki, yokan, mature seeds	260	3	0	61	1.32	0.02
Beans, baked, canned, plain or vegetarian	94	5	0	21	-0.78	-0.04
Beans, baked, canned, with beef	121	6	3	17	-1.83	-0.11
Beans, baked, canned, with franks	142	7	7	15	0.86	0.06
Beans, baked, canned, with pork	106	5	2	20	-1.52	-0.08
Beans, baked, canned, with pork and sweet sauce	112	5	1	21	-0.67	-0.03
Beans, baked, canned, with pork and tomato sauce	94	5	1	19	-0.99	-0.05
Beans, baked, home prepared	151	6	5	22	-2.68	-0.12
Beans, black turtle soup, mature seeds, canned	91	6	0	17	-0.88	-0.05
Beans, black turtle soup, mature seeds, cooked, boiled, with salt	130	8	0	24	-1.45	-0.06
Beans, black turtle soup, mature seeds, cooked, boiled, without salt	130	8	0	24	-1.45	-0.06
Beans, black turtle soup, mature seeds, raw	339	21	1	63	-11.04	-0.18
Beans, black, mature seeds, cooked, boiled, with salt	132	9	1	24	-0.10	0
Beans, black, mature seeds, cooked, boiled, without salt	132	9	1	24	-0.10	0
Beans, black, mature seeds, raw	341	22	1	62	-13.58	-0.22
Beans, chili, barbecue, ranch style, cooked	97	5	1	17	-2.87	-0.17
Beans, cranberry (roman), mature seeds, canned	83	6	0	15	-0.83	-0.06
Beans, cranberry (roman), mature seeds, cooked, boiled, with salt	136	9	0	24	-0.50	-0.02
Beans, cranberry (roman), mature seeds, cooked, boiled, without salt	136	9	0	24	-0.50	-0.02
Beans, cranberry (roman), mature seeds, raw	335	23	1	60	-8.63	-0.14
Beans, French, mature seeds, cooked, boiled, with salt	129	7	1	24	-2.81	-0.12
Beans, French, mature seeds, cooked, boiled, without salt	129	7	1	24	-2.81	-0.12
Beans, French, mature seeds, raw	343	19	2	64	-14.47	-0.23
Beans, great northern, mature seeds, canned	114	7	0	21	-0.74	-0.04
Beans, great northern, mature seeds, cooked, boiled, with salt	118	8	0	21	-0.20	-0.01
Beans, great northern, mature seeds, cooked, boiled, without salt	118	8	0	21	-0.20	-0.01
Beans, great northern, mature seeds, raw	339	22	1	62	-9.06	-0.15
Beans, kidney, all types, mature seeds, canned	84	5	1	16	-0.23	-0.01

Legumes and Legume Products

Food Description	Kcals	Protein	Fat	Carbs	PRAL	Alkali Density
Beans, kidney, all types, mature seeds, cooked, boiled, with salt	127	9	0	23	-0.49	-0.02
Beans, kidney, all types, mature seeds, cooked, boiled, without salt	127	9	0	23	-0.69	-0.03
Beans, kidney, all types, mature seeds, raw	333	43	2	110	-8.41	-0.08
Beans, kidney, California red, mature seeds, cooked, boiled, with salt	124	9	0	22	-1.36	-0.06
Beans, kidney, California red, mature seeds, cooked, boiled, without salt	124	9	0	22	-1.36	-0.06
Beans, kidney, California red, mature seeds, raw	330	24	0	60	-11.05	-0.18
Beans, kidney, red, mature seeds, canned	85	5	0	16	-0.38	-0.02
Beans, kidney, red, mature seeds, cooked, boiled, with salt	127	9	0	23	-0.49	-0.02
Beans, kidney, red, mature seeds, cooked, boiled, without salt	127	9	0	23	-0.49	-0.02
Beans, kidney, red, mature seeds, raw	337	23	1	61	-7.14	-0.12
Beans, kidney, royal red, mature seeds, cooked, boiled with salt	123	9	0	22	0.30	0.01
Beans, kidney, royal red, mature seeds, cooked, boiled, without salt	123	9	0	22	0.30	0.01
Beans, kidney, royal red, mature seeds, raw	329	25	0	58	-6.12	-0.11
Beans, liquid from stewed kidney beans	47	2	3	3	-5.56	-1.85
Beans, navy, mature seeds, canned	113	8	0	20	0.76	0.04
Beans, navy, mature seeds, cooked, boiled, with salt	140	8	1	26	-1.08	-0.04
Beans, navy, mature seeds, cooked, boiled, without salt	140	8	1	26	-1.08	-0.04
Beans, navy, mature seeds, raw	339	22	1	61	-6.63	-0.11
Beans, pink, mature seeds, cooked, boiled, with salt	149	9	0	28	-2.49	-0.09
Beans, pink, mature seeds, cooked, boiled, without salt	149	9	0	28	-2.49	-0.09
Beans, pink, mature seeds, raw	343	21	1	64	-11.54	-0.18
Beans, pinto, mature seeds, canned	86	5	1	15	-0.57	-0.04
Beans, pinto, mature seeds, cooked, boiled, with salt	143	9	1	26	-1.20	-0.05
Beans, pinto, mature seeds, cooked, boiled, without salt	143	9	1	26	-1.20	-0.05
Beans, pinto, mature seeds, raw	347	21	1	63	-9.59	-0.15
Beans, small white, mature seeds, cooked, boiled, with salt	142	9	1	26	-1.79	-0.07
Beans, small white, mature seeds, cooked, boiled, without salt	142	9	1	26	-1.79	-0.07
Beans, small white, mature seeds, raw	336	21	1	62	-12.58	-0.20
Beans, white, mature seeds, canned	114	7	0	21	-4.88	-0.23
Beans, white, mature seeds, cooked, boiled, with salt	139	10	0	25	-5.64	-0.23
Beans, white, mature seeds, cooked, boiled, without salt	139	10	0	25	-5.64	-0.23
Beans, white, mature seeds, raw	333	23	1	60	-23.17	-0.39
Beans, winged, mature seeds, cooked, boiled, without salt	147	11	6	15	1.73	0.12
Beans, yellow, mature seeds, cooked, boiled, with salt	144	9	1	25	1.70	0.07

Legumes and Legume Products

Food Description	Kcals	Protein	Fat	Carbs	PRAL	Alkali Density
Beans, yellow, mature seeds, cooked, boiled, without salt	144	9	1	25	1.70	0.07
Beans, yellow, mature seeds, raw	345	22	3	61	-0.97	-0.02
Broadbeans (fava beans), mature seeds, canned	71	5	0	12	-0.64	-0.05
Broadbeans (fava beans), mature seeds, cooked, boiled, with salt	110	8	0	20	1.13	0.06
Broadbeans (fava beans), mature seeds, cooked, boiled, without salt	110	8	0	20	1.13	0.06
Broadbeans (fava beans), mature seeds, raw	341	26	2	58	-0.25	0
Carob flour	222	5	1	89	-18.10	-0.20
Chicken, meatless	224	24	13	4	21.94	5.49
Chicken, meatless, breaded, fried	234	21	13	9	12.33	1.37
Chickpea flour (besan)	387	22	7	58	0.07	0
Chickpeas (garbanzo beans, Bengal gram), mature seeds, canned	119	5	1	23	0.97	0.04
Chickpeas (garbanzo beans, Bengal gram), mature seeds, cooked, boiled, with salt	164	9	3	27	2.56	0.09
Chickpeas (garbanzo beans, Bengal gram), mature seeds, cooked, boiled, without salt	164	9	3	27	2.56	0.09
Chickpeas (garbanzo beans, Bengal gram), mature seeds, raw	364	19	6	61	0.26	0
Chili with beans, canned	112	6	5	12	-0.95	-0.08
Cowpeas, catjang, mature seeds, cooked, boiled, with salt	117	8	1	20	-1.47	-0.07
Cowpeas, catjang, mature seeds, cooked, boiled, without salt	117	8	1	20	-1.47	-0.07
Cowpeas, catjang, mature seeds, raw	343	24	2	60	-10.74	-0.18
Cowpeas, common (blackeyes, crowder, southern), mature seeds, canned with pork	83	3	2	17	-0.18	-0.01
Cowpeas, common (blackeyes, crowder, southern), mature seeds, canned, plain	77	5	1	14	0.31	0.02
Cowpeas, common (blackeyes, crowder, southern), mature seeds, cooked, boiled, with salt	116	8	1	21	2.03	0.10
Cowpeas, common (blackeyes, crowder, southern), mature seeds, cooked, boiled, without salt	116	8	1	21	2.03	0.10
Cowpeas, common (blackeyes, crowder, southern), mature seeds, raw	336	24	1	60	-2.35	-0.04
ENSURE FIBER WITH FOS, liquid	97	3	2	16	0.23	0.01
Falafel, home-prepared	333	13	18	32	-1.49	-0.05
Fish sticks, meatless	290	23	18	9	13.48	1.50
Frankfurter, meatless	233	20	14	8	19.38	2.42
GREEN GIANT, HARVEST BURGER, Original Flavor, All Vegetable Protein Patties, frozen	153	20	5	8	5.47	0.68
Hummus, commercial	166	8	10	14	3.25	0.23
Hummus, home prepared	177	5	9	20	1.42	0.07
Hyacinth beans, mature seeds, cooked, boiled, with salt	117	8	1	21	-1.30	-0.06
Hyacinth beans, mature seeds, cooked, boiled, without salt	117	8	1	21	-1.30	-0.06
Hyacinth beans, mature seeds, raw	344	24	2	61	-9.50	-0.16
Lentils, mature seeds, cooked, boiled, with salt	114	9	0	20	2.14	0.11

Legumes and Legume Products

Food Description	Kcals	Protein	Fat	Carbs	PRAL	Alkali Density
Lentils, mature seeds, cooked, boiled, without salt	116	9	0	20	2.14	0.11
Lentils, pink, raw	345	25	2	59	8.56	0.15
Lentils, raw	353	26	1	60	5.37	0.09
Lima beans, large, mature seeds, canned	79	5	0	15	-0.75	-0.05
Lima beans, large, mature seeds, cooked, boiled, with salt	115	8	0	21	-4.07	-0.19
Lima beans, large, mature seeds, cooked, boiled, without salt	115	8	0	21	-4.07	-0.19
Lima beans, large, mature seeds, raw	338	21	1	63	-18.32	-0.29
Lima beans, thin seeded (baby), mature seeds, cooked, boiled, with salt	126	8	0	23	-1.53	-0.07
Lima beans, thin seeded (baby), mature seeds, cooked, boiled, without salt	126	8	0	23	-1.53	-0.07
Lima beans, thin seeded (baby), mature seeds, raw	335	21	1	63	-11.61	-0.18
Luncheon slices, meatless	189	18	11	4	19.73	4.93
Lupins, mature seeds, cooked, boiled, with salt	116	16	3	9	5.15	0.57
Lupins, mature seeds, cooked, boiled, without salt	119	26	5	16	5.15	0.32
Lupins, mature seeds, raw	371	10	3	11	5.29	0.48
Meat extender	313	38	3	38	-5.89	-0.16
Meatballs, meatless	197	30	13	12	18.44	1.54
Miso	199	12	6	26	5.21	0.20
MORI-NU, Tofu, silken, extra firm	55	7	2	2	2.98	1.49
MORI-NU, Tofu, silken, firm	62	7	3	2	1.51	0.76
MORI-NU, Tofu, silken, lite extra firm	38	7	1	1	4.48	4.48
MORI-NU, Tofu, silken, soft	55	5	3	3	-0.29	-0.10
MOR-NU, Tofu, silken, lite firm	37	6	1	1	4.03	4.03
Mothbeans, mature seeds, cooked, boiled, with salt	117	8	1	21	0.25	0.01
Mothbeans, mature seeds, cooked, boiled, without salt	117	8	1	21	0.25	0.01
Mothbeans, mature seeds, raw	343	23	2	62	-7.53	-0.12
Mung beans, mature seeds, cooked, boiled, with salt	105	7	0	19	-0.08	0
Mung beans, mature seeds, cooked, boiled, without salt	105	7	0	19	-0.08	0
Mung beans, mature seeds, raw	347	24	1	63	-7.52	-0.12
Mungo beans, mature seeds, cooked, boiled, with salt	105	8	1	18	2.28	0.13
Mungo beans, mature seeds, cooked, boiled, without salt	105	8	1	18	2.28	0.13
Mungo beans, mature seeds, raw	341	25	2	59	-3	-0.05
Natto	212	18	11	14	-5.99	-0.43
Noodles, Chinese, cellophane or long rice (mung beans), dehydrated	351	0	0	86	0.64	0.01
Papad	371	26	3	60	-3.13	-0.05
Peanut butter, chunk style, with salt	589	24	50	22	3.20	0.15
Peanut butter, chunk style, without salt	589	24	50	22	3.20	0.15

Legumes and Legume Products

Food Description	Kcals	Protein	Fat	Carbs	PRAL	Alkali Density
Peanut butter, chunky, vitamin and mineral fortified	593	26	51	18	-1.47	-0.08
Peanut butter, reduced sodium	633	24	50	22	3.13	0.14
Peanut butter, smooth style, with salt	588	25	50	20	7.34	0.37
Peanut butter, smooth style, without salt	588	25	50	20	7.34	0.37
Peanut butter, smooth, reduced fat	520	26	34	36	7.42	0.21
Peanut butter, smooth, vitamin and mineral fortified	591	26	51	19	2.37	0.12
Peanut flour, defatted	327	51	1	35	15.16	0.43
Peanut flour, low fat	428	34	22	31	3.90	0.13
Peanut spread, reduced sugar	650	25	55	14	2.72	0.19
Peanuts, all types, cooked, boiled, with salt	318	13	22	21	6.79	0.32
Peanuts, all types, dry-roasted, with salt	585	24	50	22	5.75	0.26
Peanuts, all types, dry-roasted, without salt	585	24	50	22	5.75	0.26
Peanuts, all types, oil-roasted, with salt	599	28	53	15	7.80	0.52
Peanuts, all types, oil-roasted, without salt	581	26	49	18	11.76	0.65
Peanuts, all types, raw	567	26	49	16	6.18	0.39
Peanuts, Spanish, oil-roasted, with salt	579	28	49	17	6.08	0.36
Peanuts, Spanish, oil-roasted, without salt	579	28	49	17	6.08	0.36
Peanuts, Spanish, raw	570	26	50	16	5.28	0.33
Peanuts, Valencia, oil-roasted, with salt	589	27	51	16	7.33	0.46
Peanuts, Valencia, oil-roasted, without salt	589	27	51	16	7.33	0.46
Peanuts, Valencia, raw	570	25	48	21	12.16	0.58
Peanuts, Virginia, oil-roasted, with salt	578	26	49	20	11.70	0.59
Peanuts, Virginia, oil-roasted, without salt	578	26	49	20	11.70	0.59
Peanuts, Virginia, raw	563	25	49	17	6.31	0.37
Peas, split, mature seeds, cooked, boiled, with salt	116	8	0	21	-0.97	-0.05
Peas, split, mature seeds, cooked, boiled, without salt	118	8	0	21	-0.97	-0.05
Peas, split, mature seeds, raw	341	25	1	60	1.26	0.02
Pigeon peas (red gram), mature seeds, cooked, boiled, with salt	121	7	0	23	-2.10	-0.09
Pigeon peas (red gram), mature seeds, cooked, boiled, without salt	121	7	0	23	-2.10	-0.09
Pigeon peas (red gram), mature seeds, raw	343	22	1	63	-11.46	-0.18
Refried beans, canned (includes USDA commodity) *	94	5	1	15	-1.04	-0.07
Sandwich spread, meatless	149	8	9	9	1.04	0.12
Sausage, meatless	257	19	18	10	10.79	1.08
Soy flour, defatted	330	47	1	38	-12.76	-0.34
Soy flour, defatted, crude protein basis (N x 6.25)	327	50	9	31	-10.58	-0.34
Soy flour, full-fat, raw	436	35	21	35	-31.44	-0.90
Soy flour, full-fat, raw, crude protein basis (N x 6.25)	434	38	21	32	-29.84	-0.93

Legumes and Legume Products

Food Description	Kcals	Protein	Fat	Carbs	PRAL	Alkali Density
Soy flour, full-fat, roasted	441	35	22	44	-20.23	-0.46
Soy flour, full-fat, roasted, crude protein basis (N x 6.25)	439	38	22	30	-18.62	-0.62
Soy flour, low-fat	372	46	9	35	-17.62	-0.50
Soy flour, low-fat, crude protein basis (N x 6.25)	369	51	7	34	-15.47	-0.46
Soy meal, defatted, raw	339	45	2	40	-15.45	-0.39
Soy meal, defatted, raw, crude protein basis (N x 6.25)	337	49	2	36	-13.37	-0.37
Soy protein concentrate, crude protein basis (N x 6.25), produced by acid wash	328	64	0	25	44.41	1.78
Soy protein concentrate, produced by acid wash	331	58	0	31	41.71	1.35
Soy protein concentrate, produced by alcohol extraction	331	16	0	9	0.37	0.04
Soy protein isolate	338	81	3	7	63.22	9.03
Soy protein isolate, potassium type	326	81	1	10	31.53	3.15
Soy protein isolate, potassium type, crude protein basis	321	88	1	3	35.27	11.76
Soy sauce made from hydrolyzed vegetable protein	40	2	0	8	1.21	0.15
Soy sauce made from soy (tamari)	60	11	0	6	4.20	0.70
Soy sauce made from soy and wheat (shoyu)	53	13	0	22	1.78	0.08
Soy sauce made from soy and wheat (shoyu), low sodium	53	13	0	22	1.71	0.08
Soybean, curd cheese	151	13	8	7	1.78	0.25
Soybeans, mature cooked, boiled, without salt	173	17	9	10	2.84	0.28
Soybeans, mature seeds, cooked, boiled, with salt	173	17	9	10	2.84	0.28
Soybeans, mature seeds, dry roasted	451	40	22	33	7.01	0.21
Soybeans, mature seeds, raw	416	36	20	30	-4.69	-0.16
Soybeans, mature seeds, roasted, no salt added	471	26	25	34	-5.74	-0.17
Soybeans, mature seeds, roasted, salted	471	26	25	34	-5.74	-0.17
Soyburger	194	16	6	14	18.39	1.31
Tempeh	193	19	11	9	6.72	0.75
Tempeh, cooked	196	18	11	9	6.60	0.73
Tofu yogurt	94	4	2	16	-0.44	-0.03
Tofu, dried-frozen (koyadofu)	480	48	30	16	34.67	2.17
Tofu, dried-frozen (koyadofu), prepared with calcium sulfate	472	48	30	13	8.49	0.65
Tofu, extra firm, prepared with nigari	91	10	6	2	3.45	1.73
Tofu, firm, prepared with calcium sulfate and magnesium chloride (nigari)	70	8	4	2	1.80	0.90
Tofu, fried	271	17	20	10	9.58	0.96
Tofu, fried, prepared with calcium sulfate	271	17	20	10	1.01	0.10
Tofu, hard, prepared with nigari	146	13	10	4	5.83	1.46
Tofu, okara	77	3	2	13	-2.39	-0.18
Tofu, raw, firm, prepared with calcium sulfate	145	16	9	4	-0.60	-0.15
Tofu, raw, regular, prepared with calcium sulfate	76	8	5	2	-0.32	-0.16

Legumes and Legume Products

Food Description	Kcals	Protein	Fat	Carbs	PRAL	Alkali Density
Tofu, salted and fermented (fuyu)	116	8	8	5	3.17	0.63
Tofu, salted and fermented (fuyu), prepared with calcium sulfate	116	8	8	5	-12.36	-2.47
Tofu, soft, prepared with calcium sulfate and magnesium chloride (nigari)	61	7	4	2	1.94	0.97
USDA Commodity, Peanut Butter, smooth	630	22	50	24	5.35	0.22
Vegetarian fillets	290	23	18	9	13.48	1.50
Vegetarian meatloaf or patties	197	21	9	8	18.39	2.30
Vegetarian stew	123	17	3	7	10.24	1.46
Veggie burgers, unprepared	177	16	6	14	5.09	0.36
Vermicelli, made from soy	330	0	0	82	-0.04	0
Winged beans, mature seeds, cooked, boiled, with salt	147	11	6	15	1.73	0.12
Winged beans, mature seeds, raw	409	30	16	42	0.32	0.01
Yardlong beans, mature seeds, cooked, boiled, without salt	118	8	0	21	1.05	0.05
Yardlong beans, mature seeds, raw	347	24	1	62	-2.27	-0.04
Yardlong beans, yardlong, mature seeds, cooked, boiled, with salt	118	8	0	21	1.05	0.05

Finfish and Shellfish Products

Food Description	Kcals	Protein	Fat	Carbs	PRAL	Acid Density
Crustaceans, crab, Alaska king, cooked, moist heat	97	19	2	0	11.93	0.63
Crustaceans, crab, Alaska king, imitation, made from surimi	95	6	0	13	10.99	1.83
Crustaceans, crab, Alaska king, raw	84	8	0	15	10.90	1.36
Crustaceans, crab, blue, canned	99	21	1	0	9.49	0.45
Crustaceans, crab, blue, cooked, moist heat	102	20	2	0	8.50	0.43
Crustaceans, crab, blue, crab cakes	155	12	5	0	8.75	0.73
Crustaceans, crab, blue, raw	87	18	1	0	8.37	0.47
Crustaceans, crab, Dungeness, cooked, moist heat	110	22	1	1	6.56	0.30
Crustaceans, crab, Dungeness, raw	86	17	1	1	6.06	0.36
Crustaceans, crab, queen, cooked, moist heat	115	24	2	0	10.09	0.42
Crustaceans, crab, queen, raw	90	18	1	0	8.74	0.49
Crustaceans, crayfish, mixed species, farmed, cooked, moist heat	87	18	1	0	10.98	0.61
Crustaceans, crayfish, mixed species, farmed, raw	72	15	1	0	8.75	0.58
Crustaceans, crayfish, mixed species, wild, cooked, moist heat	82	17	1	0	10.35	0.61
Crustaceans, crayfish, mixed species, wild, raw	77	16	1	0	9.90	0.62
Crustaceans, lobster, northern, cooked, moist heat	98	21	1	1	7.79	0.37
Crustaceans, lobster, northern, raw	90	19	1	0	7.43	0.39
Crustaceans, shrimp, mixed species, canned	100	20	1	0	12.79	0.64
Crustaceans, shrimp, mixed species, cooked, breaded and fried	242	21	12	11	11.91	0.57
Crustaceans, shrimp, mixed species, cooked, moist heat	99	21	1	0	10.10	0.48
Crustaceans, shrimp, mixed species, imitation, made from surimi	101	12	1	9	13.27	1.11
Crustaceans, shrimp, mixed species, raw	106	20	2	1	12.01	0.60
Crustaceans, spiny lobster, mixed species, cooked, moist heat	143	26	2	3	14.90	0.57
Crustaceans, spiny lobster, mixed species, raw	112	21	2	2	13.44	0.64
Fish, anchovy, European, canned in oil, drained solids	210	29	10	0	7.24	0.25
Fish, anchovy, European, raw	131	20	5	0	5.39	0.27
Fish, bass, fresh water, mixed species, raw	114	19	4	0	7.34	0.39
Fish, bass, freshwater, mixed species, cooked, dry heat	146	24	5	0	9.41	0.39
Fish, bass, striped, cooked, dry heat	124	23	3	0	12.07	0.52
Fish, bass, striped, raw	97	18	2	0	9.40	0.52
Fish, bluefish, cooked, dry heat	159	26	5	0	12.12	0.47
Fish, bluefish, raw	124	20	4	0	9.45	0.47
Fish, burbot, cooked, dry heat	115	25	1	0	8.82	0.35
Fish, burbot, raw	90	19	1	0	6.89	0.36
Fish, butterfish, cooked, dry heat	187	22	10	0	10.95	0.50
Fish, butterfish, raw	146	17	8	0	8.53	0.50
Fish, carp, cooked, dry heat	162	23	7	0	20.21	0.88

Finfish and Shellfish Products

Food Description	Kcals	Protein	Fat	Carbs	PRAL	Acid Density
Fish, carp, raw	127	18	6	0	15.81	0.88
Fish, catfish, channel, cooked, breaded and fried	229	18	13	8	8.44	0.47
Fish, catfish, channel, farmed, cooked, dry heat	152	19	8	0	10.70	0.56
Fish, catfish, channel, farmed, raw	135	16	8	0	8.10	0.51
Fish, catfish, channel, wild, cooked, dry heat	105	18	3	0	10.62	0.59
Fish, catfish, channel, wild, raw	95	16	3	0	7.46	0.47
Fish, caviar, black and red, granular	252	25	18	4	10.05	0.40
Fish, cisco, raw	98	19	2	0	6.89	0.36
Fish, cisco, smoked	177	16	12	0	6.63	0.41
Fish, cod, Atlantic, canned, solids and liquid	105	23	1	0	8.34	0.36
Fish, cod, Atlantic, cooked, dry heat	105	23	1	0	9.89	0.43
Fish, cod, Atlantic, dried and salted	290	63	2	0	29.77	0.47
Fish, cod, Atlantic, raw	82	18	1	0	6.52	0.36
Fish, cod, Pacific, cooked, dry heat	105	23	1	0	7.71	0.34
Fish, cod, Pacific, raw	82	18	1	0	6.03	0.34
Fish, croaker, Atlantic, cooked, breaded and fried	221	18	13	8	8.29	0.46
Fish, croaker, Atlantic, raw	104	18	3	0	8	0.44
Fish, cusk, cooked, dry heat	112	24	1	0	9.85	0.41
Fish, cusk, raw	87	19	1	0	7.68	0.40
Fish, dolphinfish, cooked, dry heat	109	24	1	0	5.96	0.25
Fish, dolphinfish, raw	85	18	1	0	4.64	0.26
Fish, drum, freshwater, cooked, dry heat	153	22	6	0	10.16	0.46
Fish, drum, freshwater, raw	119	18	5	0	7.92	0.44
Fish, eel, mixed species, cooked, dry heat	236	24	15	0	13.49	0.56
Fish, eel, mixed species, raw	184	18	12	0	10.53	0.59
Fish, fish portions and sticks, frozen, preheated	249	11	13	23	6.54	0.59
Fish, flatfish (flounder and sole species), cooked, dry heat	117	24	2	0	13.56	0.57
Fish, flatfish (flounder and sole species), raw	91	19	1	0	7.41	0.39
Fish, gefiltefish, commercial, sweet recipe	84	9	2	7	4.70	0.52
Fish, grouper, mixed species, cooked, dry heat	118	25	1	0	6.25	0.25
Fish, grouper, mixed species, raw	92	19	1	0	4.19	0.22
Fish, haddock, cooked, dry heat	112	24	1	0	10.57	0.44
Fish, haddock, raw	87	19	1	0	8.24	0.43
Fish, haddock, smoked	116	25	1	0	10.89	0.44
Fish, halibut, Atlantic and Pacific, cooked, dry heat	140	27	3	0	7.96	0.29
Fish, halibut, Atlantic and Pacific, raw	110	21	2	0	6.19	0.29
Fish, halibut, Greenland, cooked, dry heat	239	18	18	0	8.66	0.48
Fish, halibut, Greenland, raw	186	14	14	0	6.76	0.48
Fish, herring, Atlantic, cooked, dry heat	203	23	12	0	11.66	0.51

Finfish and Shellfish Products

Food Description	Kcals	Protein	Fat	Carbs	PRAL	Acid Density
Fish, herring, Atlantic, kippered	217	25	12	0	12.39	0.50
Fish, herring, Atlantic, pickled	262	14	18	10	7.58	0.54
Fish, herring, Atlantic, raw	158	18	9	0	9.09	0.51
Fish, herring, Pacific, cooked, dry heat	250	21	18	0	7.27	0.35
Fish, herring, Pacific, raw	195	16	14	0	5.67	0.35
Fish, ling, cooked, dry heat	111	24	1	0	8.44	0.35
Fish, ling, raw	87	19	1	0	6.59	0.35
Fish, lingcod, cooked, dry heat	109	23	1	0	7.78	0.34
Fish, lingcod, raw	85	18	1	0	6.05	0.34
Fish, mackerel, Atlantic, cooked, dry heat	262	24	18	0	10.83	0.45
Fish, mackerel, Atlantic, raw	205	19	14	0	8.41	0.44
Fish, mackerel, jack, canned, drained solids	156	23	6	0	14.33	0.62
Fish, mackerel, king, cooked, dry heat	134	26	3	0	11.20	0.43
Fish, mackerel, king, raw	105	20	2	0	8.74	0.44
Fish, mackerel, Pacific and jack, mixed species, cooked, dry heat	201	26	10	0	6.27	0.24
Fish, mackerel, Pacific and jack, mixed species, raw	158	20	8	0	4.90	0.25
Fish, mackerel, salted	305	18	25	0	5.12	0.28
Fish, mackerel, Spanish, cooked, dry heat	158	24	6	0	8.79	0.37
Fish, mackerel, Spanish, raw	139	19	6	0	6.67	0.35
Fish, milkfish, cooked, dry heat	190	26	9	0	10.90	0.42
Fish, milkfish, raw	148	21	7	0	8.47	0.40
Fish, monkfish, cooked, dry heat	97	19	2	0	6.96	0.37
Fish, monkfish, raw	76	14	2	0	5.44	0.39
Fish, mullet, striped, cooked, dry heat	150	25	5	0	10.30	0.41
Fish, mullet, striped, raw	117	19	4	0	8.87	0.47
Fish, ocean perch, Atlantic, cooked, dry heat	121	24	2	0	11.80	0.49
Fish, ocean perch, Atlantic, raw	94	19	2	0	9.21	0.48
Fish, perch, mixed species, cooked, dry heat	117	25	1	0	12.15	0.49
Fish, perch, mixed species, raw	91	19	1	0	9.43	0.50
Fish, pike, northern, cooked, dry heat	113	25	1	0	13.59	0.54
Fish, pike, northern, raw	88	19	1	0	10.59	0.56
Fish, pike, walleye, cooked, dry heat	119	25	2	0	8.67	0.35
Fish, pike, walleye, raw	93	19	1	0	6.77	0.36
Fish, pollock, Atlantic, cooked, dry heat	118	25	1	0	9.86	0.39
Fish, pollock, Atlantic, raw	92	19	1	0	7.70	0.41
Fish, pollock, walleye, cooked, dry heat	113	24	1	0	19.25	0.80
Fish, pollock, walleye, raw	81	17	1	0	13.93	0.82
Fish, pompano, Florida, cooked, dry heat	211	24	12	0	9.50	0.40
Fish, pompano, Florida, raw	164	18	9	0	7.28	0.40

Finfish and Shellfish Products

Food Description	Kcals	Protein	Fat	Carbs	PRAL	Acid Density
Fish, pout, ocean, cooked, dry heat	102	21	1	0	8.54	0.41
Fish, pout, ocean, raw	79	17	1	0	6.68	0.39
Fish, rockfish, Pacific, mixed species, cooked, dry heat	121	24	2	0	8.25	0.34
Fish, rockfish, Pacific, mixed species, raw	94	19	2	0	6.47	0.34
Fish, roe, mixed species, cooked, dry heat	204	29	8	2	26.09	0.90
Fish, roe, mixed species, raw	140	22	6	1	20.36	0.93
Fish, roughy, orange, cooked, dry heat	105	23	1	0	10.45	0.45
Fish, roughy, orange, raw	76	16	1	0	7.93	0.50
Fish, sablefish, cooked, dry heat	250	17	20	0	4.30	0.25
Fish, sablefish, raw	195	13	15	0	3.38	0.26
Fish, sablefish, smoked	257	18	20	0	4.39	0.24
Fish, salmon, Atlantic, farmed, cooked, dry heat	206	22	12	0	11.11	0.51
Fish, salmon, Atlantic, farmed, raw	183	20	13	0	9.88	0.49
Fish, salmon, Atlantic, wild, cooked, dry heat	182	25	8	0	7.59	0.30
Fish, salmon, Atlantic, wild, raw	142	20	6	0	5.92	0.30
Fish, salmon, Chinook, cooked, dry heat	231	26	13	0	12.18	0.47
Fish, salmon, Chinook, raw	179	20	10	0	9.37	0.47
Fish, salmon, Chinook, smoked	117	18	4	0	10.73	0.60
Fish, salmon, Chinook, smoked, (lox), regular	117	18	4	0	10.73	0.60
Fish, salmon, chum, canned, without salt, drained solids with bone	141	21	5	0	13.28	0.63
Fish, salmon, chum, cooked, dry heat	154	26	5	0	13.62	0.52
Fish, salmon, chum, drained solids with bone	141	21	5	0	13.28	0.63
Fish, salmon, chum, raw	120	20	4	0	10.61	0.53
Fish, salmon, Coho, farmed, cooked, dry heat	178	24	8	0	13.49	0.56
Fish, salmon, Coho, farmed, raw	160	34	12	0	10.81	0.32
Fish, salmon, Coho, wild, cooked, dry heat	139	23	4	0	12.84	0.56
Fish, salmon, Coho, wild, cooked, moist heat	184	27	8	0	13.36	0.49
Fish, salmon, Coho, wild, raw	146	22	6	0	10.13	0.46
Fish, salmon, pink, canned, drained solids with bone	136	23	5	0	13.79	0.60
Fish, salmon, pink, canned, solids with bone and liquid	139	20	6	0	11.36	0.57
Fish, salmon, pink, canned, without salt, solids with bone and liquid	139	20	6	0	11.36	0.57
Fish, salmon, pink, cooked, dry heat	149	26	4	0	13.66	0.53
Fish, salmon, pink, raw	116	20	3	0	10.65	0.53
Fish, salmon, sockeye, canned, drained solids with bone	166	23	7	0	13.36	0.58
Fish, salmon, sockeye, canned, without salt, drained solids with bone	153	20	7	0	10.31	0.52
Fish, salmon, sockeye, cooked, dry heat	216	27	11	0	14.82	0.55
Fish, salmon, sockeye, raw	168	21	9	0	9.47	0.45

Finfish and Shellfish Products

Food Description	Kcals	Protein	Fat	Carbs	PRAL	Acid Density
Fish, sardine, Pacific, canned in tomato sauce, drained solids with bone	186	21	10	1	12.59	0.60
Fish, scup, cooked, dry heat	135	24	4	0	11.48	0.48
Fish, scup, raw	105	19	3	0	8.95	0.47
Fish, sea bass, mixed species, cooked, dry heat	124	24	3	0	12.32	0.51
Fish, sea bass, mixed species, raw	97	18	2	0	9.63	0.54
Fish, seatrout, mixed species, cooked, dry heat	133	21	5	0	11.88	0.57
Fish, seatrout, mixed species, raw	104	17	4	0	9.26	0.54
Fish, shad, American, cooked, dry heat	252	22	18	0	11.45	0.52
Fish, shad, American, raw	197	17	14	0	8.90	0.52
Fish, shark, mixed species, cooked, batter-dipped and fried	228	19	14	6	11.27	0.59
Fish, shark, mixed species, raw	130	21	5	0	12.97	0.62
Fish, sheepshead, cooked, dry heat	126	26	2	0	13.55	0.52
Fish, sheepshead, raw	108	20	2	0	11.89	0.59
Fish, smelt, rainbow, cooked, dry heat	124	23	3	0	12.18	0.53
Fish, smelt, rainbow, raw	97	18	2	0	9.49	0.53
Fish, snapper, mixed species, cooked, dry heat	128	26	2	0	7.88	0.30
Fish, snapper, mixed species, raw	100	21	1	0	7.37	0.35
Fish, spot, cooked, dry heat	158	24	6	0	5.44	0.23
Fish, spot, raw	123	19	5	0	4.26	0.22
Fish, sturgeon, mixed species, cooked, dry heat	135	21	5	0	11.13	0.53
Fish, sturgeon, mixed species, raw	105	16	4	0	8.67	0.54
Fish, sturgeon, mixed species, smoked	173	31	4	0	16.28	0.53
Fish, sucker, white, cooked, dry heat	119	21	3	0	8.09	0.39
Fish, sucker, white, raw	92	17	2	0	6.31	0.37
Fish, sunfish, pumpkin seed, cooked, dry heat	114	25	1	0	8.97	0.36
Fish, sunfish, pumpkin seed, raw	89	19	1	0	6.99	0.37
Fish, surimi	99	15	1	7	14.28	0.95
Fish, swordfish, cooked, dry heat	155	25	5	0	16.19	0.65
Fish, swordfish, raw	121	20	4	0	12.63	0.63
Fish, tilapia, cooked, dry heat	128	26	3	0	11.31	0.44
Fish, tilapia, raw	96	20	2	0	8.95	0.45
Fish, tilefish, cooked, dry heat	147	24	5	0	8.78	0.37
Fish, tilefish, raw	96	17	2	0	5.33	0.31
Fish, trout, mixed species, cooked, dry heat	190	27	8	0	13.50	0.50
Fish, trout, mixed species, raw	148	21	7	0	10.53	0.50
Fish, trout, rainbow, farmed, cooked, dry heat	169	24	7	0	10.52	0.44
Fish, trout, rainbow, farmed, raw	138	21	5	0	9.48	0.45
Fish, trout, rainbow, wild, cooked, dry heat	150	23	6	0	9.85	0.43

Finfish and Shellfish Products

Food Description	Kcals	Protein	Fat	Carbs	PRAL	Acid Density
Fish, trout, rainbow, wild, raw	119	20	3	0	8.28	0.41
Fish, tuna salad	187	16	9	9	9.99	0.62
Fish, tuna, fresh, bluefin, cooked, dry heat	184	30	6	0	18.14	0.60
Fish, tuna, fresh, bluefin, raw	144	23	5	0	14.13	0.61
Fish, tuna, fresh, skipjack, raw	103	18	5	0	9.18	0.51
Fish, tuna, fresh, yellowfin, raw	108	0	0	39	7.69	
Fish, tuna, light, canned in oil, drained solids	198	29	8	0	20.45	0.71
Fish, tuna, light, canned in oil, without salt, drained solids	198	29	8	0	20.45	0.71
Fish, tuna, light, canned in water, drained solids	116	26	1	0	12.70	0.49
Fish, tuna, light, canned in water, without salt, drained solids	116	26	1	0	12.70	0.49
Fish, tuna, skipjack, fresh, cooked, dry heat	132	28	1	0	11.78	0.42
Fish, tuna, white, canned in oil, drained solids	186	27	8	0	14.95	0.55
Fish, tuna, white, canned in oil, without salt, drained solids	186	27	8	0	14.95	0.55
Fish, tuna, white, canned in water, drained solids	128	24	3	0	13.58	0.57
Fish, tuna, white, canned in water, without salt, drained solids	128	24	3	0	13.58	0.57
Fish, tuna, yellowfin, fresh, cooked, dry heat	139	30	1	0	9.86	0.33
Fish, turbot, European, cooked, dry heat	122	21	4	0	7.79	0.37
Fish, turbot, European, raw	95	16	3	0	6.08	0.38
Fish, whitefish, mixed species, cooked, dry heat	172	24	8	0	14.74	0.61
Fish, whitefish, mixed species, raw	134	19	6	0	11.49	0.60
Fish, whitefish, mixed species, smoked	108	23	1	0	6.63	0.29
Fish, whiting, mixed species, cooked, dry heat	116	23	2	0	11.42	0.50
Fish, whiting, mixed species, raw	90	18	1	0	10.78	0.60
Fish, wolffish, Atlantic, cooked, dry heat	123	22	3	0	11.29	0.51
Fish, wolffish, Atlantic, raw	96	17	2	0	8.81	0.52
Fish, yellowtail, mixed species, cooked, dry heat	187	30	7	0	9.31	0.31
Fish, yellowtail, mixed species, raw	146	20	4	0	7.24	0.36
Frog legs, raw	73	16	0	0	6.73	0.42
Jellyfish, dried, salted	36	5	1	0	3.29	0.66
Mollusks, abalone, mixed species, cooked, fried	189	20	7	11	9.74	0.49
Mollusks, abalone, mixed species, raw	105	17	1	6	8.50	0.50
Mollusks, clam, mixed species, canned, drained solids	148	26	2	5	10.17	0.39
Mollusks, clam, mixed species, canned, liquid	2	0	0	0	0.83	
Mollusks, clam, mixed species, cooked, breaded and fried	202	14	11	10	5.90	0.42
Mollusks, clam, mixed species, cooked, moist heat	148	26	2	5	10.17	0.39
Mollusks, clam, mixed species, raw	74	13	1	3	5.08	0.39
Mollusks, conch, baked or broiled	130	26	1	2	10.03	0.39
Mollusks, cuttlefish, mixed species, cooked, moist heat	158	32	1	2	20.09	0.63

Finfish and Shellfish Products

Food Description	Kcals	Protein	Fat	Carbs	PRAL	Acid Density
Mollusks, cuttlefish, mixed species, raw	79	16	1	1	12.89	0.81
Mollusks, mussel, blue, cooked, moist heat	172	24	4	7	15.18	0.63
Mollusks, mussel, blue, raw	86	12	2	4	5.17	0.43
Mollusks, octopus, common, cooked, moist heat	164	30	2	4	8.76	0.29
Mollusks, octopus, common, raw	82	15	1	2	5.36	0.36
Mollusks, oyster, eastern, canned	69	7	2	4	1.80	0.26
Mollusks, oyster, eastern, cooked, breaded and fried	197	9	13	12	2.74	0.30
Mollusks, oyster, eastern, farmed, cooked, dry heat	79	7	2	7	2.90	0.41
Mollusks, oyster, eastern, farmed, raw	59	5	2	6	1.96	0.39
Mollusks, oyster, eastern, wild, cooked, dry heat	72	8	2	5	3.76	0.47
Mollusks, oyster, eastern, wild, cooked, moist heat	137	14	5	8	4.87	0.35
Mollusks, oyster, eastern, wild, raw	68	7	2	4	3.36	0.48
Mollusks, oyster, Pacific, cooked, moist heat	163	19	5	10	10.55	0.56
Mollusks, oyster, Pacific, raw	81	9	2	5	6.42	0.71
Mollusks, scallop, (bay and sea), cooked, steamed	112	23	1	0	10.95	0.48
Mollusks, scallop, mixed species, cooked, breaded and fried	215	18	11	10	8.51	0.47
Mollusks, scallop, mixed species, imitation, made from surimi	99	13	0	11	13.30	1.02
Mollusks, scallop, mixed species, raw	88	17	1	2	7.79	0.46
Mollusks, snail, raw	90	16	1	2	3.30	0.21
Mollusks, squid, mixed species, cooked, fried	175	18	7	8	10.72	0.60
Mollusks, squid, mixed species, raw	92	16	1	3	9.37	0.59
Mollusks, whelk, unspecified, cooked, moist heat	275	48	1	16	13.28	0.28
Mollusks, whelk, unspecified, raw	137	24	0	8	6.63	0.28
Turtle, green, raw	89	20	0	0	9.47	0.47
USDA Commodity, salmon nuggets, breaded, frozen, heated	212	13	12	14	8.64	0.66
USDA Commodity, salmon nuggets, cooked as purchased, unheated	189	12	10	12	8.24	0.69

Beverages

Food Description	Kcals	Protein	Fat	Carbs	PRAL	Alkali Density
Alcoholic beverage, beer, light	29	0	2	0	-0.06	
Alcoholic beverage, beer, light, BUD LIGHT	31	0	0	2	-0.23	-0.12
Alcoholic beverage, beer, light, MICHELOB ULTRA	27	0	0	1	-0.13	-0.13
Alcoholic beverage, beer, regular, all	43	0	0	4	-0.03	-0.01
Alcoholic beverage, beer, regular, BUDWEISER	41	0	0	3	-0.27	-0.09
Alcoholic beverage, crème de menthe, 72 proof	371	0	0	42	0	0
Alcoholic beverage, daiquiri, canned	125	0	0	16	-0.18	-0.01
Alcoholic beverage, daiquiri, prepared-from-recipe	186	0	0	7	-0.31	-0.04
Alcoholic beverage, distilled, all (gin, rum, vodka, whiskey) 100 proof	295	0	0	0	0.10	
Alcoholic beverage, distilled, all (gin, rum, vodka, whiskey) 80 proof	231	0	0	0	0.10	
Alcoholic beverage, distilled, all (gin, rum, vodka, whiskey) 86 proof	250	0	0	0	0.10	
Alcoholic beverage, distilled, all (gin, rum, vodka, whiskey) 90 proof	263	0	0	0	0.10	
Alcoholic beverage, distilled, all (gin, rum, vodka, whiskey) 94 proof	275	0	0	0	0.10	
Alcoholic beverage, distilled, gin, 90 proof	263	0	0	0	0	
Alcoholic beverage, distilled, rum, 80 proof	231	0	0	0	0.14	
Alcoholic beverage, distilled, vodka, 80 proof	231	0	0	0	0.16	
Alcoholic beverage, distilled, whiskey, 86 proof	250	0	0	0	0.09	
Alcoholic beverage, liqueur, coffee with cream, 34 proof	327	3	16	21	2.29	0.11
Alcoholic beverage, liqueur, coffee, 53 proof	336	0	0	47	-0.45	-0.01
Alcoholic beverage, liqueur, coffee, 63 proof	308	0	0	32	-0.45	-0.01
Alcoholic beverage, pina colada, canned	237	1	8	28	-0.28	-0.01
Alcoholic beverage, pina colada, prepared-from-recipe	174	0	2	23	-1.33	-0.06
Alcoholic beverage, rice (sake)	134	0	0	5	-0.27	-0.05
Alcoholic beverage, tequila sunrise, canned	110	0	0	3	0.12	0.04
Alcoholic beverage, whiskey sour, canned	119	0	0	13	-0.03	0
Alcoholic beverage, whiskey sour, prepared from item 14028	153	0	0	13	-0.20	-0.02
Alcoholic beverage, whiskey sour, prepared from item 14530	149	0	0	13	0.07	0.01
Alcoholic beverage, whiskey sour, prepared with water, whiskey and powder mix	164	0	0	16	-0.55	-0.03
Alcoholic beverage, wine, cooking	50	0	0	6	-1.42	-0.24
Alcoholic beverage, wine, dessert, dry	152	0	0	12	-1.83	-0.15
Alcoholic beverage, wine, dessert, sweet	160	0	0	14	-1.83	-0.13
Alcoholic beverage, wine, light	50	0	0	1	-1.63	-1.63
Alcoholic beverage, wine, table, all	84	0	0	3	-1.69	-0.56
Alcoholic beverage, wine, table, red	85	0	0	3	-2.19	-0.73
Alcoholic Beverage, wine, table, red, Merlot	84	0	0	3	-2.19	-0.73
Alcoholic beverage, wine, table, white	83	0	0	3	-1.16	-0.39

Beverages

Food Description	Kcals	Protein	Fat	Carbs	PRAL	Alkali Density
Apple cider-flavored drink, powder, added vitamin C and sugar	395	0	0	99	-1.38	-0.01
Apple cider-flavored drink, powder, low calorie, with vitamin C, prepared	1	0	0	0	0.27	
Beef broth and tomato juice, canned	37	1	0	8	-1.46	-0.18
Carbonated beverage, chocolate-flavored soda	42	c	0	11	-1.09	-0.10
Carbonated beverage, club soda	0	0	0	0	-0.13	
Carbonated beverage, cola, contains caffeine	37	0	0	10	0.33	0.03
Carbonated beverage, cola, with higher caffeine	41	0	0	11	0.31	0.03
Carbonated beverage, cola, without caffeine	41	0	0	11	0.31	0.03
Carbonated beverage, cream soda	51	0	0	13	-0.11	-0.01
Carbonated beverage, ginger ale	34	0	0	9	-0.08	-0.01
Carbonated beverage, grape soda	43	0	0	11	-0.08	-0.01
Carbonated beverage, lemon-lime soda, contains caffeine	41	0	0	10	-0.02	0
Carbonated beverage, low calorie, cola or pepper-type, with aspartame, contains caffeine	2	0	0	0	0.15	
Carbonated beverage, low calorie, cola or pepper-type, with aspartame, without caffeine	1	0	0	0	0.24	
Carbonated beverage, low calorie, cola or pepper-types, with sodium saccharin, contains caffeine	0	0	0	0	0.24	
Carbonated beverage, low calorie, other than cola or pepper, without caffeine	0	0	0	0	-0.07	
Carbonated beverage, low calorie, other than cola or pepper, with aspartame, contains caffeine	0	0	0	0	-0.07	
Carbonated beverage, low calorie, other than cola or pepper, with sodium saccharin, without caffeine	0	0	0	0	-0.12	
Carbonated beverage, orange	48	0	0	12	-0.09	-0.01
Carbonated beverage, pepper-type, contains caffeine	41	0	0	10	0.34	0.03
Carbonated beverage, reduced sugar, cola, contains caffeine and sweeteners	20	0	0	5	0.31	0.06
Carbonated beverage, root beer	41	0	0	11	-0.11	-0.01
Carbonated beverage, SPRITE, lemon-lime, without caffeine	40	0	0	10	-0.04	0
Carbonated beverage, tonic water	34	0	0	9	-0.01	0
Carob-flavor beverage mix, powder	372	2	0	93	-1.58	-0.02
Carob-flavor beverage mix, powder, prepared with whole milk	75	3	3	9	0.22	0.02
Chocolate syrup	279	2	1	65	-0.77	-0.01
Chocolate syrup, prepared with whole milk	90	2	1	65	0.16	0
Chocolate-flavor beverage mix for milk, powder, with added nutrients	400	5	2	90	-7.76	-0.09
Chocolate-flavor beverage mix for milk, powder, with added nutrients, prepared with whole milk	88	3	3	12	-0.35	-0.03
Chocolate-flavor beverage mix for milk, powder, without added nutrients	349	3	3	91	-9.08	-0.10
Chocolate-flavor beverage mix, powder, prepared with whole milk	85	3	3	12	-0.47	-0.04
Chocolate-flavored drink, whey and milk based	49	1	0	11	-2.04	-0.19

Beverages

Food Description	Kcals	Protein	Fat	Carbs	PRAL	Alkali Density
Citrus fruit juice drink, frozen concentrate	162	1	0	40	-7.17	-0.18
Citrus fruit juice drink, frozen concentrate, prepared with water	50	0	0	11	-0.96	-0.09
Clam and tomato juice, canned	48	1	0	11	-1.40	-0.13
Cocktail mix, non-alcoholic, concentrated, frozen	287	0	0	72	-0.42	-0.01
Cocoa mix, no sugar added, powder	377	15	3	72	-29	-0.40
Cocoa mix, powder	398	7	4	84	-3.91	-0.05
Cocoa mix, powder, prepared with water	55	1	1	12	-0.66	-0.06
Cocoa mix, with aspartame, low calorie, powder, with added calcium phosphorus, without added sodium or vitamin A	359	25	3	58	-8.26	-0.14
Cocoa mix, with aspartame, powder, prepared from item 14196	29	1	0	6	-2.27	-0.38
Coffee and cocoa (mocha) powder, with whitener and low calorie sweetener	257	9	13	71	-21.83	-0.31
Coffee and cocoa (mocha) powder, with whitener and low calorie sweetener, decaffeinated	257	9	13	71	-21.83	-0.31
Coffee substitute, cereal grain beverage, powder	360	6	3	78	-33.91	-0.43
Coffee substitute, cereal grain beverage, powder, prepared with whole milk	65	3	3	6	-0.29	-0.05
Coffee substitute, cereal grain beverage, prepared with water	6	0	0	1	-0.61	-0.61
Coffee, brewed from grounds, prepared with tap water	1	0	0	0	-0.96	
Coffee, brewed from grounds, prepared with tap water, decaffeinated	0	0	0	0	-1.20	
Coffee, brewed, espresso, restaurant-prepared	2	0	0	0	-4.20	
Coffee, brewed, espresso, restaurant-prepared, decaffeinated	0	0	0	0	-4.21	
Coffee, dry, powder, with whitener, reduced calorie	509	2	29	60	-13.42	-0.22
Coffee, instant, decaffeinated, powder	224	12	0	43	-67.16	-1.56
Coffee, instant, decaffeinated, powder, prepared with water	2	0	0	0	-0.92	
Coffee, instant, regular, powder	241	12	0	41	-67.38	-1.64
Coffee, instant, regular, powder, half the caffeine	350	14	0	71	-66.29	-0.93
Coffee, instant, regular, prepared with water	2	0	0	0	-0.60	
Coffee, instant, with chicory, powder	351	9	0	74	-63.58	-0.86
Coffee, instant, with chicory, prepared with water	3	0	0	1	-0.67	-0.67
Coffee, instant, with sugar, cappuccino-flavor powder	406	3	6	86	-12	-0.14
Coffee, instant, with sugar, French-flavor, powder	484	5	23	66	-10.70	-0.16
Coffee, instant, with sugar, mocha-flavor, powder	460	5	16	74	-15.10	-0.20
Corn beverage	29	1	0	9	-0.59	-0.07
Cranberry juice cocktail, bottled	54	0	0	14	-0.32	-0.02
Cranberry juice cocktail, bottled, low calorie, with calcium, saccharin and corn sweetener	19	0	0	6	-0.64	-0.11
Cranberry juice cocktail, frozen concentrate	201	0	0	51	-1.09	-0.02

Beverages

Food Description	Kcals	Protein	Fat	Carbs	PRAL	Alkali Density
Cranberry juice cocktail, frozen concentrate, prepared with water	55	0	0	12	-0.37	-0.03
Cranberry-apple juice drink, bottled	63	0	0	16	-0.34	-0.02
Cranberry-apple juice drink, low calorie, with vitamin C added	19	0	0	5	-1.06	-0.21
Cranberry-apricot juice drink, bottled	64	0	0	16	-1.19	-0.07
Cranberry-grape juice drink, bottled	56	0	0	14	-0.44	-0.03
Dairy drink mix, chocolate, reduced calorie, with aspartame, powder	298	25	3	51	-25.56	-0.50
Dairy drink mix, chocolate, reduced calorie, with aspartame, powder, prepared with water	31	2	0	5	-2.18	-0.44
Drink mix, QUAKER OATS, GATORADE, orange flavor, powder	388	0	1	94	3.26	0.03
Eggnog-flavor mix, powder, prepared with whole milk	95	3	3	14	0.28	0.02
Energy drink, RED BULL, sugar free, with added caffeine, niacin, pantothenic acid, vitamins B6 and B12	5	0	0	1	-0.18	-0.18
Energy drink, RED BULL, with added caffeine, niacin, pantothenic acid, vitamins B6 and B12	45	0	0	11	-0.18	-0.02
Fruit punch drink, frozen concentrate	162	0	0	41	-1.01	-0.02
Fruit punch drink, frozen concentrate, prepared with water	46	0	0	12	-0.31	-0.03
Fruit punch drink, with added nutrients, canned	47	0	0	12	-0.72	-0.06
Fruit punch drink, without added nutrients, canned	48	0	0	12	-0.59	-0.05
Fruit punch juice drink, frozen concentrate	175	0	1	43	-5.62	-0.13
Fruit punch juice drink, frozen concentrate, prepared with water	50	0	0	10	-1.76	-0.18
Fruit punch-flavor drink, powder, without added sodium	382	0	0	98	-1.95	-0.02
Fruit punch-flavor drink, powder, without added sodium, prepared with water	37	0	0	9	-0.28	-0.03
Fruit-flavored drink mix, powder, unsweetened	226	0	0	91	4.44	0.05
Fruit-flavored drink, dry powdered mix, low calorie, with aspartame	217	0	0	87	21.91	0.25
Fruit-flavored drink, powder, with high vitamin C, low calorie	227	0	0	91	-51.28	-0.56
Grape drink, canned	61	0	0	16	-0.95	-0.06
Grape juice drink, canned	57	0	0	15	-0.71	-0.05
Lemonade, frozen concentrate, pink	181	0	0	47	-1.14	-0.02
Lemonade, frozen concentrate, pink, prepared with water	40	0	0	10	-0.28	-0.03
Lemonade, frozen concentrate, white	181	0	0	47	-1.14	-0.02
Lemonade, frozen concentrate, white, prepared with water	53	0	0	10	-0.36	-0.04
Lemonade, low calorie, with aspartame, powder	332	4	0	84	18.39	0.22
Lemonade, low calorie, with aspartame, powder, prepared with water	2	0	0	1	0.06	0.06
Lemonade, powder	389	0	0	94	-1.03	-0.01
Lemonade, powder, prepared with water	39	0	0	10	-0.14	-0.01
Lemonade-flavor drink, powder	389	0	0	94	-0.78	-0.01

Beverages

Food Description	Kcals	Protein	Fat	Carbs	PRAL	Alkali Density
Lemonade-flavor drink, powder, prepared with water	42	0	0	7	-0.15	-0.02
Limeade, frozen concentrate	247	0	0	62	-0.92	-0.01
Limeade, frozen concentrate, prepared with water	42	0	0	14	-0.19	-0.01
Malt beverage	37	0	0	8	0.25	0.03
Malted drink mix, chocolate, powder	411	5	5	87	-6.60	-0.08
Malted drink mix, chocolate, powder, prepared with whole milk	85	3	3	11	-0.25	-0.02
Malted drink mix, chocolate, with added nutrients, powder	389	5	3	85	-34.76	-0.41
Malted drink mix, chocolate, with added nutrients, powder, prepared with whole milk	84	3	3	2	-1	-0.50
Malted drink mix, natural, powder	429	14	10	71	-1.96	-0.03
Malted drink mix, natural, with added nutrients, powder	376	9	1	84	-8.43	-0.10
Malted drink mix, natural, with added nutrients, powder, prepared with whole milk	86	4	3	11	-0.43	-0.04
Mixed vegetable and fruit juice drink, with added nutrients	29	0	0	7	-0.37	-0.05
Orange and apricot juice drink, canned	51	0	0	13	-1.43	-0.11
Orange breakfast drink, ready-to-drink	43	0	0	11	-0.88	-0.08
Orange breakfast drink, ready-to-drink, with added nutrients	53	0	0	13	-2.91	-0.22
Orange drink, breakfast type, with juice and pulp, frozen concentrate, prepared with water	45	0	0	11	-4.02	-0.37
Orange drink, breakfast type, with juice and pulp, frozen concentrate	153	0	0	39	-11.38	-0.29
Orange drink, canned, with added vitamin C	49	0	0	12	-0.45	-0.04
Orange juice drink	54	0	0	13	-0.74	-0.06
Orange-flavor drink, breakfast type, low calorie, powder	217	4	0	86	-65.79	-0.77
Orange-flavor drink, breakfast type, powder	386	0	0	99	-3.40	-0.03
Orange-flavor drink, breakfast type, powder, prepared with water	49	0	0	13	-0.49	-0.04
Orange-flavor drink, breakfast type, with pulp, frozen concentrate, prepared with water	49	0	0	12	-2.30	-0.19
Orange-flavor drink, breakfast type, with pulp, frozen concentrate	172	0	0	43	-8.01	-0.19
Pineapple and grapefruit juice drink, canned	47	0	0	12	-1.20	-0.10
Pineapple and orange juice drink, canned	50	1	0	12	-0.40	-0.03
QUAKER OATS, PROPEL Fitness Water, fruit-flavored, non-carbonated	5	0	0	1	-0.34	-0.34
Shake, fast food, chocolate	127	3	4	21	-0.67	-0.03
Shake, fast food, strawberry	113	3	3	19	-0.26	-0.01
Shake, fast food, vanilla	148	3	7	20	-0.04	0
Sports drink, COCA-COLA, POWERADE, lemon-lime flavored, ready-to-drink	32	0	0	32	-0.35	-0.01
Sports drink, fruit-flavored, low calorie, ready-to-drink	11	0	0	3	0.09	0.03
Sports drink, QUAKER OATS, GATORADE, fruit-flavored, ready-to-drink	26	0	0	6	0	0
Strawberry-flavor beverage mix, powder	389	0	0	99	0.03	0

Beverages

Food Description	Kcals	Protein	Fat	Carbs	PRAL	Alkali Density
Tea, brewed, prepared with distilled water	1	0	0	0	-0.43	
Tea, brewed, prepared with tap water	1	0	0	0	-0.81	
Tea, brewed, prepared with tap water, decaffeinated	1	0	0	0	-0.81	
Tea, herb, chamomile, brewed	1	0	0	0	-0.24	
Tea, herb, other than chamomile, brewed	1	0	0	0	-0.24	
Tea, instant, sweetened with sodium saccharin, lemon-flavored, powder	338	3	1	85	-50.27	-0.59
Tea, instant, sweetened with sodium saccharin, lemon-flavored, powder, decaffeinated	338	3	1	85	-50.27	-0.59
Tea, instant, sweetened with sodium saccharin, lemon-flavored, prepared	2	0	0	0	-0.29	
Tea, instant, sweetened with sugar, lemon-flavored, with added ascorbic acid, powder	385	1	0	98	-4.07	-0.04
Tea, instant, sweetened with sugar, lemon-flavored, without added ascorbic acid, powder, prepared	35	0	0	9	-0.36	-0.04
Tea, instant, sweetened with sugar, lemon-flavored, without added ascorbic acid, powder	401	0	1	99	-3.52	-0.04
Tea, instant, sweetened with sugar, lemon-flavored, without added ascorbic acid, powder, decaffeinated	385	0	1	99	-3.52	-0.04
Tea, instant, unsweetened, lemon-flavored, powder	346	7	0	78	-68.90	-0.88
Tea, instant, unsweetened, powder	315	20	0	59	-116.70	-1.98
Tea, instant, unsweetened, powder, decaffeinated	315	20	0	59	-116.70	-1.98
Tea, instant, unsweetened, powder, prepared	1	0	0	0	-0.37	
Tea, ready-to-drink, ARIZONA iced tea, with lemon flavor	39	0	0	10	-0.23	-0.02
Tea, ready-to-drink, LIPTON BRISK iced tea, with lemon flavor	35	0	0	9	0.55	0.06
Tea, ready-to-drink, NESTLE, COOL NESTEA ice tea lemon flavor	36	0	0	9	0.86	0.10
Tea, ready-to-drink, unsweetened, WENDY'S, fast food, without ice	1	0	0	0	-0.20	
Water, bottled, generic	0	0	0	0	-0.18	
Water, bottled, non-carbonated, DANNON	0	0	0	0	-0.06	
Water, bottled, non-carbonated, DANNON Fluoride To Go	0	0	0	0	-0.06	
Water, bottled, non-carbonated, DASANI	0	0	0	0	0	
Water, bottled, non-carbonated, EVIAN	0	0	0	0	-0.15	
Water, bottled, non-carbonated, PEPSI, AQUAFINA	0	0	0	0	0	
Water, bottled, PERRIER	0	0	0	0	-0.18	
Water, bottled, POLAND SPRING	0	0	0	0	-0.03	
Water, tap, drinking	0	0	0	0	-0.06	
Water, tap, municipal	0	0	0	0	-0.08	
Water, tap, well	0	0	0	0	-0.06	
Whiskey sour mix, bottled	87	0	21	0	-0.36	
Whiskey sour mix, bottled, with added potassium and sodium	84	0	21	0	0.07	

Beverages

Food Description	Kcals	Protein	Fat	Carbs	PRAL	Alkali Density
Whiskey sour mix, powder	383	1	0	97	-3.65	-0.04
Wine, non-alcoholic	6	0	1	0	-1.42	

Beef Products

Food Description	Kcals	Protein	Fat	Carbs	PRAL	Acid Density
Beef, bottom sirloin, tri-tip roast, separable lean and fat, trimmed to 0" fat, choice, raw	172	21	10	0	9.44	0.45
Beef, bottom sirloin, tri-tip roast, separable lean and fat, trimmed to 0" fat, all grades, raw	164	21	9	0	9.57	0.46
Beef, bottom sirloin, tri-tip roast, separable lean and fat, trimmed to 0" fat, select, raw	157	21	8	0	9.69	0.46
Beef, bottom sirloin, tri-tip roast, separable lean and fat, trimmed to 0" fat, choice, cooked, roasted	218	26	12	0	12.35	0.48
Beef, bottom sirloin, tri-tip roast, separable lean and fat, trimmed to 0" fat, all grades, cooked, roasted	208	26	11	0	12.60	0.48
Beef, bottom sirloin, tri-tip roast, separable lean and fat, trimmed to 0" fat, select, cooked, roasted	198	26	10	0	12.83	0.49
Beef, bottom sirloin, tri-tip, separable lean only, trimmed to 0" fat, choice, raw	154	21	7	0	9.80	0.47
Beef, bottom sirloin, tri-tip, separable lean only, trimmed to 0" fat, all grades, raw	142	21	6	0	9.87	0.47
Beef, bottom sirloin, tri-tip, separable lean only, trimmed to 0" fat, select, raw	129	21	4	0	9.89	0.47
Beef, bottom sirloin, tri-tip, separable lean only, trimmed to 0" fat, select, cooked, roasted	179	27	7	0	13.10	0.49
Beef, bottom sirloin, tri-tip, separable lean only, trimmed to 0" fat, choice, cooked, roasted	193	26	10	0	12.81	0.49
Beef, brisket, flat half, separable lean and fat, trimmed to 0" fat, select, cooked, braised	205	34	7	0	17.54	0.52
Beef, brisket, flat half, separable lean and fat, trimmed to 0" fat, all grades, cooked, braised	213	33	8	0	17.18	0.52
Beef, brisket, flat half, separable lean and fat, trimmed to 0" fat, choice, cooked, braised	221	32	9	0	16.74	0.52
Beef, brisket, flat half, separable lean and fat, trimmed to 1/8" fat, select, raw	276	18	22	0	8.39	0.47
Beef, brisket, flat half, separable lean and fat, trimmed to 1/8" fat, all grades, raw	277	18	22	0	8.42	0.47
Beef, brisket, flat half, separable lean and fat, trimmed to 1/8" fat, choice, raw	277	18	22	0	8.43	0.47
Beef, brisket, flat half, separable lean and fat, trimmed to 1/8" fat, choice, cooked, braised	298	29	19	0	14.92	0.51
Beef, brisket, flat half, separable lean and fat, trimmed to 1/8" fat, all grades, cooked, braised	289	29	18	0	15.02	0.52
Beef, brisket, flat half, separable lean and fat, trimmed to 1/8" fat, select, cooked, braised	280	29	17	0	15.16	0.52
Beef, brisket, flat half, separable lean only, trimmed to 0" fat, choice, cooked, braised	212	33	8	0	17.20	0.52
Beef, brisket, flat half, separable lean only, trimmed to 0" fat, select, cooked, braised	198	34	6	0	17.85	0.53
Beef, brisket, flat half, separable lean only, trimmed to 0" fat, all grades, cooked, braised	205	33	7	0	17.49	0.53
Beef, brisket, flat half, separable lean only, trimmed to 1/8" fat, all grades, raw	127	22	4	0	10.18	0.46
Beef, brisket, flat half, separable lean only, trimmed to 1/8" fat, choice, raw	129	22	4	0	10.31	0.47
Beef, brisket, flat half, separable lean only, trimmed to 1/8" fat, select, raw	124	21	4	0	10.11	0.48
Beef, brisket, flat half, separable lean only, trimmed to 1/8" fat, all grades, cooked, braised	196	33	6	0	17.42	0.53
Beef, brisket, flat half, separable lean only, trimmed to 1/8" fat, select, cooked, braised	189	33	5	0	17.46	0.53
Beef, brisket, flat half, separable lean only, trimmed to 1/8" fat, choice, cooked, braised	203	33	7	0	17.47	0.53
Beef, brisket, point half, separable lean and fat, trimmed to 0" fat, all grades, cooked, braised	358	24	28	0	12.98	0.54

Beef Products

Food Description	Kcals	Protein	Fat	Carbs	PRAL	Acid Density
Beef, brisket, point half, separable lean and fat, trimmed to 1/8" fat, all grades, raw	265	18	21	0	8.70	0.48
Beef, brisket, point half, separable lean and fat, trimmed to 1/8" fat, all grades, cooked, braised	349	24	27	0	13.47	0.56
Beef, brisket, point half, separable lean only, trimmed to 0" fat, all grades, cooked, braised	244	28	14	0	15.72	0.56
Beef, brisket, whole, separable lean and fat, trimmed to 0" fat, all grades, cooked, braised	291	27	20	0	15.04	0.56
Beef, brisket, whole, separable lean and fat, trimmed to 1/8" fat, all grades, raw	251	18	19	0	9.08	0.50
Beef, brisket, whole, separable lean and fat, trimmed to 1/8" fat, all grades, cooked, braised	331	26	24	0	14.44	0.56
Beef, brisket, whole, separable lean only, all grades, raw	155	21	7	0	9.99	0.48
Beef, brisket, whole, separable lean only, trimmed to 0" fat, all grades, cooked, braised	218	30	10	0	16.83	0.56
Beef, carcass, separable lean and fat, choice, raw	291	17	24	0	8.03	0.47
Beef, carcass, separable lean and fat, select, raw	278	17	23	0	8.10	0.48
Beef, chuck, arm pot roast, separable lean and fat, trimmed to 0" fat, all grades, cooked, braised	297	29	19	0	15.06	0.52
Beef, chuck, arm pot roast, separable lean and fat, trimmed to 0" fat, select, cooked, braised	283	29	18	0	15.25	0.53
Beef, chuck, arm pot roast, separable lean and fat, trimmed to 1/8" fat, choice, raw	249	19	19	0	8.91	0.47
Beef, chuck, arm pot roast, separable lean and fat, trimmed to 1/8" fat, all grades, raw	244	19	18	0	9.05	0.48
Beef, chuck, arm pot roast, separable lean and fat, trimmed to 1/8" fat, select, raw	239	19	17	0	9.16	0.48
Beef, chuck, arm pot roast, separable lean and fat, trimmed to 1/8" fat, select, cooked, braised	295	30	18	0	15.67	0.52
Beef, chuck, arm pot roast, separable lean and fat, trimmed to 1/8" fat, all grades, cooked, braised	302	30	19	0	15.70	0.52
Beef, chuck, arm pot roast, separable lean and fat, trimmed to 1/8" fat, choice, cooked, braised	309	30	20	0	15.74	0.52
Beef, chuck, arm pot roast, separable lean only, trimmed to 0" fat, select, cooked, braised	195	33	6	0	17.54	0.53
Beef, chuck, arm pot roast, separable lean only, trimmed to 0" fat, choice, cooked, braised	212	33	8	0	17.56	0.53
Beef, chuck, arm pot roast, separable lean only, trimmed to 1/8" fat, choice, raw	139	22	5	0	10.43	0.47
Beef, chuck, arm pot roast, separable lean only, trimmed to 1/8" fat, all grades, raw	132	22	4	0	10.46	0.48
Beef, chuck, arm pot roast, separable lean only, trimmed to 1/8" fat, select, raw	125	22	3	0	10.50	0.48
Beef, chuck, arm pot roast, separable lean only, trimmed to 1/8" fat, select, cooked, braised	205	35	6	0	18.18	0.52
Beef, chuck, arm pot roast, separable lean only, trimmed to 1/8" fat, all grades, cooked, braised	214	35	17	0	18.24	0.52
Beef, chuck, arm pot roast, separable lean only, trimmed to 1/8" fat, choice, cooked, braised	224	35	8	0	18.32	0.52
Beef, chuck, blade roast, separable lean and fat, trimmed to 0" fat, select, cooked, braised	313	28	22	0	15.50	0.55
Beef, chuck, blade roast, separable lean and fat, trimmed to 0" fat, choice, cooked, braised	348	27	26	0	15.12	0.56
Beef, chuck, blade roast, separable lean and fat, trimmed to 1/8" fat, choice, raw	265	17	21	0	8.06	0.47
Beef, chuck, blade roast, separable lean and fat, trimmed to 1/8" fat, all grades, raw	248	17	19	0	8.13	0.48
Beef, chuck, blade roast, separable lean and fat, trimmed to 1/8" fat, select, raw	230	17	17	0	8.21	0.48

Beef Products

Food Description	Kcals	Protein	Fat	Carbs	PRAL	Acid Density
Beef, chuck, blade roast, separable lean and fat, trimmed to 1/8" fat, all grades, cooked, braised	341	27	25	0	15.04	0.56
Beef, chuck, blade roast, separable lean and fat, trimmed to 1/8" fat, choice, cooked, braised	359	26	27	0	14.75	0.57
Beef, chuck, blade roast, separable lean and fat, trimmed to 1/8" fat, select, cooked, braised	318	27	22	0	15.34	0.57
Beef, chuck, blade roast, separable lean only, trimmed to 0" fat, all grades, cooked, braised	253	31	13	0	17.62	0.57
Beef, chuck, blade roast, separable lean only, trimmed to 0" fat, choice, cooked, braised	265	31	15	0	17.62	0.57
Beef, chuck, blade roast, separable lean only, trimmed to 0" fat, select, cooked, braised	238	31	12	0	17.62	0.57
Beef, chuck, clod roast, separable lean and fat, trimmed to 0" fat, USDA choice, cooked, roasted	216	25	12	0	11.58	0.46
Beef, chuck, clod roast, separable lean and fat, trimmed to 0" fat, all grades, cooked, roasted	207	26	11	0	12.09	0.47
Beef, chuck, clod roast, separable lean and fat, trimmed to 0" fat, USDA select, cooked, roasted	196	27	9	0	12.88	0.48
Beef, chuck, clod roast, separable lean only, trimmed to 0" fat, all grades, cooked, roasted	172	27	6	0	12.60	0.47
Beef, chuck, clod roast, separable lean only, trimmed to 0" fat, USDA choice, cooked, roasted	171	26	7	0	12.19	0.47
Beef, chuck, clod roast, separable lean only, trimmed to 0" fat, USDA select, cooked, roasted	172	28	6	0	13.25	0.47
Beef, chuck, clod steak, separable lean and fat, trimmed to 0" fat, USDA choice, cooked, braised	231	28	12	0	13.89	0.50
Beef, chuck, clod steak, separable lean and fat, trimmed to 0" fat, all grades, cooked, braised	220	29	11	0	15.39	0.53
Beef, chuck, clod steak, separable lean and fat, trimmed to 0" fat, USDA select, cooked, braised	205	30	9	0	17.58	0.59
Beef, chuck, clod steak, separable lean only, trimmed to 0" fat, USDA choice, cooked, braised	193	30	7	0	14.63	0.49
Beef, chuck, clod steak, separable lean only, trimmed to 0" fat, all grades, cooked, braised	192	30	7	0	15.98	0.53
Beef, chuck, clod steak, separable lean only, trimmed to 0" fat, USDA select, cooked, braised	191	30	7	0	17.90	0.60
Beef, chuck, mock tender steak, separable lean and fat, trimmed to 0" fat, USDA select, cooked, broiled	159	26	5	0	13.96	0.54
Beef, chuck, mock tender steak, separable lean and fat, trimmed to 0" fat, all grades, cooked, broiled	160	26	6	0	14.22	0.55
Beef, chuck, mock tender steak, separable lean and fat, trimmed to 0" fat, USDA choice, cooked, broiled	161	26	6	0	14.41	0.55
Beef, chuck, mock tender steak, separable lean only, trimmed to 0" fat, USDA select, cooked, broiled	157	26	5	0	13.99	0.54
Beef, chuck, mock tender steak, separable lean only, trimmed to 0" fat, all grades, cooked, broiled	160	26	5	0	14.23	0.55
Beef, chuck, mock tender steak, separable lean only, trimmed to 0" fat, USDA choice, cooked, broiled	161	26	6	0	14.41	0.55
Beef, chuck, shoulder clod, shoulder tender, medallion, separable lean and fat, trimmed to 0" fat, choice, raw	145	21	6	0	9.66	0.46
Beef, chuck, shoulder clod, shoulder tender, medallion, separable lean and fat, trimmed to 0" fat, all grades, raw	144	21	6	0	9.78	0.47

Beef Products

Food Description	Kcals	Protein	Fat	Carbs	PRAL	Acid Density
Beef, chuck, shoulder clod, shoulder tender, medallion, separable lean and fat, trimmed to 0" fat, select, raw	142	21	6	0	9.95	0.47
Beef, chuck, shoulder clod, shoulder tender, medallion, separable lean and fat, trimmed to 0" fat, choice, cooked, grilled	181	26	8	0	12.87	0.50
Beef, chuck, shoulder clod, shoulder tender, medallion, separable lean and fat, trimmed to 0" fat, all grades, cooked, grilled	177	26	7	0	12.98	0.50
Beef, chuck, shoulder clod, shoulder tender, medallion, separable lean and fat, trimmed to 0" fat, select, cooked, grilled	172	26	6	0	13.21	0.51
Beef, chuck, shoulder clod, shoulder top and center steaks, steak, separable lean and fat, trimmed to 0" fat, select, raw	140	21	6	0	10.05	0.48
Beef, chuck, shoulder clod, shoulder top and center steaks, steak, separable lean and fat, trimmed to 0" fat, select, cooked, grilled	176	27	7	0	13.06	0.48
Beef, chuck, shoulder clod, shoulder top and center steaks, steak, separable lean and fat, trimmed to 0" fat, choice, raw	143	20	6	0	9.87	0.49
Beef, chuck, shoulder clod, shoulder top and center steaks, steak, separable lean and fat, trimmed to 0" fat, all grades, cooked, grilled	182	26	8	0	13.14	0.51
Beef, chuck, shoulder clod, shoulder top and center steaks, steak, separable lean and fat, trimmed to 0" fat, choice, cooked, grilled	184	26	8	0	13.15	0.51
Beef, chuck, shoulder clod, top and center steaks, steak, separable lean and fat, trimmed to 0" fat, all grades, raw	141	21	6	0	9.95	0.47
Beef, chuck, shoulder clod, top blade, steak, separable lean and fat, trimmed to 0" fat, choice, raw	182	19	11	0	8.84	0.47
Beef, chuck, shoulder clod, top blade, steak, separable lean and fat, trimmed to 0" fat, all grades, raw	176	19	11	0	9	0.47
Beef, chuck, shoulder clod, top blade, steak, separable lean and fat, trimmed to 0" fat, choice, cooked, grilled	228	25	14	0	12.13	0.49
Beef, chuck, shoulder clod, top blade, steak, separable lean and fat, trimmed to 0" fat, all grades, cooked, grilled	222	25	13	0	12.28	0.49
Beef, chuck, shoulder clod, top blade, steak, separable lean and fat, trimmed to 0" fat, select, raw	166	19	9	0	9.34	0.49
Beef, chuck, shoulder clod, top blade, steak, separable lean and fat, trimmed to 0" fat, select, cooked, grilled	212	25	12	0	12.50	0.50
Beef, chuck, top blade, separable lean and fat, trimmed to 0" fat, USDA select, cooked, broiled	200	26	10	0	13.44	0.52
Beef, chuck, top blade, separable lean and fat, trimmed to 0" fat, all grades, cooked, broiled	216	26	12	0	13.53	0.52
Beef, chuck, top blade, separable lean and fat, trimmed to 0" fat, USDA choice, cooked, broiled	227	26	13	0	13.56	0.52
Beef, chuck, top blade, separable lean only, trimmed to 0" fat, all grades, cooked, broiled	203	26	10	0	13.73	0.53
Beef, chuck, top blade, separable lean only, trimmed to 0" fat, USDA choice, cooked, broiled	217	28	12	0	13.76	0.49
Beef, chuck, top blade, separable lean only, trimmed to 0" fat, USDA select, cooked, broiled	184	26	8	0	13.74	0.53
Beef, composite of trimmed retail cuts, separable lean and fat, trimmed to 1/8" fat, prime, raw	265	19	20	0	8.63	0.45

Beef Products

Food Description	Kcals	Protein	Fat	Carbs	PRAL	Acid Density
Beef, composite of trimmed retail cuts, separable lean and fat, trimmed to 1/8" fat, choice, raw	243	19	18	0	8.64	0.45
Beef, composite of trimmed retail cuts, separable lean and fat, trimmed to 1/8" fat, all grades, raw	234	19	17	0	8.69	0.46
Beef, composite of trimmed retail cuts, separable lean and fat, trimmed to 1/8" fat, select, raw	223	19	16	0	8.75	0.46
Beef, composite of trimmed retail cuts, separable lean and fat, trimmed to 1/8" fat, prime, cooked	299	26	21	0	12.14	0.47
Beef, composite of trimmed retail cuts, separable lean and fat, trimmed to 1/8" fat, select, cooked	278	27	18	0	13.32	0.49
Beef, composite of trimmed retail cuts, separable lean and fat, trimmed to 1/8" fat, choice, cooked	301	26	21	0	13.09	0.50
Beef, composite of trimmed retail cuts, separable lean and fat, trimmed to 0" fat, choice, cooked	283	27	19	0	13.62	0.50
Beef, composite of trimmed retail cuts, separable lean and fat, trimmed to 0" fat, all grades, cooked	273	27	17	0	13.70	0.51
Beef, composite of trimmed retail cuts, separable lean and fat, trimmed to 1/8" fat, all grades, cooked	291	26	20	0	13.22	0.51
Beef, composite of trimmed retail cuts, separable lean and fat, trimmed to 0" fat, select, cooked	261	27	16	0	13.76	0.51
Beef, composite of trimmed retail cuts, separable lean only, trimmed to 0" fat, all grades, cooked	211	30	9	0	14.95	0.50
Beef, composite of trimmed retail cuts, separable lean only, trimmed to 0" fat, choice, cooked	219	30	10	0	14.95	0.50
Beef, composite of trimmed retail cuts, separable lean only, trimmed to 0" fat, select, cooked	201	30	8	0	14.97	0.50
Beef, cured, breakfast strips, cooked	449	31	34	1	14.59	0.47
Beef, cured, breakfast strips, raw or unheated	406	13	39	1	6.27	0.48
Beef, cured, corned beef, brisket, cooked	251	18	19	0	10.06	0.56
Beef, cured, corned beef, brisket, raw	198	15	15	0	4.83	0.32
Beef, flank, separable lean and fat, trimmed to 0" fat, all grades, raw	155	21	7	0	9.82	0.47
Beef, flank, separable lean and fat, trimmed to 0" fat, all grades, cooked, broiled	188	28	8	0	13.34	0.48
Beef, flank, separable lean and fat, trimmed to 0" fat, choice, cooked, broiled	202	28	9	0	13.28	0.47
Beef, flank, separable lean and fat, trimmed to 0" fat, choice, raw	165	21	8	0	9.68	0.46
Beef, flank, separable lean and fat, trimmed to 0" fat, select, cooked, broiled	179	28	7	0	13.47	0.48
Beef, flank, separable lean and fat, trimmed to 0" fat, select, raw	145	21	6	0	9.95	0.47
Beef, flank, separable lean only, trimmed to 0" fat, all grades, raw	141	22	5	0	9.99	0.45
Beef, flank, separable lean only, trimmed to 0" fat, all grades, cooked, broiled	186	28	7	0	13.51	0.48
Beef, flank, separable lean only, trimmed to 0" fat, choice, cooked, broiled	194	28	8	0	13.54	0.48
Beef, flank, separable lean only, trimmed to 0" fat, choice, cooked, braised	237	28	13	0	15.53	0.55
Beef, flank, separable lean only, trimmed to 0" fat, choice, raw	149	22	6	0	10.08	0.46
Beef, flank, separable lean only, trimmed to 0" fat, select, cooked, broiled	178	28	6	0	13.51	0.48
Beef, flank, separable lean only, trimmed to 0" fat, select, raw	137	21	5	0	9.96	0.47
Beef, ground, 70% lean meat / 30% fat, crumbles, cooked, pan-browned	270	26	18	0	12.05	0.46

Beef Products

Food Description	Kcals	Protein	Fat	Carbs	PRAL	Acid Density
Beef, ground, 70% lean meat / 30% fat, loaf, cooked, baked	241	24	15	0	11.90	0.50
Beef, ground, 70% lean meat / 30% fat, patty cooked, pan-broiled	238	23	16	0	10.91	0.47
Beef, ground, 70% lean meat / 30% fat, patty, cooked, broiled	273	25	18	0	12.55	0.50
Beef, ground, 70% lean meat / 30% fat, raw	332	14	30	0	6.66	0.48
Beef, ground, 75% lean meat / 25% fat, crumbles, cooked, pan-browned	277	26	18	0	12.34	0.47
Beef, ground, 75% lean meat / 25% fat, loaf, cooked, baked	254	25	17	0	12.19	0.49
Beef, ground, 75% lean meat / 25% fat, patty, cooked, broiled	278	26	19	0	12.53	0.48
Beef, ground, 75% lean meat / 25% fat, patty, cooked, pan-broiled	248	23	16	0	11.15	0.48
Beef, ground, 75% lean meat / 25% fat, raw	293	16	25	0	7.30	0.46
Beef, ground, 80% lean meat / 20% fat, crumbles, cooked, pan-browned	272	27	17	0	12.65	0.47
Beef, ground, 80% lean meat / 20% fat, loaf, cooked, baked	254	25	16	0	12.51	0.50
Beef, ground, 80% lean meat / 20% fat, patty, cooked, broiled	271	26	18	0	12.58	0.48
Beef, ground, 80% lean meat / 20% fat, patty, cooked, pan-broiled	246	24	16	0	11.44	0.48
Beef, ground, 80% lean meat / 20% fat, raw	254	17	20	0	7.91	0.47
Beef, ground, 85% lean meat / 15% fat, crumbles, cooked, pan-browned	256	28	15	0	12.91	0.46
Beef, ground, 85% lean meat / 15% fat, loaf, cooked, baked	240	26	14	0	12.82	0.49
Beef, ground, 85% lean meat / 15% fat, patty, cooked, broiled	250	26	15	0	12.57	0.48
Beef, ground, 85% lean meat / 15% fat, patty, cooked, pan-broiled	232	25	14	0	11.71	0.47
Beef, ground, 85% lean meat / 15% fat, raw	215	19	15	0	8.57	0.45
Beef, ground, 90% lean meat / 10% fat, crumbles, cooked, pan-browned	230	28	12	0	13.18	0.47
Beef, ground, 90% lean meat / 10% fat, loaf, cooked, baked	214	27	11	0	13.17	0.49
Beef, ground, 90% lean meat / 10% fat, patty, cooked, broiled	217	26	12	0	12.53	0.48
Beef, ground, 90% lean meat / 10% fat, patty, cooked, pan-broiled	204	25	11	0	11.92	0.48
Beef, ground, 90% lean meat / 10% fat, raw	176	20	10	0	9.19	0.46
Beef, ground, 95% lean meat / 5% fat, crumbles, cooked, pan-browned	193	29	8	0	13.54	0.47
Beef, ground, 95% lean meat / 5% fat, loaf, cooked, baked	174	27	6	0	13.45	0.50
Beef, ground, 95% lean meat / 5% fat, patty, cooked, broiled	171	26	7	9	12.53	0.48
Beef, ground, 95% lean meat / 5% fat, patty, cooked, pan-broiled	164	26	6	0	12.21	0.47
Beef, ground, 95% lean meat / 5% fat, raw	137	21	5	0	9.86	0.47
Beef, loin, bottom sirloin butt, tri-tip roast, separable lean only, trimmed to 0" fat, all grades, cooked, roasted	182	27	8	0	12.95	0.48
Beef, loin, bottom sirloin butt, tri-tip steak, separable lean and fat, trimmed to 0" fat, all grades, cooked, broiled	265	30	15	0	14.48	0.48

Beef Products

Food Description	Kcals	Protein	Fat	Carbs	PRAL	Acid Density
Beef, loin, bottom sirloin butt, tri-tip steak, separable lean only, trimmed 0" fat, all grades, cooked, broiled	250	31	13	0	14.83	0.48
Beef, plate, inside skirt steak, separable lean and fat, trimmed to 0" fat, all grades, cooked, broiled	220	26	12	0	14.47	0.56
Beef, plate, inside skirt steak, separable lean only, trimmed to 0" fat, all grades, cooked, broiled	205	27	10	0	14.83	0.55
Beef, plate, outside skirt steak, separable lean and fat, trimmed to 0" fat, all grades, cooked, broiled	255	24	17	0	10.71	0.45
Beef, plate, outside skirt steak, separable lean only, trimmed to 0" fat, all grades, cooked, broiled	233	24	14	0	10.99	0.46
Beef, retail cuts, separable fat, cooked	680	11	70	0	5.10	0.46
Beef, retail cuts, separable fat, raw	674	8	71	0	3.79	0.47
Beef, rib eye, small end (ribs 10-12), separable lean and fat, trimmed to 0" fat, select, cooked, broiled	230	28	13	0	13.58	0.49
Beef, rib eye, small end (ribs 10-12), separable lean and fat, trimmed to 0" fat, all grades, cooked, broiled	247	27	15	0	13.20	0.49
Beef, rib, eye, small end (ribs 10- 12) separable lean only, trimmed to 0" fat, select, cooked, broiled	182	30	6	0	14.43	0.48
Beef, rib, eye, small end (ribs 10-12), separable lean and fat, trimmed to 0" fat, choice, raw	274	18	22	0	7.79	0.43
Beef, rib, eye, small end (ribs 10-12), separable lean and fat, trimmed to 0" fat, choice, cooked, broiled	265	27	17	0	12.80	0.47
Beef, rib, eye, small end (ribs 10-12), separable lean only, trimmed to 0" fat, choice, raw	161	20	8	0	8.58	0.43
Beef, rib, eye, small end (ribs 10-12), separable lean only, trimmed to 0" fat, choice, cooked, broiled	205	29	9	0	14.06	0.48
Beef, rib, large end (ribs 6-9), separable lean and fat, trimmed to 1/8" fat, prime, cooked, broiled	404	21	35	0	9.30	0.44
Beef, rib, large end (ribs 6-9), separable lean and fat, trimmed to 1/8" fat, select, raw	295	17	25	0	7.72	0.45
Beef, rib, large end (ribs 6-9), separable lean and fat, trimmed to 1/8" fat, all grades, cooked, broiled	338	22	27	0	10.18	0.46
Beef, rib, large end (ribs 6-9), separable lean and fat, trimmed to 1/8" fat, select, cooked, broiled	324	22	26	0	10.18	0.46
Beef, rib, large end (ribs 6-9), separable lean and fat, trimmed to 1/8" fat, prime, raw	367	16	33	0	7.46	0.47
Beef, rib, large end (ribs 6-9), separable lean and fat, trimmed to 0" fat, choice, cooked, roasted	372	23	30	0	10.79	0.47
Beef, rib, large end (ribs 6-9), separable lean and fat, trimmed to 1/8" fat, choice, cooked, broiled	370	21	31	0	9.86	0.47
Beef, rib, large end (ribs 6-9), separable lean and fat, trimmed to 1/8" fat, prime, cooked, roasted	393	23	33	0	10.80	0.47
Beef, rib, large end (ribs 6-9), separable lean and fat, trimmed to 1/8" fat, all grades, cooked, roasted	355	23	29	0	10.87	0.47
Beef, rib, large end (ribs 6-9), separable lean and fat, trimmed to 1/8" fat, choice, raw	333	16	29	0	7.57	0.47
Beef, rib, large end (ribs 6-9), separable lean and fat, trimmed to 1/8" fat, all grades, raw	316	16	27	0	7.64	0.48
Beef, rib, large end (ribs 6-9), separable lean and fat, trimmed to 1/8" fat, select, cooked, roasted	333	23	26	0	11.06	0.48

Beef Products

Food Description	Kcals	Protein	Fat	Carbs	PRAL	Acid Density
Beef, rib, large end (ribs 6-9), separable lean and fat, trimmed to 0" fat, select, cooked, roasted	331	23	26	0	11.11	0.48
Beef, rib, large end (ribs 6-9), separable lean and fat, trimmed to 1/8" fat, choice, cooked, roasted	378	22	31	0	10.64	0.48
Beef, rib, large end (ribs 6-9), separable lean only, trimmed to 0" fat, all grades, cooked, roasted	238	28	13	0	12.97	0.46
Beef, rib, large end (ribs 6-9), separable lean only, trimmed to 0" fat, choice, cooked, roasted	253	28	15	0	12.97	0.46
Beef, rib, large end (ribs 6-9), separable lean only, trimmed to 0" fat, select, cooked, roasted	220	28	11	0	12.97	0.46
Beef, rib, shortribs, separable lean and fat, choice, cooked, braised	471	22	42	0	11.31	0.51
Beef, rib, shortribs, separable lean and fat, choice, raw	388	14	36	0	6.77	0.48
Beef, rib, shortribs, separable lean only, choice, cooked, braised	295	31	18	0	16.47	0.53
Beef, rib, shortribs, separable lean only, choice, raw	173	19	10	0	8.19	0.43
Beef, rib, small end (ribs 10-12), separable lean and fat, trimmed to 0" fat, choice, cooked, broiled	312	25	23	0	10.94	0.44
Beef, rib, small end (ribs 10-12), separable lean and fat, trimmed to 0" fat, select, cooked, broiled	285	25	20	0	11.02	0.44
Beef, rib, small end (ribs 10-12), separable lean and fat, trimmed to 1/8" fat, prime, raw	335	17	29	0	7.54	0.44
Beef, rib, small end (ribs 10-12), separable lean and fat, trimmed to 1/8" fat, prime, cooked, broiled	354	24	28	0	10.69	0.45
Beef, rib, small end (ribs 10-12), separable lean and fat, trimmed to 1/8" fat, all grades, cooked, roasted	341	23	27	0	10.32	0.45
Beef, rib, small end (ribs 10-12), separable lean and fat, trimmed to 1/8" fat, prime, cooked, roasted	411	22	35	0	9.96	0.45
Beef, rib, small end (ribs 10-12), separable lean and fat, trimmed to 1/8" fat, select, cooked, roasted	323	23	25	0	10.42	0.45
Beef, rib, small end (ribs 10-12), separable lean and fat, trimmed to 1/8" fat, select, raw	246	20	18	0	9.20	0.46
Beef, rib, small end (ribs 10-12), separable lean and fat, trimmed to 1/8" fat, choice, raw	263	19	20	0	8.75	0.46
Beef, rib, small end (ribs 10-12), separable lean and fat, trimmed to 1/8" fat, choice, cooked, roasted	359	22	29	0	10.22	0.46
Beef, rib, small end (ribs 10-12), separable lean and fat, trimmed to 1/8" fat, choice, cooked, broiled	304	25	22	0	11.80	0.47
Beef, rib, small end (ribs 10-12), separable lean and fat, trimmed to 1/8" fat, all grades, raw	254	19	19	0	8.97	0.47
Beef, rib, small end (ribs 10-12), separable lean and fat, trimmed to 1/8" fat, all grades, cooked, broiled	291	26	20	0	12.50	0.48
Beef, rib, small end (ribs 10-12), separable lean and fat, trimmed to 0" fat, all grades, cooked, broiled	249	27	15	0	13.20	0.49
Beef, rib, small end (ribs 10-12), separable lean and fat, trimmed to 1/8" fat, select, cooked, broiled	278	27	18	0	13.20	0.49
Beef, rib, small end (ribs 10-12), separable lean only, trimmed to 0" fat, choice, cooked, broiled	225	28	12	0	12.29	0.44
Beef, rib, small end (ribs 10-12), separable lean only, trimmed to 0" fat, select, cooked, broiled	198	28	9	0	12.29	0.44

Beef Products

Food Description	Kcals	Protein	Fat	Carbs	PRAL	Acid Density
Beef, rib, small end (ribs 10-12), separable lean only, trimmed to 1/8" fat, select, raw	134	23	4	0	10.47	0.46
Beef, rib, small end (ribs 10-12), separable lean only, trimmed to 1/8" fat, choice, raw	148	22	6	0	10.26	0.47
Beef, rib, small end (ribs 10-12), separable lean only, trimmed to 1/8" fat, all grades, raw	141	22	5	0	10.36	0.47
Beef, rib, small end (ribs 10-12), separable lean only, trimmed to 1/8" fat, all grades, cooked, broiled	195	30	8	0	14.35	0.48
Beef, rib, small end (ribs 10-12), separable lean only, trimmed to 1/8" fat, select, cooked, broiled	188	31	6	0	14.91	0.48
Beef, rib, small end (ribs 10-12), separable lean only, trimmed to 0" fat, all grades, cooked, broiled	193	29	8	0	14.23	0.49
Beef, rib, small end (ribs 10-12), separable lean only, trimmed to 1/8"fat, choice, cooked, broiled	202	28	9	0	13.74	0.49
Beef, rib, whole (ribs 6-12), separable lean and fat, trimmed to 1/8" fat, prime, cooked, broiled	386	22	32	0	9.83	0.45
Beef, rib, whole (ribs 6-12), separable lean and fat, trimmed to 1/8" fat, all grades, raw	306	17	26	0	7.62	0.45
Beef, rib, whole (ribs 6-12), separable lean and fat, trimmed to 1/8" fat, select, raw	288	17	24	0	7.69	0.45
Beef, rib, whole (ribs 6-12), separable lean and fat, trimmed to 1/8" fat, select, cooked, broiled	315	23	24	0	10.46	0.45
Beef, rib, whole (ribs 6-12), separable lean and fat, trimmed to 1/8" fat, prime, cooked, roasted	400	23	34	0	10.48	0.46
Beef, rib, whole (ribs 6-12), separable lean and fat, trimmed to 1/8" fat, choice, cooked, roasted	365	23	30	0	10.58	0.46
Beef, rib, whole (ribs 6-12), separable lean and fat, trimmed to 1/8" fat, all grades, cooked, roasted	351	23	28	0	10.63	0.46
Beef, rib, whole (ribs 6-12), separable lean and fat, trimmed to 1/8" fat, choice, cooked, broiled	352	22	28	0	10.25	0.47
Beef, rib, whole (ribs 6-12), separable lean and fat, trimmed to 1/8" fat, prime, raw	355	16	32	0	7.48	0.47
Beef, rib, whole (ribs 6-12), separable lean and fat, trimmed to 1/8" fat, all grades, cooked, broiled	337	22	27	0	10.33	0.47
Beef, rib, whole (ribs 6-12), separable lean and fat, trimmed to 1/8" fat, select, cooked, roasted	330	23	26	0	10.80	0.47
Beef, rib, whole (ribs 6-12), separable lean and fat, trimmed to 1/8" fat, choice, raw	322	16	28	0	7.56	0.47
Beef, round, bottom round , separable lean only, trimmed to 1/8" fat, select, cooked, roasted	164	28	5	0	15.14	0.54
Beef, round, bottom round roast, separable lean only, trimmed to 0" fat, select, cooked, roasted	169	28	5	0	15.06	0.54
Beef, round, bottom round, separable lean and fat, trimmed to 0" fat, choice, cooked, roasted	199	27	9	0	14.07	0.52
Beef, round, bottom round, separable lean and fat, trimmed to 0" fat, choice, cooked, braised	230	33	10	0	17.22	0.52
Beef, round, bottom round, separable lean and fat, trimmed to 0" fat, all grades, cooked, braised	223	34	9	0	17.77	0.52
Beef, round, bottom round, separable lean and fat, trimmed to 0" fat, select, cooked, roasted	175	28	6	0	14.92	0.53
Beef, round, bottom round, separable lean and fat, trimmed to 0" fat, all grades, cooked, roasted	187	27	8	0	14.52	0.54
Beef, round, bottom round, separable lean and fat, trimmed to 0" fat, select, cooked, braised	217	34	8	0	18.29	0.54
Beef, round, bottom round, separable lean and fat, trimmed to 1/8" fat, select, raw	187	21	12	0	9.66	0.46
Beef, round, bottom round, separable lean and fat, trimmed to 1/8" fat, all grades, raw	192	21	12	0	9.80	0.47

Beef Products

Food Description	Kcals	Protein	Fat	Carbs	PRAL	Acid Density
Beef, round, bottom round, separable lean and fat, trimmed to 1/8" fat, choice, raw	198	21	12	0	9.95	0.47
Beef, round, bottom round, separable lean and fat, trimmed to 1/8" fat, choice, cooked, braised	254	33	13	0	17.30	0.52
Beef, round, bottom round, separable lean and fat, trimmed to 1/8" fat, all grades, cooked, braised	247	33	12	0	17.36	0.53
Beef, round, bottom round, separable lean and fat, trimmed to 1/8" fat, select, cooked, braised	240	33	11	0	17.37	0.53
Beef, round, bottom round, separable lean and fat, trimmed to 1/8" fat, choice, cooked, roasted	223	26	12	0	13.71	0.53
Beef, round, bottom round, separable lean and fat, trimmed to 1/8" fat, select, cooked, roasted	212	27	11	0	14.24	0.53
Beef, round, bottom round, separable lean and fat, trimmed to 1/8" fat, all grades, cooked, roasted	218	26	12	0	13.99	0.54
Beef, round, bottom round, separable lean only, trimmed to 0" fat, all grades, cooked, roasted	177	28	6	0	14.75	0.53
Beef, round, bottom round, separable lean only, trimmed to 0" fat, select, cooked, braised	206	35	6	0	18.57	0.53
Beef, round, bottom round, separable lean only, trimmed to 0" fat, all grades, cooked, braised	214	34	8	0	18.05	0.53
Beef, round, bottom round, separable lean only, trimmed to 0" fat, choice, cooked, braised	223	33	9	0	17.58	0.53
Beef, round, bottom round, separable lean only, trimmed to 0" fat, choice, cooked, roasted	185	27	8	0	14.49	0.54
Beef, round, bottom round, separable lean only, trimmed to 1/8" fat, select, raw	128	22	4	0	10.41	0.47
Beef, round, bottom round, separable lean only, trimmed to 1/8" fat, all grades, raw	128	22	4	0	10.55	0.48
Beef, round, bottom round, separable lean only, trimmed to 1/8" fat, choice, raw	140	22	5	0	10.81	0.49
Beef, round, bottom round, separable lean only, trimmed to 1/8" fat, choice, cooked, roasted	179	28	7	0	14.64	0.52
Beef, round, bottom round, separable lean only, trimmed to 1/8" fat, all grades, cooked	163	28	6	0	14.86	0.53
Beef, round, bottom round, separable lean only, trimmed to 1/8" fat, choice, cooked, braised	228	34	9	0	18.19	0.54
Beef, round, bottom round, separable lean only, trimmed to 1/8" fat, all grades, cooked, braised	216	34	8	0	18.24	0.54
Beef, round, bottom round, separable lean only, trimmed to 1/8" fat, select, cooked, braised	205	34	6	0	18.34	0.54
Beef, round, eye of round, separable lean only, trimmed to 1/8" fat, choice, cooked, roasted	175	30	5	0	15.89	0.53
Beef, round, eye of round roast, separable lean only, trimmed to 1/8" fat, select, cooked, roasted	163	30	4	0	15.71	0.52
Beef, round, eye of round, separable lean and fat, trimmed to 0" fat, choice, cooked, roasted	166	29	5	0	15.08	0.52
Beef, round, eye of round, separable lean and fat, trimmed to 0" fat, select, cooked, roasted	169	30	5	0	15.77	0.53
Beef, round, eye of round, separable lean and fat, trimmed to 0" fat, all grades, cooked, roasted	168	29	5	0	15.41	0.53
Beef, round, eye of round, separable lean and fat, trimmed to 1/8" fat, choice, raw	173	22	9	0	10.42	0.47
Beef, round, eye of round, separable lean and fat, trimmed to 1/8" fat, select, raw	159	21	8	0	9.95	0.47
Beef, round, eye of round, separable lean and fat, trimmed to 1/8" fat, all grades, raw	166	21	8	0	10.19	0.49
Beef, round, eye of round, separable lean and fat, trimmed to 1/8" fat, choice, cooked, roasted	212	28	10	0	14.96	0.53
Beef, round, eye of round, separable lean and fat, trimmed to 1/8" fat, all grades, cooked, roasted	208	28	10	0	14.98	0.54

Beef Products

Food Description	Kcals	Protein	Fat	Carbs	PRAL	Acid Density
Beef, round, eye of round, separable lean and fat, trimmed to 1/8" fat, select, cooked, roasted	204	28	9	0	14.98	0.54
Beef, round, eye of round, separable lean only, trimmed to 0" fat, choice, cooked, roasted	162	29	4	0	15.28	0.53
Beef, round, eye of round, separable lean only, trimmed to 0" fat, select, cooked, roasted	163	30	4	0	15.89	0.53
Beef, round, eye of round, separable lean only, trimmed to 0" fat, all grades, cooked, roasted	162	29	4	0	15.58	0.54
Beef, round, eye of round, separable lean only, trimmed to 1/8" fat, all grades, raw	124	23	3	0	10.77	0.47
Beef, round, eye of round, separable lean only, trimmed to 1/8" fat, select, raw	119	22	3	0	10.45	0.48
Beef, round, eye of round, separable lean only, trimmed to 1/8" fat, choice, raw	128	23	3	0	11.10	0.48
Beef, round, eye of round, separable lean only, trimmed to 1/8" fat, all grades, cooked, roasted	169	30	5	0	15.79	0.53
Beef, round, full cut, separable lean and fat, trimmed to 1/8" fat, choice, raw	195	21	12	0	9.63	0.46
Beef, round, full cut, separable lean and fat, trimmed to 1/8" fat, select, raw	184	21	11	0	9.63	0.46
Beef, round, full cut, separable lean and fat, trimmed to 1/8" fat, choice, cooked, broiled	235	28	13	0	13.32	0.48
Beef, round, full cut, separable lean and fat, trimmed to 1/8" fat, select, cooked, broiled	218	28	11	0	13.34	0.48
Beef, round, knuckle, tip center, steak, separable lean and fat, trimmed to 0" fat, choice, raw	150	21	7	0	9.72	0.46
Beef, round, knuckle, tip center, steak, separable lean and fat, trimmed to 0" fat, all grades, raw	143	21	6	0	9.89	0.47
Beef, round, knuckle, tip center, steak, separable lean and fat, trimmed to 0" fat, select, cooked, grilled	162	27	5	0	13.18	0.49
Beef, round, knuckle, tip center, steak, separable lean and fat, trimmed to 0" fat, choice, cooked, grilled	188	27	8	0	13.40	0.50
Beef, round, knuckle, tip center, steak, separable lean and fat, trimmed to 0" fat, all grades, cooked, grilled	177	27	7	0	13.51	0.50
Beef, round, knuckle, tip side, steak, separable lean and fat, trimmed to 0" fat, select, raw	124	22	3	0	10.04	0.46
Beef, round, knuckle, tip side, steak, separable lean and fat, trimmed to 0" fat, all grades, raw	129	22	4	0	9.89	0.45
Beef, round, knuckle, tip side, steak, separable lean and fat, trimmed to 0" fat, choice, raw	133	21	5	0	9.74	0.46
Beef, round, knuckle, tip side, steak, separable lean and fat, trimmed to 0" fat, choice, cooked, grilled	174	29	6	0	14.43	0.50
Beef, round, knuckle, tip side, steak, separable lean and fat, trimmed to 0" fat, all grades, cooked, grilled	168	29	5	0	14.68	0.51
Beef, round, knuckle, tip side, steak, separable lean and fat, trimmed to 0" fat, select, cooked, grilled	160	29	4	0	14.96	0.52
Beef, round, outside round, bottom round, steak, separable lean and fat, trimmed to 0" fat, all grades, raw	142	22	6	0	10.45	0.48
Beef, round, outside round, bottom round, steak, separable lean and fat, trimmed to 0" fat, select, raw	129	22	4	0	10.63	0.48
Beef, round, outside round, bottom round, steak, separable lean and fat, trimmed to 0" fat, all grades, cooked, grilled	182	28	7	0	13.76	0.49

Beef Products

Food Description	Kcals	Protein	Fat	Carbs	PRAL	Acid Density
Beef, round, outside round, bottom round, steak, separable lean and fat, trimmed to 0" fat, choice, raw	150	21	7	0	10.35	0.49
Beef, round, outside round, bottom round, steak, separable lean and fat, trimmed to 0" fat, select, cooked, grilled	166	28	5	0	14.02	0.50
Beef, round, outside round, bottom round, steak, separable lean and fat, trimmed to 0" fat, choice, cooked, grilled	191	27	8	0	13.62	0.50
Beef, round, tip round, separable lean and fat, trimmed to 0" fat, select, raw	145	21	6	0	9.70	0.46
Beef, round, tip round, separable lean and fat, trimmed to 0" fat, all grades, raw	151	20	7	0	9.71	0.49
Beef, round, tip round, separable lean and fat, trimmed to 0" fat, choice, raw	156	20	8	0	9.71	0.49
Beef, round, tip round, separable lean and fat, trimmed to 0" fat, select, cooked, roasted	181	27	8	0	14.13	0.52
Beef, round, tip round, separable lean and fat, trimmed to 0" fat, all grades, cooked, roasted	188	27	8	0	14.19	0.53
Beef, round, tip round, separable lean and fat, trimmed to 0" fat, choice, cooked, roasted	196	27	9	0	14.24	0.53
Beef, round, tip round, separable lean and fat, trimmed to 1/8" fat, all grades, raw	189	20	12	0	9.19	0.46
Beef, round, tip round, separable lean and fat, trimmed to 1/8" fat, select, raw	178	20	10	0	9.27	0.46
Beef, round, tip round, separable lean and fat, trimmed to 1/8" fat, choice, raw	199	19	13	0	9.19	0.48
Beef, round, tip round, separable lean and fat, trimmed to 1/8" fat, select, cooked, roasted	210	28	10	0	13.59	0.49
Beef, round, tip round, separable lean and fat, trimmed to 1/8" fat, choice, cooked, roasted	228	27	12	0	13.44	0.50
Beef, round, tip round, separable lean and fat, trimmed to 1/8" fat, all grades, cooked, roasted	219	27	11	0	13.50	0.50
Beef, round, tip round, separable lean only, trimmed to 0" fat, all grades, raw	126	21	4	0	10.06	0.48
Beef, round, tip round, separable lean only, trimmed to 0" fat, all grades, cooked, roasted	174	28	6	0	14.63	0.52
Beef, round, tip round, separable lean only, trimmed to 0" fat, choice, raw	130	21	5	0	10.06	0.48
Beef, round, tip round, separable lean only, trimmed to 0" fat, choice, cooked, roasted	176	28	6	0	14.70	0.53
Beef, round, tip round, separable lean only, trimmed to 0" fat, select, raw	122	21	3	0	10.05	0.48
Beef, round, tip round, separable lean only, trimmed to 0" fat, select, cooked, roasted	149	27	4	0	14.58	0.54
Beef, round, top round , separable lean only, trimmed to 1/8" fat, choice, raw	140	23	5	0	11.03	0.48
Beef, round, top round, separable lean and fat, trimmed to 0" fat, all grades, cooked, braised	209	36	6	0	18.07	0.50
Beef, round, top round, separable lean and fat, trimmed to 0" fat, choice, cooked, braised	216	36	6	0	18.07	0.50
Beef, round, top round, separable lean and fat, trimmed to 0" fat, select, cooked, braised	200	36	5	0	18.07	0.50
Beef, round, top round, separable lean and fat, trimmed to 0" fat, choice, cooked, broiled	200	32	6	0	16.66	0.52
Beef, round, top round, separable lean and fat, trimmed to 0" fat, all grades, cooked, broiled	186	32	6	0	16.72	0.52
Beef, round, top round, separable lean and fat, trimmed to 0" fat, select, cooked, broiled	177	32	5	0	16.82	0.53
Beef, round, top round, separable lean and fat, trimmed to 1/8" fat, prime, cooked, broiled	225	31	10	0	14.29	0.46

Beef Products

Food Description	Kcals	Protein	Fat	Carbs	PRAL	Acid Density
Beef, round, top round, separable lean and fat, trimmed to 1/8" fat, choice, cooked, pan-fried	266	33	14	0	15.28	0.46
Beef, round, top round, separable lean and fat, trimmed to 1/8" fat, prime, raw	173	22	9	0	10.32	0.47
Beef, round, top round, separable lean and fat, trimmed to 1/8" fat, select, raw	164	22	8	0	10.34	0.47
Beef, round, top round, separable lean and fat, trimmed to 1/8" fat, all grades, raw	166	22	8	0	10.42	0.47
Beef, round, top round, separable lean and fat, trimmed to 1/8" fat, choice, raw	168	22	8	0	10.55	0.48
Beef, round, top round, separable lean and fat, trimmed to 1/8" fat, select, cooked, braised	225	35	9	0	17.54	0.50
Beef, round, top round, separable lean and fat, trimmed to 1/8" fat, choice, cooked, braised	250	34	12	0	17.27	0.51
Beef, round, top round, separable lean and fat, trimmed to 1/8" fat, all grades, cooked, braised	238	34	10	0	17.39	0.51
Beef, round, top round, separable lean and fat, trimmed to 1/8" fat, choice, cooked, broiled	224	31	10	0	16.14	0.52
Beef, round, top round, separable lean and fat, trimmed to 1/8" fat, select, cooked, broiled	201	31	8	0	16.30	0.53
Beef, round, top round, separable lean only, trimmed to 0" fat, all grades, cooked, broiled	186	88	6	0	16.86	0.19
Beef, round, top round, separable lean only, trimmed to 0" fat, all grades, cooked, braised	199	36	5	0	18.31	0.51
Beef, round, top round, separable lean only, trimmed to 0" fat, choice, cooked, braised	207	36	6	0	18.31	0.51
Beef, round, top round, separable lean only, trimmed to 0" fat, choice, cooked, broiled	197	32	7	0	16.89	0.53
Beef, round, top round, separable lean only, trimmed to 0" fat, select, cooked, braised	190	36	4	0	18.31	0.51
Beef, round, top round, separable lean only, trimmed to 0" fat, select, cooked, broiled	176	32	4	0	16.84	0.53
Beef, round, top round, separable lean only, trimmed to 1/8" fat, select, raw	129	23	3	0	10.85	0.47
Beef, round, top round, separable lean only, trimmed to 1/8" fat, all grades, raw	135	23	4	0	10.92	0.47
Beef, round, top round, separable lean only, trimmed to 1/8" fat, select, cooked, broiled	177	32	5	0	16.81	0.53
Beef, round, top round, separable lean only, trimmed to 1/8" fat, all grades, cooked, broiled	185	32	5	0	16.95	0.53
Beef, round, top round, separable lean only, trimmed to 1/8" fat, choice, cooked, broiled	193	32	6	0	17.02	0.53
Beef, sandwich steaks, flaked, chopped, formed and thinly sliced, raw	309	17	27	0	7.54	0.44
Beef, short loin, porterhouse steak, separable lean and fat, trimmed to 1/8" fat, select, raw	222	21	15	0	9.50	0.45
Beef, short loin, porterhouse steak, separable lean and fat, trimmed to 1/8" fat, all grades, raw	247	19	19	0	8.65	0.46
Beef, short loin, porterhouse steak, separable lean and fat, trimmed to 1/8" fat, all grades, cooked, broiled	297	24	22	0	10.99	0.46
Beef, short loin, porterhouse steak, separable lean and fat, trimmed to 1/8" fat, choice, raw	258	18	20	0	8.25	0.46
Beef, short loin, porterhouse steak, separable lean and fat, trimmed to 1/8" fat, select, cooked, broiled	294	24	21	0	11.24	0.47
Beef, short loin, porterhouse steak, separable lean and fat, trimmed to 1/8" fat, choice, cooked, broiled	299	23	22	0	10.85	0.47
Beef, short loin, porterhouse steak, separable lean and fat, trimmed to 0" fat, USDA select, cooked, broiled	267	24	18	0	11.46	0.48

Beef Products

Food Description	Kcals	Protein	Fat	Carbs	PRAL	Acid Density
Beef, short loin, porterhouse steak, separable lean and fat, trimmed to 0" fat, all grades, cooked, broiled	276	24	19	0	11.93	0.50
Beef, short loin, porterhouse steak, separable lean and fat, trimmed to 0" fat, USDA choice, cooked, broiled	283	24	20	0	12.24	0.51
Beef, short loin, porterhouse steak, separable lean only, trimmed to 0" fat, USDA select, cooked, broiled	194	27	9	0	12.54	0.46
Beef, short loin, porterhouse steak, separable lean only, trimmed to 0" fat, all grades, cooked, broiled	212	26	11	0	12.96	0.50
Beef, short loin, porterhouse steak, separable lean only, trimmed to 0" fat, USDA choice, cooked, broiled	224	26	13	0	13.25	0.51
Beef, short loin, t-bone steak, separable lean and fat, trimmed to 1/8" fat, select, raw	192	20	12	0	9.03	0.45
Beef, short loin, t-bone steak, separable lean and fat, trimmed to 1/8" fat, choice, raw	232	19	17	0	8.59	0.45
Beef, short loin, t-bone steak, separable lean and fat, trimmed to 1/8" fat, all grades, raw	220	19	15	0	8.74	0.46
Beef, short loin, t-bone steak, separable lean and fat, trimmed to 1/8" fat, choice, cooked, broiled	286	24	20	0	11.10	0.46
Beef, short loin, t-bone steak, separable lean and fat, trimmed to 1/8" fat, select, cooked, broiled	265	25	18	0	11.57	0.46
Beef, short loin, t-bone steak, separable lean and fat, trimmed to 1/8" fat, all grades, cooked, broiled	280	24	19	0	11.27	0.47
Beef, short loin, t-bone steak, separable lean and fat, trimmed to 0" fat, USDA choice, cooked, broiled	258	24	17	0	12.08	0.50
Beef, short loin, t-bone steak, separable lean and fat, trimmed to 0" fat, all grades, cooked, broiled	247	24	16	0	12.18	0.51
Beef, short loin, t-bone steak, separable lean and fat, trimmed to 0" fat, USDA select, cooked, broiled	230	24	14	0	12.25	0.51
Beef, short loin, t-bone steak, separable lean only, trimmed to 0" fat, all grades, cooked, broiled	189	26	9	0	13.09	0.50
Beef, short loin, t-bone steak, separable lean only, trimmed to 0" fat, USDA choice, cooked, broiled	198	26	10	0	13.09	0.50
Beef, short loin, t-bone steak, separable lean only, trimmed to 0" fat, USDA select, cooked, broiled	177	26	7	0	13.10	0.50
Beef, short loin, top loin , separable lean only, trimmed to 1/8" fat, choice, raw	155	23	6	0	10.54	0.46
Beef, short loin, top loin , separable lean only, trimmed to 1/8" fat, choice, cooked, broiled	201	29	8	0	14.19	0.49
Beef, short loin, top loin, separable lean and fat, trimmed to 0" fat, all grades, cooked, broiled	193	29	8	0	13.95	0.48
Beef, short loin, top loin, separable lean and fat, trimmed to 0" fat, choice, cooked, broiled	205	28	9	0	13.69	0.49
Beef, short loin, top loin, separable lean and fat, trimmed to 0" fat, select, cooked, broiled	180	29	6	0	14.21	0.49
Beef, short loin, top loin, separable lean and fat, trimmed to 1/8" fat, choice, raw	232	21	16	0	9.47	0.45
Beef, short loin, top loin, separable lean and fat, trimmed to 1/8" fat, prime, raw	281	19	22	0	8.60	0.45
Beef, short loin, top loin, separable lean and fat, trimmed to 1/8" fat, prime, cooked, broiled	310	26	22	0	11.81	0.45
Beef, short loin, top loin, separable lean and fat, trimmed to 1/8" fat, all grades, raw	228	21	15	0	9.55	0.45
Beef, short loin, top loin, separable lean and fat, trimmed to 1/8" fat, select, raw	224	21	15	0	9.66	0.46

Beef Products

Food Description	Kcals	Protein	Fat	Carbs	PRAL	Acid Density
Beef, short loin, top loin, separable lean and fat, trimmed to 1/8" fat, select, cooked, broiled	250	27	15	0	12.95	0.48
Beef, short loin, top loin, separable lean and fat, trimmed to 1/8" fat, choice, cooked, broiled	278	26	18	0	12.63	0.49
Beef, short loin, top loin, separable lean and fat, trimmed to 1/8" fat, all grades, cooked, broiled	264	26	17	0	12.79	0.49
Beef, short loin, top loin, separable lean only, trimmed to 0" fat, select, cooked, broiled	172	30	5	0	14.27	0.48
Beef, short loin, top loin, separable lean only, trimmed to 0" fat, choice, cooked, broiled	192	29	8	0	14.07	0.49
Beef, short loin, top loin, separable lean only, trimmed to 0" fat, all grades, cooked, broiled	182	29	6	0	14.13	0.49
Beef, short loin, top loin, separable lean only, trimmed to 1/8" fat, all grades, raw	138	23	5	0	10.66	0.46
Beef, short loin, top loin, separable lean only, trimmed to 1/8" fat, select, raw	133	23	4	0	10.71	0.47
Beef, short loin, top loin, separable lean only, trimmed to 1/8" fat, select, cooked, broiled	177	29	6	0	14.24	0.49
Beef, tenderloin, separable lean and fat, trimmed to 0" fat, all grades, cooked, broiled	218	28	11	0	13.33	0.48
Beef, tenderloin, separable lean and fat, trimmed to 0" fat, choice, cooked, broiled	231	28	12	0	13.50	0.48
Beef, tenderloin, separable lean and fat, trimmed to 0" fat, select, cooked, broiled	205	27	10	0	13.19	0.49
Beef, tenderloin, separable lean and fat, trimmed to 1/8" fat, all grades, raw	247	20	18	0	9.10	0.46
Beef, tenderloin, separable lean and fat, trimmed to 1/8" fat, all grades, cooked, roasted	324	24	25	0	11.58	0.48
Beef, tenderloin, separable lean and fat, trimmed to 1/8" fat, all grades, cooked, broiled	267	26	17	0	12.82	0.49
Beef, tenderloin, separable lean and fat, trimmed to 1/8" fat, choice, raw	246	20	18	0	9.05	0.45
Beef, tenderloin, separable lean and fat, trimmed to 1/8" fat, choice, cooked, roasted	331	24	25	0	11.10	0.46
Beef, tenderloin, separable lean and fat, trimmed to 1/8" fat, choice, cooked, broiled	273	26	18	0	12.75	0.49
Beef, tenderloin, separable lean and fat, trimmed to 1/8" fat, prime, cooked, broiled	308	25	22	0	11.63	0.47
Beef, tenderloin, separable lean and fat, trimmed to 1/8" fat, prime, raw	274	18	22	0	8.59	0.48
Beef, tenderloin, separable lean and fat, trimmed to 1/8" fat, prime, cooked, roasted	343	24	27	0	11.53	0.48
Beef, tenderloin, separable lean and fat, trimmed to 1/8" fat, select, raw	249	19	18	0	9.11	0.48
Beef, tenderloin, separable lean and fat, trimmed to 1/8" fat, select, cooked, roasted	316	24	24	0	11.58	0.48
Beef, tenderloin, separable lean and fat, trimmed to 1/8" fat, select, cooked, broiled	262	26	17	0	12.86	0.49
Beef, tenderloin, separable lean only, trimmed to 0" fat, all grades, cooked, broiled	193	29	8	0	13.83	0.48
Beef, tenderloin, separable lean only, trimmed to 0" fat, choice, cooked, broiled	206	29	9	0	14.10	0.49
Beef, tenderloin, separable lean only, trimmed to 0" fat, select, cooked, broiled	179	28	7	0	13.56	0.48
Beef, tenderloin, separable lean only, trimmed to 1/8" fat, all grades, raw	152	22	7	0	10.26	0.47
Beef, tenderloin, separable lean only, trimmed to 1/8" fat, all grades, cooked, broiled	200	29	8	0	14.07	0.49
Beef, tenderloin, separable lean only, trimmed to 1/8" fat, choice, raw	158	22	7	0	10.30	0.47
Beef, tenderloin, separable lean only, trimmed to 1/8" fat, choice, cooked, broiled	206	29	9	0	14.11	0.49

Beef Products

Food Description	Kcals	Protein	Fat	Carbs	PRAL	Acid Density
Beef, tenderloin, separable lean only, trimmed to 1/8" fat, select, raw	148	22	6	0	10.22	0.46
Beef, tenderloin, separable lean only, trimmed to 1/8" fat, select, cooked, broiled	194	29	8	0	14.02	0.48
Beef, top sirloin, separable lean and fat, trimmed to 0" fat, all grades, cooked, broiled	212	29	10	0	14.18	0.49
Beef, top sirloin, separable lean and fat, trimmed to 0" fat, choice, cooked, broiled	219	29	11	0	13.96	0.48
Beef, top sirloin, separable lean and fat, trimmed to 0" fat, select, cooked, broiled	206	30	9	0	14.38	0.48
Beef, top sirloin, separable lean and fat, trimmed to 1/4" fat, choice, cooked, pan-fried	326	29	21	0	13.04	0.45
Beef, top sirloin, separable lean and fat, trimmed to 1/8" fat, all grades, raw	201	20	13	0	9.39	0.47
Beef, top sirloin, separable lean and fat, trimmed to 1/8" fat, all grades, cooked, broiled	243	27	14	0	13.05	0.48
Beef, top sirloin, separable lean and fat, trimmed to 1/8" fat, choice, raw	214	20	14	0	9.12	0.46
Beef, top sirloin, separable lean and fat, trimmed to 1/8" fat, choice, cooked, pan-fried	313	29	21	0	13.38	0.46
Beef, top sirloin, separable lean and fat, trimmed to 1/8" fat, choice, cooked, broiled	257	27	16	0	12.89	0.48
Beef, top sirloin, separable lean and fat, trimmed to 1/8" fat, select, raw	189	21	11	0	9.71	0.46
Beef, top sirloin, separable lean and fat, trimmed to 1/8" fat, select, cooked, broiled	230	27	13	0	13.18	0.49
Beef, top sirloin, separable lean only, trimmed to 0" fat, all grades, cooked, broiled	183	31	6	0	14.80	0.48
Beef, top sirloin, separable lean only, trimmed to 0" fat, choice, cooked, broiled	188	30	7	0	14.73	0.49
Beef, top sirloin, separable lean only, trimmed to 0" fat, select, cooked, broiled	177	31	5	0	14.85	0.48
Beef, top sirloin, separable lean only, trimmed to 1/8" fat, all grades, raw	131	22	4	0	10.23	0.47
Beef, top sirloin, separable lean only, trimmed to 1/8" fat, all grades, cooked, broiled	178	29	6	0	14.24	0.49
Beef, top sirloin, separable lean only, trimmed to 1/8" fat, choice, raw	135	22	5	0	10.17	0.46
Beef, top sirloin, separable lean only, trimmed to 1/8" fat, choice, cooked, broiled	187	30	7	0	14.38	0.48
Beef, top sirloin, separable lean only, trimmed to 1/8" fat, select, raw	127	22	4	0	10.33	0.47
Beef, top sirloin, separable lean only, trimmed to 1/8" fat, select, cooked, broiled	170	29	5	0	14.15	0.49
Beef, variety meats and by-products, brain, cooked, pan-fried	196	13	16	0	12.50	0.96
Beef, variety meats and by-products, brain, cooked, simmered	151	12	11	1	12.56	1.05
Beef, variety meats and by-products, brain, raw	143	11	10	1	12.06	1.10
Beef, variety meats and by-products, heart, cooked, simmered	165	28	5	0	18.14	0.65
Beef, variety meats and by-products, heart, raw	112	18	4	0	9.86	0.55
Beef, variety meats and by-products, kidneys, cooked, simmered	158	23	5	0	21.21	0.92
Beef, variety meats and by-products, kidneys, raw	103	17	3	0	11.92	0.70
Beef, variety meats and by-products, liver, cooked, braised	191	29	5	5	24.62	0.85
Beef, variety meats and by-products, liver, cooked, pan-fried	175	27	5	5	22.91	0.85

Beef Products

Food Description	Kcals	Protein	Fat	Carbs	PRAL	Acid Density
Beef, variety meats and by-products, liver, raw	135	20	4	0	17.18	0.86
Beef, variety meats and by-products, lungs, cooked, braised	120	20	4	0	12.54	0.63
Beef, variety meats and by-products, lungs, raw	92	16	3	0	8.59	0.54
Beef, variety meats and by-products, mechanically separated beef, raw	276	15	24	0	6.75	0.45
Beef, variety meats and by-products, pancreas, cooked, braised	271	27	17	0	24.12	0.89
Beef, variety meats and by-products, pancreas, raw	235	16	19	0	13.41	0.84
Beef, variety meats and by-products, spleen, cooked, braised	145	25	4	0	16.97	0.68
Beef, variety meats and by-products, spleen, raw	105	18	3	0	10.22	0.57
Beef, variety meats and by-products, suet, raw - PDS READY- 7/2006	854	1	94	0	0.90	0.90
Beef, variety meats and by-products, thymus, cooked, braised	319	22	25	0	14.69	0.67
Beef, variety meats and by-products, thymus, raw	236	12	20	0	12.49	1.04
Beef, variety meats and by-products, tongue, cooked, simmered	284	19	22	0	10.49	0.55
Beef, variety meats and by-products, tongue, raw	224	15	16	4	5.11	0.34
Beef, variety meats and by-products, tripe, cooked, simmered	94	12	4	2	5.85	0.49
Beef, variety meats and by-products, tripe, raw	85	12	4	0	5.64	0.47
USDA Commodity, beef patties with VPP, frozen, cooked	247	16	17	8	7.75	0.48
USDA Commodity, beef patties with VPP, frozen, raw	225	15	16	4	6.99	0.47
USDA Commodity, beef, ground bulk/coarse ground, frozen, cooked	259	26	16	0	13.21	0.51
USDA Commodity, beef, ground, bulk/coarse ground, frozen, raw	228	17	17	0	7.32	0.43
USDA Commodity, beef, patties (100%), frozen, cooked	249	23	16	1	12.54	0.55
USDA Commodity, beef, patties (100%), frozen, raw	204	15	16	0	6.32	0.42

Fruits and Fruit Juices

Food Description	Kcals	Protein	Fat	Carbs	PRAL	Alkali Density
Abiyuch, raw	69	1	0	18	-4.63	-0.26
Acerola juice, raw	23	0	5	0	-1.95	
Acerola, (West Indian cherry), raw	32	0	0	8	-3.08	-0.39
Apple juice, canned or bottled, unsweetened, with added ascorbic acid	47	0	0	11	-2.38	-0.22
Apple juice, canned or bottled, unsweetened, without added ascorbic acid	47	0	0	11	-2.38	-0.22
Apple juice, frozen concentrate, unsweetened, diluted with 3 volume water without added ascorbic acid	47	0	0	11	-2.52	-0.23
Apple juice, frozen concentrate, unsweetened, diluted with 3 volume water, with added ascorbic acid	47	0	0	11	-2.52	-0.23
Apple juice, frozen concentrate, unsweetened, undiluted, with added ascorbic acid	166	1	0	41	-8.93	-0.22
Apple juice, frozen concentrate, unsweetened, undiluted, without added ascorbic acid	166	1	0	41	-8.93	-0.22
Apples, canned, sweetened, sliced, drained, heated	67	0	0	17	-1.29	-0.08
Apples, canned, sweetened, sliced, drained, unheated	67	0	0	17	-1.25	-0.07
Apples, dehydrated (low moisture), sulfured, stewed	74	0	0	20	-2.45	-0.12
Apples, dehydrated (low moisture), sulfured, uncooked	346	1	1	94	-11.57	-0.12
Apples, dried, sulfured, stewed, with added sugar	83	0	0	21	-1.78	-0.08
Apples, dried, sulfured, stewed, without added sugar	57	0	0	15	-1.90	-0.13
Apples, dried, sulfured, uncooked	243	1	0	66	-8.18	-0.12
Apples, frozen, unsweetened, heated	47	0	0	12	-1.30	-0.11
Apples, frozen, unsweetened, unheated	48	0	0	12	-1.31	-0.11
Apples, raw, with skin	52	0	0	14	-1.92	-0.14
Apples, raw, without skin	48	0	0	13	-1.52	-0.12
Apples, raw, without skin, cooked, boiled	53	0	0	14	-1.56	-0.11
Apples, raw, without skin, cooked, microwave	56	0	0	14	-1.66	-0.12
Applesauce, canned, sweetened, with salt	76	0	20	0	-1.06	
Applesauce, canned, sweetened, without salt	76	0	20	0	-1.06	
Applesauce, canned, unsweetened, with added ascorbic acid	43	0	0	11	-1.35	-0.12
Applesauce, canned, unsweetened, without added ascorbic acid	43	0	0	11	-1.35	-0.12
Apricot nectar, canned, with added ascorbic acid	56	0	0	14	-2.10	-0.15
Apricot nectar, canned, without added ascorbic acid	56	0	0	14	-2.10	-0.15
Apricots, canned, extra heavy syrup pack, without skin, solids and liquids	96	1	0	25	-2.13	-0.09
Apricots, canned, extra light syrup pack, with skin, solids and liquids	49	1	0	13	-2.48	-0.19
Apricots, canned, heavy syrup pack, with skin, solids and liquids	83	1	0	21	-2.53	-0.12
Apricots, canned, heavy syrup pack, without skin, solids and liquids	83	1	0	21	-2.40	-0.11
Apricots, canned, heavy syrup, drained	83	1	0	21	-2.52	-0.12

Fruits and Fruit Juices

Food Description	Kcals	Protein	Fat	Carbs	PRAL	Alkali Density
Apricots, canned, juice pack, with skin, solids and liquids	48	1	0	12	-2.83	-0.24
Apricots, canned, light syrup pack, with skin, solids and liquids	63	1	0	16	-2.50	-0.16
Apricots, canned, water pack, with skin, solids and liquids	27	1	0	6	-3.48	-0.58
Apricots, canned, water pack, without skin, solids and liquids	22	1	0	5	-2.64	-0.53
Apricots, dehydrated (low-moisture), sulfured, stewed	126	2	0	33	-13.01	-0.39
Apricots, dehydrated (low-moisture), sulfured, uncooked	320	5	1	83	-33.07	-0.40
Apricots, dried, sulfured, stewed, with added sugar	113	3	0	29	-7.90	-0.27
Apricots, dried, sulfured, stewed, without added sugar	85	1	0	22	-7.65	-0.35
Apricots, dried, sulfured, uncooked	241	3	1	63	-21.66	-0.34
Apricots, frozen, sweetened	98	1	0	25	-4.12	-0.16
Apricots, raw	48	1	0	11	-4.33	-0.39
Avocados, raw, all commercial varieties	160	2	15	9	-8.19	-0.91
Avocados, raw, California	167	2	15	9	-8.61	-0.96
Avocados, raw, Florida	120	2	10	8	-5.55	-0.69
Bananas, dehydrated, or banana powder	346	4	2	88	-29.76	-0.34
Bananas, raw	89	1	0	23	-6.93	-0.30
Blackberries, canned, heavy syrup, solids and liquids	92	1	0	23	-1.63	-0.07
Blackberries, frozen, unsweetened	64	1	0	16	-2.20	-0.14
Blackberries, raw	43	1	0	10	-2.80	-0.28
Blackberry juice, canned	38	0	1	8	-2.94	-0.37
Blueberries, canned, heavy syrup, solids and liquids	88	1	0	22	-0.32	-0.01
Blueberries, frozen, sweetened	81	0	0	22	-0.93	-0.04
Blueberries, frozen, unsweetened	51	0	1	12	-0.75	-0.06
Blueberries, raw	57	1	0	14	-1.04	-0.07
Boysenberries, canned, heavy syrup	88	1	0	22	-1.55	-0.07
Boysenberries, frozen, unsweetened	50	1	0	12	-2.14	-0.18
Breadfruit, raw	103	1	0	27	-9.52	-0.35
Candied fruit	321	0	0	83	-1.17	-0.01
Carambola, (starfruit), raw	31	1	0	7	-2.13	-0.30
Carissa, (natal-plum), raw	62	0	1	14	-5.51	-0.39
Cherimoya, raw	74	2	1	18	-4.39	-0.24
Cherries, sour, red, canned, extra heavy syrup pack, solids and liquids	114	1	0	29	-1.49	-0.05
Cherries, sour, red, canned, heavy syrup pack, solids and liquids	91	1	0	23	-1.51	-0.07
Cherries, sour, red, canned, light syrup pack, solids and liquids	75	1	0	19	-1.54	-0.08
Cherries, sour, red, canned, water pack, solids and liquids (includes USDA commodity red tart cherries, canned)	36	1	0	9	-1.61	-0.18

Fruits and Fruit Juices

Food Description	Kcals	Protein	Fat	Carbs	PRAL	Alkali Density
Cherries, sour, red, frozen, unsweetened	46	1	0	11	-1.96	-0.18
Cherries, sour, red, raw	50	1	0	12	-3.03	-0.25
Cherries, sweet, canned, extra heavy syrup pack, solids and liquids	102	1	0	26	-2.38	-0.09
Cherries, sweet, canned, heavy syrup pack, solids and liquids	83	1	0	21	-2.43	-0.12
Cherries, sweet, canned, heavy syrup, drained	83	1	0	21	-2.37	-0.11
Cherries, sweet, canned, juice pack, solids and liquids	54	1	0	14	-1.98	-0.14
Cherries, sweet, canned, light syrup pack, solids and liquids	67	1	0	17	-2.49	-0.15
Cherries, sweet, canned, water pack, solids and liquids	46	1	0	12	-2.19	-0.18
Cherries, sweet, frozen, sweetened	89	1	0	22	-3.44	-0.16
Cherries, sweet, raw	63	1	0	16	-3.82	-0.24
Clementines, raw	47	1	0	12	-3.17	-0.26
Crabapples, raw	76	0	0	20	-3.73	-0.19
Cranberries, dried, sweetened	308	0	1	82	-0.77	-0.01
Cranberries, raw	46	0	0	12	-1.37	-0.11
Cranberry juice, unsweetened	46	0	0	12	-1.20	-0.10
Cranberry sauce, canned, sweetened	151	0	0	39	-0.35	-0.01
Cranberry-orange relish, canned	178	0	0	46	-0.60	-0.01
Currants, European black, raw	63	1	0	15	-5.23	-0.35
Currants, red and white, raw	56	1	0	14	-4.22	-0.30
Currants, zante, dried	283	4	0	74	-14.29	-0.19
Custard-apple, (bullock's-heart), raw	101	2	1	25	-7.27	-0.29
Dates, deglet noor	282	2	0	75	-11.90	-0.16
Dates, medjool	277	2	0	75	-13.67	-0.18
Durian, raw or frozen	147	1	5	27	-7.85	-0.29
Elderberries, raw	73	1	0	18	-4.73	-0.26
Feijoa, raw	49	1	1	11	-2.36	-0.21
Figs, canned, extra heavy syrup pack, solids and liquids	107	0	0	28	-2.07	-0.07
Figs, canned, heavy syrup pack, solids and liquids	88	0	0	23	-2.13	-0.09
Figs, canned, light syrup pack, solids and liquids	69	0	0	18	-2.19	-0.12
Figs, canned, water pack, solids and liquids	53	0	0	14	-2.22	-0.16
Figs, dried, stewed	107	1	0	28	-6.06	-0.22
Figs, dried, uncooked	249	3	1	64	-14.05	-0.22
Figs, raw	74	1	0	19	-4.88	-0.26
Fruit cocktail, (peach and pineapple and pear and grape and cherry), canned, water pack, solids and liquids	32	0	0	9	-1.60	-0.18
Fruit cocktail, (peach and pineapple and pear and grape and cherry), canned, extra light syrup, solids and liquids	45	0	0	12	-1.80	-0.15

Fruits and Fruit Juices

Food Description	Kcals	Protein	Fat	Carbs	PRAL	Alkali Density
Fruit cocktail, (peach and pineapple and pear and grape and cherry), canned, juice pack, solids and liquids	46	0	0	12	-1.53	-0.13
Fruit cocktail, (peach and pineapple and pear and grape and cherry), canned, light syrup, solids and liquids	57	0	0	15	-1.47	-0.10
Fruit cocktail, (peach and pineapple and pear and grape and cherry), canned, heavy syrup, solids and liquids	73	0	0	19	-1.45	-0.08
Fruit cocktail, (peach and pineapple and pear and grape and cherry), canned, extra heavy syrup, solids and liquids	88	0	0	23	-1.41	-0.06
Fruit cocktail, canned, heavy syrup, drained	70	0	0	19	-1.43	-0.08
Fruit salad, (peach and pear and apricot and pineapple and cherry), canned, water pack, solids and liquids	30	0	0	8	-1.35	-0.17
Fruit salad, (peach and pear and apricot and pineapple and cherry), canned, juice pack, solids and liquids	50	1	0	13	-2.01	-0.15
Fruit salad, (peach and pear and apricot and pineapple and cherry), canned, light syrup, solids and liquids	58	0	0	15	-1.44	-0.10
Fruit salad, (peach and pear and apricot and pineapple and cherry), canned, heavy syrup, solids and liquids	73	0	0	19	-1.38	-0.07
Fruit salad, (peach and pear and apricot and pineapple and cherry), canned, extra heavy syrup, solids and liquids	88	0	0	23	-1.39	-0.06
Fruit salad, (pineapple and papaya and banana and guava), tropical, canned, heavy syrup, solids and liquids	86	0	0	22	-2.79	-0.13
Fruit, mixed, (peach and cherry-sweet and -sour and raspberry and grape and boysenberry), frozen, sweetened	98	1	0	24	-1.85	-0.08
Fruit, mixed, (peach and pear and pineapple), canned, heavy syrup, solids and liquids	72	0	0	19	-1.35	-0.07
Fruit, mixed, (prune and apricot and pear), dried	243	2	0	64	-14.17	-0.22
Gooseberries, canned, light syrup pack, solids and liquids	73	1	0	19	-1.40	-0.07
Gooseberries, raw	44	1	1	10	-3.31	-0.33
Grape juice, canned or bottled, unsweetened, without added vitamin C	61	0	0	15	-2.46	-0.16
Grape juice, frozen concentrate, sweetened, diluted with 3 volume water, with added vitamin C	51	0	0	13	-0.35	-0.03
Grape juice, frozen concentrate, sweetened, undiluted, with added vitamin C	179	1	0	44	-1.24	-0.03
Grapefruit juice, pink, raw	39	0	0	9	-3.03	-0.34
Grapefruit juice, white, canned, sweetened	46	1	0	11	-3.07	-0.28
Grapefruit juice, white, canned, unsweetened	38	1	0	9	-2.90	-0.32
Grapefruit juice, white, frozen concentrate, unsweetened, diluted with 3 volume water	41	1	0	10	-2.45	-0.25
Grapefruit juice, white, frozen concentrate, unsweetened, undiluted	146	2	0	35	-8.72	-0.25
Grapefruit juice, white, raw	39	0	0	9	-3.03	-0.34
Grapefruit, raw, pink and red and white, all areas	32	1	0	8	-2.67	-0.33

Fruits and Fruit Juices

Food Description	Kcals	Protein	Fat	Carbs	PRAL	Alkali Density
Grapefruit, raw, pink and red, all areas	42	1	0	11	-2.31	-0.21
Grapefruit, raw, pink and red, California and Arizona	37	0	0	10	-2.77	-0.28
Grapefruit, raw, pink and red, Florida	30	1	0	8	-2.46	-0.31
Grapefruit, raw, white, all areas	33	1	0	8	-2.86	-0.36
Grapefruit, raw, white, California	37	1	0	9	-2.51	-0.28
Grapefruit, raw, white, Florida	32	1	0	8	-3.01	-0.38
Grapefruit, sections, canned, juice pack, solids and liquids	37	1	0	9	-3.24	-0.36
Grapefruit, sections, canned, light syrup pack, solids and liquids	60	1	0	15	-2.50	-0.17
Grapefruit, sections, canned, water pack, solids and liquids	36	1	0	9	-2.57	-0.29
Grapes, American type (slip skin), raw	67	1	0	17	-3.64	-0.21
Grapes, canned, thompson seedless, heavy syrup pack, solids and liquids	73	0	0	20	-1.58	-0.08
Grapes, canned, thompson seedless, water pack, solids and liquids	40	0	0	10	-1.62	-0.16
Grapes, red or green (European type, such as Thompson seedless), raw	69	1	0	18	-3.23	-0.18
Guanabana nectar, canned	59	0	0	15	-0.56	-0.04
Guava nectar, canned	57	0	0	15	-0.90	-0.06
Guava sauce, cooked	36	0	0	9	-4.43	-0.49
Guavas, common, raw	68	3	1	14	-6.83	-0.49
Guavas, strawberry, raw	69	1	1	17	-5.56	-0.33
Jackfruit, canned, syrup pack	92	0	24	0	-2.45	
Jackfruit, raw	94	1	0	24	-5.71	-0.24
Java-plum, (jambolan), raw	60	1	0	16	-1.31	-0.08
Jujube, dried	287	4	1	74	-7.62	-0.10
Jujube, raw	79	1	0	20	-4.34	-0.22
Kiwi fruit, (Chinese gooseberries), fresh, raw	61	1	1	15	-5.61	-0.37
Kiwifruit, (Chinese gooseberries), held in storage, raw	61	1	0	15	-6.12	-0.41
Kumquats, raw	71	2	1	16	-3.60	-0.23
Lemon juice, canned or bottled	21	0	0	6	-1.96	-0.33
Lemon juice, frozen, unsweetened, single strength	22	0	0	6	-1.66	-0.28
Lemon juice, raw	25	0	0	9	-2.44	-0.27
Lemon peel, raw	47	1	0	16	-4.31	-0.27
Lemons, raw, with peel	20	1	0	11	-3	-0.27
Lemons, raw, without peel	29	1	0	9	-2.31	-0.26
Lime juice, canned or bottled, unsweetened	21	0	0	7	-1.42	-0.20
Lime juice, raw	25	0	0	8	-2.12	-0.27
Limes, raw	30	1	0	11	-1.71	-0.16
Litchis, dried	277	4	1	71	-16.27	-0.23
Litchis, raw	66	1	0	17	-2.36	-0.14

Fruits and Fruit Juices

Food Description	Kcals	Protein	Fat	Carbs	PRAL	Alkali Density
Loganberries, frozen	55	2	0	13	-2.22	-0.17
Longans, dried	286	5	0	74	-5.94	-0.08
Longans, raw	60	1	0	15	-4.44	-0.30
Loquats, raw	47	0	0	12	-4.92	-0.41
Mammy-apple, (mamey), raw	51	0	0	13	-0.89	-0.07
Mango nectar, canned	51	0	0	13	-0.67	-0.05
Mangos, raw	65	1	0	17	-2.98	-0.18
Mangosteen, canned, syrup pack	73	0	1	18	-1	-0.06
Maraschino cherries, canned, drained	165	0	0	42	-1.02	-0.02
Melon balls, frozen	33	1	0	8	-5.51	-0.69
Melons, cantaloupe, raw	34	1	0	9	-5.06	-0.56
Melons, casaba, raw	28	1	0	7	-3.52	-0.50
Melons, honeydew, raw	36	1	0	9	-4.45	-0.49
Mulberries, raw	43	1	0	10	-2.93	-0.29
Nectarines, raw	44	1	0	11	-3.05	-0.28
Oheloberries, raw	28	0	0	7	-0.48	-0.07
Olives, pickled, canned or bottled, green	145	1	15	4	-1.19	-0.30
Olives, ripe, canned (jumbo-super colossal)	81	1	7	6	-0.92	-0.15
Olives, ripe, canned (small-extra large)	115	1	11	6	-0.89	-0.15
Orange juice, California, chilled, includes from concentrate	44	1	0	10	-3.60	-0.36
Orange juice, canned, unsweetened	42	1	0	11	-3.25	-0.30
Orange juice, chilled, includes from concentrate	44	1	0	10	-3.60	-0.36
Orange juice, chilled, includes from concentrate, fortified with calcium and vitamin D	44	1	0	10	-5.31	-0.53
Orange juice, frozen concentrate, unsweetened, diluted with 3 volume water	45	1	0	11	-3.44	-0.31
Orange juice, frozen concentrate, unsweetened, undiluted	159	2	0	38	-12.17	-0.32
Orange juice, raw	45	1	0	10	-3.65	-0.37
Orange peel, raw	97	1	0	25	-5.60	-0.22
Orange-grapefruit juice, canned, unsweetened	43	1	0	10	-2.87	-0.29
Oranges, raw, all commercial varieties	47	1	0	12	-3.60	-0.30
Oranges, raw, California, Valencia's	49	1	0	12	-3.40	-0.28
Oranges, raw, Florida	46	1	0	12	-3.58	-0.30
Oranges, raw, navels	49	1	0	13	-3.03	-0.23
Oranges, raw, with peel	63	1	0	15	-3.93	-0.26
Orange-strawberry-banana juice	46	0	0	12	-1.85	-0.15
Papaya nectar, canned	57	0	0	15	-0.77	-0.05
Papayas, raw	39	1	0	10	-5.48	-0.55
Passion-fruit juice, purple, raw	51	0	0	14	-5.66	-0.40
Passion-fruit juice, yellow, raw	60	1	0	14	-5.07	-0.36

Fruits and Fruit Juices

Food Description	Kcals	Protein	Fat	Carbs	PRAL	Alkali Density
Passion-fruit, (granadilla), purple, raw	97	2	1	23	-4.62	-0.20
Peach nectar, canned, with added ascorbic acid	54	0	0	14	-0.65	-0.05
Peach nectar, canned, without added ascorbic acid	54	0	0	14	-0.65	-0.05
Peaches, canned, extra heavy syrup pack, solids and liquids	96	0	0	26	-1.27	-0.05
Peaches, canned, extra light syrup, solids and liquids	42	0	0	11	-1.14	-0.10
Peaches, canned, heavy syrup pack, solids and liquids	74	0	0	20	-1.47	-0.07
Peaches, canned, heavy syrup, drained	77	1	0	20	-1.43	-0.07
Peaches, canned, juice pack, solids and liquids	44	1	0	12	-2.01	-0.17
Peaches, canned, light syrup pack, solids and liquids	54	0	0	15	-1.57	-0.10
Peaches, canned, water pack, solids and liquids	24	0	0	6	-1.64	-0.27
Peaches, dehydrated (low-moisture), sulfured, stewed	133	2	0	34	-9.01	-0.27
Peaches, dehydrated (low-moisture), sulfured, uncooked	325	5	1	83	-21.95	-0.26
Peaches, dried, sulfured, stewed, with added sugar	103	1	0	27	-4.73	-0.18
Peaches, dried, sulfured, stewed, without added sugar	77	1	0	20	-5.20	-0.26
Peaches, dried, sulfured, uncooked	239	4	1	61	-16.20	-0.27
Peaches, frozen, sliced, sweetened	94	1	0	24	-2.18	-0.09
Peaches, raw	39	1	0	10	-3.11	-0.31
Peaches, spiced, canned, heavy syrup pack, solids and liquids	75	0	0	20	-1.51	-0.08
Pear nectar, canned, with added ascorbic acid	60	0	0	16	-0.25	-0.02
Pear nectar, canned, without added ascorbic acid	60	0	0	16	-0.25	-0.02
Pears, Asian, raw	42	0	0	11	-2.14	-0.19
Pears, canned, extra heavy syrup pack, solids and liquids	97	0	0	25	-1.16	-0.05
Pears, canned, extra light syrup pack, solids and liquids	47	0	0	12	-0.76	-0.06
Pears, canned, heavy syrup pack, solids and liquids	74	0	0	19	-1.17	-0.06
Pears, canned, heavy syrup, drained	74	0	0	19	-1.15	-0.06
Pears, canned, juice pack, solids and liquids	50	0	0	13	-1.70	-0.13
Pears, canned, light syrup pack, solids and liquids	57	0	0	15	-1.20	-0.08
Pears, canned, water pack, solids and liquids	29	0	0	0	-0.91	
Pears, dried, sulfured, stewed, with added sugar	140	1	0	37	-4.31	-0.12
Pears, dried, sulfured, stewed, without added sugar	127	1	0	34	-4.56	-0.13
Pears, dried, sulfured, uncooked	262	2	1	70	-9.39	-0.13
Pears, raw	58	0	0	15	-2.20	-0.15
Persimmons, Japanese, dried	274	1	1	73	-14.30	-0.20
Persimmons, Japanese, raw	70	1	0	19	-2.80	-0.15
Pineapple juice, canned, unsweetened, with added ascorbic acid	53	0	0	13	-2.73	-0.21

Fruits and Fruit Juices

Food Description	Kcals	Protein	Fat	Carbs	PRAL	Alkali Density
Pineapple juice, canned, unsweetened, without added ascorbic acid	53	0	0	13	-2.73	-0.21
Pineapple juice, frozen concentrate, unsweetened, diluted with 3 volume water	52	0	0	13	-2.74	-0.21
Pineapple juice, frozen concentrate, unsweetened, undiluted	179	1	0	44	-9.65	-0.22
Pineapple, canned, extra heavy syrup pack, solids and liquids	83	0	0	22	-2.28	-0.10
Pineapple, canned, heavy syrup pack, solids and liquids	78	0	0	20	-2.35	-0.12
Pineapple, canned, juice pack, drained	60	1	0	16	-2.69	-0.17
Pineapple, canned, juice pack, solids and liquids	60	0	0	16	-2.68	-0.17
Pineapple, canned, light syrup pack, solids and liquids	52	0	0	13	-2.36	-0.18
Pineapple, canned, water pack, solids and liquids	32	0	0	8	-2.97	-0.37
Pineapple, frozen, chunks, sweetened	86	0	0	22	-2.13	-0.10
Pineapple, raw, all varieties	48	1	0	13	-2.33	-0.18
Pineapple, raw, extra sweet variety	51	1	0	13	-2.19	-0.17
Pineapple, raw, traditional varieties	45	1	0	12	-2.50	-0.21
Pitanga, (Surinam-cherry), raw	33	1	0	7	-1.79	-0.26
Plantains, cooked	116	1	0	31	-9.20	-0.30
Plantains, raw	122	1	0	32	-9.58	-0.30
Plums, canned, heavy syrup, drained	89	0	0	23	-1.44	-0.06
Plums, canned, purple, extra heavy syrup pack, solids and liquids	101	0	0	26	-1.49	-0.06
Plums, canned, purple, heavy syrup pack, solids and liquids	89	0	0	23	-1.50	-0.07
Plums, canned, purple, juice pack, solids and liquids	58	1	0	15	-2.76	-0.18
Plums, canned, purple, light syrup pack, solids and liquids	63	0	0	16	-1.53	-0.10
Plums, canned, purple, water pack, solids and liquids	41	0	0	11	-2.19	-0.20
Plums, dried (prunes), stewed, with added sugar	124	1	0	33	-5.56	-0.17
Plums, dried (prunes), stewed, without added sugar	107	1	0	28	-5.87	-0.21
Plums, dried (prunes), uncooked	240	2	0	64	-13.37	-0.21
Plums, raw	46	1	0	11	-2.62	-0.24
Pomegranates, raw	68	1	2	19	-4.79	-0.25
Prickly pears, raw	41	1	1	10	-6.31	-0.63
Prune juice, canned	71	1	0	17	-5.09	-0.30
Prunes, canned, heavy syrup pack, solids and liquids	105	1	0	28	-3.96	-0.14
Prunes, dehydrated (low-moisture), stewed	113	1	0	30	-6.29	-0.21
Prunes, dehydrated (low-moisture), uncooked	339	4	1	89	-18.86	-0.21
Pummelo, raw	38	1	0	10	-3.74	-0.37
Quinces, raw	57	0	0	15	-3.66	-0.24
Raisins, golden seedless	302	3	0	80	-11.34	-0.14

Fruits and Fruit Juices

Food Description	Kcals	Protein	Fat	Carbs	PRAL	Alkali Density
Raisins, seeded	296	3	1	78	-14.45	-0.19
Raisins, seedless	299	3	0	79	-11.97	-0.15
Rambutan, canned, syrup pack	82	1	0	21	-0.69	-0.03
Raspberries, canned, red, heavy syrup pack, solids and liquids	91	1	0	23	-1.68	-0.07
Raspberries, frozen, red, sweetened	103	1	0	26	-1.95	-0.08
Raspberries, raw	52	1	1	12	-2.40	-0.20
Rhubarb, frozen, cooked, with sugar	116	0	0	31	-3.72	-0.12
Rhubarb, frozen, uncooked	21	1	0	5	-4.54	-0.91
Rhubarb, raw	21	1	0	5	-6.51	-1.30
Rose-apples, raw	25	1	0	6	-2.50	-0.42
Roselle, raw	49	1	1	11	-6.65	-0.60
Rowal, raw	111	2	2	24	-0.72	-0.03
Sapodilla, raw	83	0	1	20	-3.97	-0.20
Sapotes, (marmalade plum), raw	134	2	1	34	-6.43	-0.19
Soursop, raw	66	1	0	17	-5.07	-0.30
Strawberries, canned, heavy syrup pack, solids and liquids	92	1	0	24	-1.46	-0.06
Strawberries, frozen, sweetened, sliced	96	1	0	26	-1.64	-0.06
Strawberries, frozen, sweetened, whole	78	1	0	21	-1.65	-0.08
Strawberries, frozen, unsweetened	35	0	0	9	-2.91	-0.32
Strawberries, raw	32	1	0	8	-2.54	-0.32
Sugar-apples, (sweetsop), raw	94	2	0	24	-3.85	-0.16
Tamarind nectar, canned	57	0	0	15	-0.68	-0.05
Tamarinds, raw	239	3	1	63	-10.98	-0.17
Tangerine juice, canned, sweetened	50	0	0	12	-3.41	-0.28
Tangerine juice, frozen concentrate, sweetened, diluted with 3 volume water	46	0	0	11	-2.17	-0.20
Tangerine juice, frozen concentrate, sweetened, undiluted	161	1	0	39	-7.57	-0.19
Tangerine juice, raw	43	0	0	10	-3.41	-0.34
Tangerines, (mandarin oranges), canned, juice pack	37	1	0	10	-2.54	-0.25
Tangerines, (mandarin oranges), canned, juice pack, drained	38	1	0	9	-2.52	-0.28
Tangerines, (mandarin oranges), canned, light syrup pack	61	1	0	16	-1.34	-0.08
Tangerines, (mandarin oranges), raw	53	1	0	13	-3.14	-0.24
USDA Commodity peaches, canned, light syrup, drained	61	1	0	16	-1.35	-0.08
USDA Commodity pears, canned, juice pack, drained	51	0	0	13	-1.87	-0.14
USDA Commodity pears, canned, light syrup, drained	62	0	0	16	-1.05	-0.07
USDA Commodity, mixed fruit (peaches, pears, grapes), canned, light syrup, drained	57	0	0	15	-1.39	-0.09
USDA Commodity, mixed fruit (peaches, pears, grapes), canned, light syrup, solids and liquids	55	0	0	14	-1.29	-0.09

Fruits and Fruit Juices

Food Description	Kcals	Protein	Fat	Carbs	PRAL	Alkali Density
Watermelon, raw	30	1	0	8	-1.99	-0.25

Pork Products

Food Description	Kcals	Protein	Fat	Carbs	PRAL	Acid Density
Pork, bacon, rendered fat, cooked	898	0	99	0	0.03	0
Pork, cured, bacon, cooked, baked	548	36	43	1	24	0.67
Pork, cured, bacon, cooked, broiled, pan-fried or roasted	541	37	42	1	25	0.68
Pork, cured, bacon, cooked, broiled, pan-fried or roasted, reduced sodium	541	37	42	1	25	0.68
Pork, cured, bacon, cooked, microwaved	505	39	37	1	25.27	0.65
Pork, cured, bacon, cooked, pan-fried	533	38	40	1	26.04	0.69
Pork, cured, bacon, raw	458	12	45	1	7.88	0.66
Pork, cured, breakfast strips, cooked	459	12	45	1	13.34	1.11
Pork, cured, breakfast strips, raw or unheated	388	12	37	1	6.12	0.51
Pork, cured, Canadian-style bacon, grilled	185	24	8	1	13.96	0.58
Pork, cured, Canadian-style bacon, unheated	157	21	7	2	11.33	0.54
Pork, cured, feet, pickled	140	12	10	0	7.94	0.66
Pork, cured, ham -- water added, rump, bone-in, separable lean and fat, heated, roasted	161	20	9	1	12.95	0.65
Pork, cured, ham -- water added, rump, bone-in, separable lean and fat, unheated	172	14	13	1	10.27	0.73
Pork, cured, ham -- water added, rump, bone-in, separable lean only, heated, roasted	121	21	4	1	13.77	0.66
Pork, cured, ham -- water added, rump, bone-in, separable lean only, unheated	95	15	3	1	11.44	0.76
Pork, cured, ham -- water added, shank, bone-in, separable lean and fat, heated, roasted	200	19	13	1	11.35	0.60
Pork, cured, ham -- water added, shank, bone-in, separable lean and fat, unheated	167	17	11	1	10.94	0.64
Pork, cured, ham -- water added, shank, bone-in, separable lean only, heated, roasted	128	21	4	1	12.59	0.60
Pork, cured, ham -- water added, shank, bone-in, separable lean only, unheated	91	19	2	1	12.24	0.64
Pork, cured, ham -- water added, slice, bone-in, separable lean and fat, heated, pan-broil	166	21	9	2	12.96	0.62
Pork, cured, ham -- water added, slice, bone-in, separable lean and fat, unheated	162	16	11	1	10.85	0.68
Pork, cured, ham -- water added, slice, bone-in, separable lean only, heated, pan-broil	131	22	4	2	13.68	0.62
Pork, cured, ham -- water added, slice, bone-in, separable lean only, unheated	91	17	2	1	12.01	0.71
Pork, cured, ham -- water added, slice, boneless, separable lean and fat, heated, pan-broil	125	19	5	2	11.84	0.62
Pork, cured, ham -- water added, slice, boneless, separable lean only, heated, pan-broil	117	19	4	2	11.99	0.63
Pork, cured, ham -- water added, whole, boneless, separable lean and fat, heated, roasted	126	18	5	2	11.43	0.64
Pork, cured, ham -- water added, whole, boneless, separable lean and fat, unheated	121	17	5	1	10.90	0.64
Pork, cured, ham -- water added, whole, boneless, separable lean only, heated, roasted	117	18	4	2	11.55	0.64
Pork, cured, ham -- water added, whole, boneless, separable lean only, unheated	110	17	4	1	11.04	0.65
Pork, cured, ham and water product, rump, bone-in, separable lean only, heated, roasted	131	21	5	1	12.43	0.59
Pork, cured, ham and water product, rump, bone-in, separable lean and fat, heated, roasted	186	19	11	1	11.48	0.60
Pork, cured, ham and water product, rump, bone-in, separable lean only, unheated	107	18	3	1	11.61	0.65

Pork Products

Food Description	Kcals	Protein	Fat	Carbs	PRAL	Acid Density
Pork, cured, ham and water product, rump, bone-in, separable lean and fat, unheated	179	16	12	1	10.43	0.65
Pork, cured, ham and water product, shank, bone-in, separable lean only, heated, roasted	132	22	4	1	12.89	0.59
Pork, cured, ham and water product, shank, bone-in, separable lean and fat, heated, roasted	234	18	17	1	11.01	0.61
Pork, cured, ham and water product, shank, bone-in, unheated, separable lean only	113	18	4	1	10.91	0.61
Pork, cured, ham and water product, shank, bone-in, unheated, separable lean and fat	243	14	20	1	8.99	0.64
Pork, cured, ham and water product, slice, bone-in, separable lean and fat, heated, pan-broil	155	20	8	1	12.43	0.62
Pork, cured, ham and water product, slice, bone-in, separable lean only, heated, pan-broil	122	21	4	1	13.06	0.62
Pork, cured, ham and water product, slice, bone-in, separable lean and fat, unheated	149	14	9	3	9.81	0.70
Pork, cured, ham and water product, slice, bone-in, separable lean only, unheated	103	14	4	3	10.43	0.75
Pork, cured, ham and water product, slice, boneless, separable lean and fat, heated, pan-broil	124	15	5	5	10.01	0.67
Pork, cured, ham and water product, slice, boneless, separable lean only, heated, pan-broil	123	15	5	5	10.01	0.67
Pork, cured, ham and water product, whole, boneless, separable lean and fat, unheated	117	14	5	4	9.16	0.65
Pork, cured, ham and water product, whole, boneless, separable lean only, unheated	116	14	5	4	9.19	0.66
Pork, cured, ham and water product, whole, boneless, separable lean and fat, heated, roasted	123	14	5	5	9.45	0.68
Pork, cured, ham and water product, whole, boneless, separable lean only, heated, roasted	123	14	5	5	9.45	0.68
Pork, cured, ham with natural juices, rump, bone-in, separable lean only, heated, roasted	137	24	4	0	10.42	0.43
Pork, cured, ham with natural juices, rump, bone-in, separable lean and fat, heated, roasted	177	22	9	1	9.93	0.45
Pork, cured, ham with natural juices, rump, bone-in, separable lean only, unheated	122	23	3	0	13.46	0.59
Pork, cured, ham with natural juices, rump, bone-in, separable lean and fat, unheated	200	20	13	0	11.76	0.59
Pork, cured, ham with natural juices, shank, bone-in, separable lean only, heated, roasted	145	25	5	0	11.40	0.46
Pork, cured, ham with natural juices, shank, bone-in, separable lean and fat, heated, roasted	191	23	11	0	10.72	0.47
Pork, cured, ham with natural juices, shank, bone-in, separable lean only, unheated	130	25	3	0	14.66	0.59
Pork, cured, ham with natural juices, shank, bone-in, separable lean and fat, unheated	191	22	11	0	13.14	0.60
Pork, cured, ham with natural juices, slice, bone-in, separable lean only, heated, pan-broil	150	28	4	0	16.09	0.57
Pork, cured, ham with natural juices, slice, bone-in, separable lean and fat, heated, pan-broil	180	26	8	0	15.23	0.59
Pork, cured, ham with natural juices, slice, bone-in, separable lean and fat, unheated	159	23	7	0	13.67	0.59
Pork, cured, ham with natural juices, slice, bone-in, separable lean only, unheated	123	24	3	0	14.53	0.61
Pork, cured, ham with natural juices, slice, boneless, separable lean and fat, heated, pan-broil	118	21	3	1	13.84	0.66
Pork, cured, ham with natural juices, slice, boneless, separable lean only, heated, pan-broil	116	21	3	1	13.88	0.66
Pork, cured, ham with natural juices, spiral slice, boneless, separable lean and fat, unheated	129	19	6	1	12.29	0.65

Pork Products

Food Description	Kcals	Protein	Fat	Carbs	PRAL	Acid Density
Pork, cured, ham with natural juices, spiral slice, boneless, separable lean and fat, heated, roasted	136	22	5	1	14.39	0.65
Pork, cured, ham with natural juices, spiral slice, boneless, separable lean only, unheated	109	19	3	1	12.67	0.67
Pork, cured, ham with natural juices, spiral slice, meat only, boneless, separable lean only, heated, roasted	126	23	4	1	14.64	0.64
Pork, cured, ham with natural juices, whole, boneless, separable lean and fat, heated, roasted	114	21	3	1	13.47	0.64
Pork, cured, ham with natural juices, whole, boneless, separable lean only, heated, roasted	113	21	3	1	13.48	0.64
Pork, cured, ham with natural juices, whole, boneless, separable lean and fat, unheated	112	19	3	1	12.78	0.67
Pork, cured, ham with natural juices, whole, boneless, separable lean only, unheated	110	19	3	1	12.82	0.67
Pork, cured, ham, boneless, extra lean (approximately 5% fat), roasted	145	21	6	1	11.01	0.52
Pork, cured, ham, boneless, extra lean and regular, roasted	165	22	8	0	11.74	0.53
Pork, cured, ham, boneless, extra lean and regular, unheated	162	18	8	2	10.88	0.60
Pork, cured, ham, boneless, low sodium, extra lean (approximately 5% fat), roasted	145	21	5	1	10.99	0.52
Pork, cured, ham, boneless, low sodium, extra lean and regular, roasted	165	22	8	0	11.75	0.53
Pork, cured, ham, boneless, regular (approximately 11% fat), roasted	178	23	9	0	12.21	0.53
Pork, cured, ham, center slice, country-style, separable lean only, raw	195	28	8	0	13.89	0.50
Pork, cured, ham, center slice, separable lean and fat, unheated	203	20	13	0	10.25	0.51
Pork, cured, ham, extra lean (approximately 4% fat), canned, roasted	136	21	5	1	10.16	0.48
Pork, cured, ham, extra lean (approximately 4% fat), canned, unheated	120	18	5	0	9.18	0.51
Pork, cured, ham, extra lean and regular, canned, roasted	167	21	8	0	10.45	0.50
Pork, cured, ham, extra lean and regular, canned, unheated	144	18	7	0	8.95	0.50
Pork, cured, ham, low sodium, lean and fat, cooked	172	22	8	0	11.97	0.54
Pork, cured, ham, patties, grilled	342	13	31	2	4.75	0.37
Pork, cured, ham, patties, unheated	315	13	28	2	6.39	0.49
Pork, cured, ham, regular (approximately 13% fat), canned, roasted	226	21	15	0	11	0.52
Pork, cured, ham, regular (approximately 13% fat), canned, unheated	190	17	13	0	7.71	0.45
Pork, cured, ham, rump, bone-in, separable lean and fat, heated, roasted	177	24	9	1	13	0.54
Pork, cured, ham, rump, bone-in, separable lean only, heated, roasted	132	26	3	1	13.92	0.54
Pork, cured, ham, rump, bone-in, separable lean only, unheated	125	24	3	0	13.06	0.54
Pork, cured, ham, separable fat, boneless, heated	507	9	52	2	5.96	0.66
Pork, cured, ham, separable fat, boneless, unheated	515	8	53	2	4.97	0.62
Pork, cured, ham, shank, bone-in, separable lean and fat, heated, roasted	183	24	9	1	13.32	0.56
Pork, cured, ham, shank, bone-in, separable lean and fat, unheated	177	22	10	0	11.86	0.54

Pork Products

Food Description	Kcals	Protein	Fat	Carbs	PRAL	Acid Density
Pork, cured, ham, shank, bone-in, separable lean only, heated, roasted	139	26	4	1	14.30	0.55
Pork, cured, ham, shank, bone-in, separable lean only, unheated	125	24	3	0	12.90	0.54
Pork, cured, ham, slice, bone-in, separable lean and fat, heated, pan-broil	180	25	8	1	13.69	0.55
Pork, cured, ham, slice, bone-in, separable lean and fat, unheated	173	22	9	0	12.21	0.56
Pork, cured, ham, slice, bone-in, separable lean only, heated, pan-broil	146	27	4	1	14.45	0.54
Pork, cured, ham, slice, bone-in, separable lean only, unheated	130	24	4	0	13.13	0.55
Pork, cured, ham, steak, boneless, extra lean, unheated	122	20	4	0	11.83	0.59
Pork, cured, ham, whole, separable lean and fat, roasted	243	22	17	0	11.89	0.54
Pork, cured, ham, whole, separable lean and fat, unheated	246	18	19	0	9.50	0.53
Pork, cured, ham, whole, separable lean only, roasted	157	25	5	0	13.37	0.53
Pork, cured, ham, whole, separable lean only, unheated	147	22	6	0	11.17	0.51
Pork, cured, salt pork, raw	748	5	81	0	2.75	0.55
Pork, cured, separable fat (from ham and arm picnic), roasted	591	8	62	0	5.88	0.74
Pork, cured, separable fat (from ham and arm picnic), unheated	579	6	61	0	3.98	0.66
Pork, cured, shoulder, arm picnic, separable lean and fat, roasted	280	20	21	0	12.27	0.61
Pork, cured, shoulder, arm picnic, separable lean only, roasted	170	25	7	0	14.52	0.58
Pork, cured, shoulder, blade roll, separable lean and fat, roasted	287	17	23	0	9.73	0.57
Pork, cured, shoulder, blade roll, separable lean and fat, unheated	269	16	22	0	8.80	0.55
Pork, fresh, backfat, raw	812	3	89	0	1.39	0.46
Pork, fresh, backribs, separable lean and fat, cooked, roasted	370	24	30	0	11.35	0.47
Pork, fresh, backribs, separable lean and fat, raw	282	16	24	0	7.46	0.47
Pork, fresh, belly, raw	518	9	53	0	4.51	0.50
Pork, fresh, carcass, separable lean and fat, raw	376	14	35	0	6.65	0.48
Pork, fresh, composite of trimmed leg, loin, shoulder, and spareribs, (includes cuts to be cured), separable lean and fat, raw	227	18	16	0	8.71	0.48
Pork, fresh, composite of trimmed retail cuts (leg, loin, and shoulder), separable lean only, cooked	212	29	10	0	14.28	0.49
Pork, fresh, composite of trimmed retail cuts (leg, loin, shoulder), separable lean only, raw	143	21	6	0	9.34	0.44
Pork, fresh, composite of trimmed retail cuts (leg, loin, shoulder, and spareribs), separable lean and fat, raw	216	19	15	0	8.85	0.47
Pork, fresh, composite of trimmed retail cuts (leg, loin, shoulder, and spareribs), separable lean and fat, cooked	273	28	17	0	13.71	0.49
Pork, fresh, composite of trimmed retail cuts (loin and shoulder blade), separable lean and fat, raw	200	20	13	0	8.60	0.43

Pork Products

Food Description	Kcals	Protein	Fat	Carbs	PRAL	Acid Density
Pork, fresh, composite of trimmed retail cuts (loin and shoulder blade), separable lean only, raw	144	21	6	0	9.25	0.44
Pork, fresh, composite of trimmed retail cuts (loin and shoulder blade), separable lean only, cooked	211	29	9	0	14.21	0.49
Pork, fresh, composite of trimmed retail cuts (loin and shoulder blade), separable lean and fat, cooked	252	26	14	0	13.47	0.52
Pork, fresh, ground, cooked	297	26	21	0	12.43	0.48
Pork, fresh, ground, raw	263	17	21	0	8.04	0.47
Pork, fresh, leg (ham), rump half, separable lean and fat, cooked, roasted	252	29	14	0	15.50	0.53
Pork, fresh, leg (ham), rump half, separable lean and fat, raw	222	19	16	0	9.23	0.49
Pork, fresh, leg (ham), rump half, separable lean only, cooked, roasted	206	31	8	0	16.65	0.54
Pork, fresh, leg (ham), rump half, separable lean only, raw	137	21	5	0	10.29	0.49
Pork, fresh, leg (ham), shank half, separable lean and fat, cooked, roasted	289	25	20	0	14.06	0.56
Pork, fresh, leg (ham), shank half, separable lean and fat, raw	263	17	21	0	8.91	0.52
Pork, fresh, leg (ham), shank half, separable lean only, cooked, roasted	215	28	11	0	15.80	0.56
Pork, fresh, leg (ham), shank half, separable lean only, raw	139	21	6	0	10.58	0.50
Pork, fresh, leg (ham), whole, separable lean and fat, cooked, roasted	273	27	18	0	14.73	0.55
Pork, fresh, leg (ham), whole, separable lean and fat, raw	245	17	19	0	8.70	0.51
Pork, fresh, leg (ham), whole, separable lean only, cooked, roasted	211	29	9	0	16.23	0.56
Pork, fresh, leg (ham), whole, separable lean only, raw	136	20	5	0	10.03	0.50
Pork, fresh, loin, blade (chops or roasts), bone-in, separable lean and fat, raw	285	16	24	0	7.12	0.45
Pork, fresh, loin, blade (chops or roasts), bone-in, separable lean only, raw	157	19	8	0	8.52	0.45
Pork, fresh, loin, blade (chops), bone-in, separable lean and fat, cooked, braised	323	22	25	0	9.55	0.43
Pork, fresh, loin, blade (chops), bone-in, separable lean and fat, cooked, broiled	320	22	25	0	10.68	0.49
Pork, fresh, loin, blade (chops), bone-in, separable lean and fat, cooked, pan-fried	342	21	28	0	10.24	0.49
Pork, fresh, loin, blade (chops), bone-in, separable lean only, cooked, braised	225	25	13	0	10.59	0.42
Pork, fresh, loin, blade (chops), bone-in, separable lean only, cooked, pan-fried	241	25	15	0	11.67	0.47
Pork, fresh, loin, blade (chops), bone-in, separable lean only, cooked, broiled	234	25	14	0	11.95	0.48
Pork, fresh, loin, blade (roasts), bone-in, separable lean and fat, cooked, roasted	323	24	25	0	11.58	0.48
Pork, fresh, loin, blade (roasts), bone-in, separable lean only, cooked, roasted	247	27	15	0	12.88	0.48
Pork, fresh, loin, center loin (chops or roasts), bone-in, separable lean only, raw	140	22	5	0	9.98	0.45
Pork, fresh, loin, center loin (chops), bone-in, separable lean and fat, cooked, braised	247	28	14	0	12.06	0.43
Pork, fresh, loin, center loin (chops), bone-in, separable lean and fat, cooked, pan-fried	277	30	17	0	14.20	0.47

Pork Products

Food Description	Kcals	Protein	Fat	Carbs	PRAL	Acid Density
Pork, fresh, loin, center loin (chops), bone-in, separable lean and fat, cooked, broiled	209	26	11	0	14.05	0.54
Pork, fresh, loin, center loin (chops), bone-in, separable lean only, cooked, braised	202	30	8	0	12.76	0.43
Pork, fresh, loin, center loin (chops), bone-in, separable lean only, cooked, pan-fried	232	32	10	0	15.23	0.48
Pork, fresh, loin, center loin (chops), bone-in, separable lean only, cooked, broiled	202	27	7	0	14.73	0.55
Pork, fresh, loin, center loin (roasts), bone-in, separable lean only, cooked, roasted	199	28	9	0	13.10	0.47
Pork, fresh, loin, center loin (roasts), bone-in, separable lean and fat, cooked, roasted	234	26	13	0	12.58	0.48
Pork, fresh, loin, center rib (chops or roasts), bone-in, separable lean only, raw	136	22	5	0	9.07	0.41
Pork, fresh, loin, center rib (chops or roasts), bone-in, separable lean and fat, raw	188	20	11	0	8.38	0.42
Pork, fresh, loin, center rib (chops or roasts), boneless, separable lean only, raw	152	22	6	0	8.86	0.40
Pork, fresh, loin, center rib (chops or roasts), boneless, separable lean and fat, raw	211	20	14	0	8.24	0.41
Pork, fresh, loin, center rib (chops), bone-in, separable lean and fat, cooked, braised	250	27	15	0	10.69	0.40
Pork, fresh, loin, center rib (chops), bone-in, separable lean and fat, cooked, pan-fried	265	26	17	0	11.61	0.45
Pork, fresh, loin, center rib (chops), bone-in, separable lean and fat, cooked, broiled	222	24	13	0	13.35	0.56
Pork, fresh, loin, center rib (chops), bone-in, separable lean only, cooked, braised	206	28	9	0	11.23	0.40
Pork, fresh, loin, center rib (chops), bone-in, separable lean only, cooked, pan-fried	218	28	11	0	12.35	0.44
Pork, fresh, loin, center rib (chops), bone-in, separable lean only, cooked, broiled	186	26	8	0	14.18	0.55
Pork, fresh, loin, center rib (chops), boneless, separable lean and fat, cooked, braised	255	26	16	0	10.61	0.41
Pork, fresh, loin, center rib (chops), boneless, separable lean and fat, cooked, pan-fried	273	26	18	0	11.33	0.44
Pork, fresh, loin, center rib (chops), boneless, separable lean and fat, cooked, broiled	260	28	16	0	12.84	0.46
Pork, fresh, loin, center rib (chops), boneless, separable lean only, cooked, braised	211	28	10	0	11.03	0.39
Pork, fresh, loin, center rib (chops), boneless, separable lean only, cooked, pan-fried	224	28	12	0	12.03	0.43
Pork, fresh, loin, center rib (chops), boneless, separable lean only, cooked, broiled	216	29	10	0	13.54	0.47
Pork, fresh, loin, center rib (roasts), bone-in, separable lean and fat, cooked, roasted	255	27	15	0	12.23	0.45
Pork, fresh, loin, center rib (roasts), bone-in, separable lean only, cooked, roasted	223	29	11	0	12.75	0.44
Pork, fresh, loin, center rib (roasts), boneless, separable lean only, cooked, roasted	214	29	10	0	14	0.48
Pork, fresh, loin, center rib (roasts), boneless, separable lean and fat, cooked, roasted	252	27	15	0	13.22	0.49
Pork, fresh, loin, country-style ribs, separable lean and fat, cooked, braised	296	26	18	0	10.16	0.39
Pork, fresh, loin, country-style ribs, separable lean and fat, cooked, roasted	328	23	25	0	11.68	0.51
Pork, fresh, loin, country-style ribs, separable lean and fat, raw	241	19	12	0	7.56	0.40
Pork, fresh, loin, country-style ribs, separable lean only, cooked, braised	234	28	14	0	10.93	0.39
Pork, fresh, loin, country-style ribs, separable lean only, cooked, roasted	247	27	15	0	12.88	0.48

Pork Products

Food Description	Kcals	Protein	Fat	Carbs	PRAL	Acid Density
Pork, fresh, loin, country-style ribs, separable lean only, raw	157	21	6	0	8.52	0.41
Pork, fresh, loin, sirloin (chops or roasts), bone-in, separable lean only, raw	142	22	4	0	9.77	0.44
Pork, fresh, loin, sirloin (chops or roasts), bone-in, separable lean and fat, raw	205	20	9	0	9.14	0.46
Pork, fresh, loin, sirloin (chops or roasts), boneless, separable lean and fat, raw	145	21	6	0	9.59	0.46
Pork, fresh, loin, sirloin (chops or roasts), boneless, separable lean only, raw	128	21	4	0	9.77	0.47
Pork, fresh, loin, sirloin (chops), bone-in, separable lean and fat, cooked, braised	245	25	15	0	11.31	0.45
Pork, fresh, loin, sirloin (chops), bone-in, separable lean and fat, cooked, broiled	259	27	16	0	13.14	0.49
Pork, fresh, loin, sirloin (chops), bone-in, separable lean only, cooked, braised	197	27	9	0	11.99	0.44
Pork, fresh, loin, sirloin (chops), bone-in, separable lean only, cooked, broiled	213	28	10	0	14.05	0.50
Pork, fresh, loin, sirloin (chops), boneless, separable lean and fat, cooked, braised	189	27	8	0	11.59	0.43
Pork, fresh, loin, sirloin (chops), boneless, separable lean and fat, cooked, broiled	208	31	9	0	15.19	0.49
Pork, fresh, loin, sirloin (chops), boneless, separable lean only, cooked, braised	175	27	7	0	11.74	0.43
Pork, fresh, loin, sirloin (chops), boneless, separable lean only, cooked, broiled	193	31	7	0	15.50	0.50
Pork, fresh, loin, sirloin (roasts), bone-in, separable lean and fat, cooked, roasted	261	27	13	0	13.21	0.49
Pork, fresh, loin, sirloin (roasts), bone-in, separable lean only, cooked, roasted	216	28	9	0	13.95	0.50
Pork, fresh, loin, sirloin (roasts), boneless, separable lean and fat, cooked, roasted	207	28	9	0	13.96	0.50
Pork, fresh, loin, sirloin (roasts), boneless, separable lean only, cooked, roasted	198	29	8	0	14.10	0.49
Pork, fresh, loin, tenderloin, separable lean and fat, cooked, broiled	201	30	8	0	15.06	0.50
Pork, fresh, loin, tenderloin, separable lean and fat, cooked, roasted	173	26	4	0	13.26	0.51
Pork, fresh, loin, tenderloin, separable lean and fat, raw	136	21	4	0	10.02	0.48
Pork, fresh, loin, tenderloin, separable lean only, cooked, broiled	187	30	6	0	15.34	0.51
Pork, fresh, loin, tenderloin, separable lean only, cooked, roasted	143	26	4	0	13.38	0.51
Pork, fresh, loin, tenderloin, separable lean only, raw	120	21	2	0	10.22	0.49
Pork, fresh, loin, top loin (chops), boneless, enhanced, separable lean only, cooked, pan-broiled	169	29	5	0	14.31	0.49
Pork, fresh, loin, top loin (chops), boneless, enhanced, separable lean and fat, cooked, pan-broiled	190	28	8	0	14.01	0.50
Pork, fresh, loin, top loin (chops), boneless, separable lean and fat, raw	185	22	7	0	8.47	0.39
Pork, fresh, loin, top loin (chops), boneless, separable lean and fat, cooked, braised	233	26	13	0	11.16	0.43
Pork, fresh, loin, top loin (chops), boneless, separable lean and fat, cooked, pan-fried	257	29	15	0	12.84	0.44
Pork, fresh, loin, top loin (chops), boneless, separable lean and fat, cooked, broiled	197	27	9	0	13.90	0.51
Pork, fresh, loin, top loin (chops), boneless, separable lean only, cooked, braised	202	29	9	0	11.46	0.40

Pork Products

Food Description	Kcals	Protein	Fat	Carbs	PRAL	Acid Density
Pork, fresh, loin, top loin (chops), boneless, separable lean only, raw	141	22	3	0	8.92	0.41
Pork, fresh, loin, top loin (chops), boneless, separable lean only, cooked, pan-fried	225	30	11	0	13.39	0.45
Pork, fresh, loin, top loin (chops), boneless, separable lean only, cooked, broiled	203	28	6	0	14.37	0.51
Pork, fresh, loin, top loin (roasts), boneless, separable lean and fat, raw	191	21	8	0	8.40	0.40
Pork, fresh, loin, top loin (roasts), boneless, separable lean and fat, cooked, roasted	226	26	9	0	14.22	0.55
Pork, fresh, loin, top loin (roasts), boneless, separable lean only, raw	141	22	4	0	8.92	0.41
Pork, fresh, loin, top loin (roasts), boneless, separable lean only, cooked, roasted	194	27	6	0	14.84	0.55
Pork, fresh, loin, whole, separable lean and fat, cooked, braised	239	27	14	0	11.41	0.42
Pork, fresh, loin, whole, separable lean and fat, cooked, broiled	242	27	14	0	12.63	0.47
Pork, fresh, loin, whole, separable lean and fat, cooked, roasted	248	27	15	0	12.73	0.47
Pork, fresh, loin, whole, separable lean and fat, raw	198	20	13	0	8.70	0.44
Pork, fresh, loin, whole, separable lean only, cooked, braised	204	29	9	0	11.88	0.41
Pork, fresh, loin, whole, separable lean only, cooked, broiled	210	29	10	0	13.18	0.45
Pork, fresh, loin, whole, separable lean only, cooked, roasted	209	29	10	0	13.35	0.46
Pork, fresh, loin, whole, separable lean only, raw	143	21	6	0	9.32	0.44
Pork, fresh, separable fat, cooked	635	9	66	0	6.16	0.68
Pork, fresh, separable fat, raw	638	6	71	0	3.28	0.55
Pork, fresh, shoulder, arm picnic, separable lean and fat, cooked, braised	329	28	23	0	13.08	0.47
Pork, fresh, shoulder, arm picnic, separable lean and fat, cooked, roasted	317	23	24	0	12.42	0.54
Pork, fresh, shoulder, arm picnic, separable lean and fat, raw	253	17	20	0	8.55	0.50
Pork, fresh, shoulder, arm picnic, separable lean only, cooked, braised	248	32	12	0	14.98	0.47
Pork, fresh, shoulder, arm picnic, separable lean only, cooked, roasted	228	27	13	0	14.20	0.53
Pork, fresh, shoulder, blade, Boston (roasts), separable lean and fat, cooked, roasted	269	23	19	0	10.80	0.47
Pork, fresh, shoulder, blade, Boston (roasts), separable lean only, cooked, roasted	232	24	14	0	10.56	0.44
Pork, fresh, shoulder, blade, Boston (steaks), separable lean and fat, cooked, braised	319	25	18	0	11.61	0.46
Pork, fresh, shoulder, blade, Boston (steaks), separable lean and fat, cooked, broiled	259	26	17	0	12.44	0.48
Pork, fresh, shoulder, blade, Boston (steaks), separable lean only, cooked, braised	273	27	13	0	12.41	0.46
Pork, fresh, shoulder, blade, Boston (steaks), separable lean only, cooked, broiled	227	27	13	0	12.98	0.48
Pork, fresh, shoulder, whole, separable lean and fat, cooked, roasted	292	23	21	0	11.56	0.50
Pork, fresh, shoulder, whole, separable lean and fat, raw	236	17	18	0	8.14	0.48
Pork, fresh, shoulder, whole, separable lean only, cooked, roasted	230	25	14	0	12.56	0.50

Pork Products

Food Description	Kcals	Protein	Fat	Carbs	PRAL	Acid Density
Pork, fresh, shoulder, whole, separable lean only, raw	148	20	7	0	9.16	0.46
Pork, fresh, spareribs, separable lean and fat, cooked, braised	397	29	30	0	15.94	0.55
Pork, fresh, spareribs, separable lean and fat, raw	286	15	23	0	10.80	0.72
Pork, fresh, variety meats and by-products, brain, cooked, braised	138	12	10	0	9.56	0.80
Pork, fresh, variety meats and by-products, brain, raw	127	10	9	0	9.55	0.96
Pork, fresh, variety meats and by-products, chitterlings, cooked, simmered	233	12	20	0	7.70	0.64
Pork, fresh, variety meats and by-products, chitterlings, raw	182	8	17	0	4.77	0.60
Pork, fresh, variety meats and by-products, ears, frozen, cooked, simmered	166	16	11	0	7.44	0.47
Pork, fresh, variety meats and by-products, ears, frozen, raw	234	22	15	1	10.90	0.50
Pork, fresh, variety meats and by-products, feet, cooked, simmered	232	22	16	0	12.96	0.59
Pork, fresh, variety meats and by-products, feet, raw	212	23	13	0	11.73	0.51
Pork, fresh, variety meats and by-products, heart, cooked, braised	148	24	5	0	13.10	0.55
Pork, fresh, variety meats and by-products, heart, raw	118	17	4	1	7.98	0.47
Pork, fresh, variety meats and by-products, jowl, raw	655	6	70	0	3.07	0.51
Pork, fresh, variety meats and by-products, kidneys, cooked, braised	151	25	5	0	17.68	0.71
Pork, fresh, variety meats and by-products, kidneys, raw	100	16	3	0	10.24	0.64
Pork, fresh, variety meats and by-products, leaf fat, raw	857	2	94	0	0.87	0.44
Pork, fresh, variety meats and by-products, liver, cooked, braised	165	26	4	4	18.02	0.69
Pork, fresh, variety meats and by-products, liver, raw	134	21	4	2	14.81	0.71
Pork, fresh, variety meats and by-products, lungs, cooked, braised	99	17	3	0	11.42	0.67
Pork, fresh, variety meats and by-products, lungs, raw	85	14	3	0	7.33	0.52
Pork, fresh, variety meats and by-products, mechanically separated, raw	304	15	27	0	3.99	0.27
Pork, fresh, variety meats and by-products, pancreas, cooked, braised	219	28	11	0	20.39	0.73
Pork, fresh, variety meats and by-products, pancreas, raw	199	19	13	0	13.03	0.69
Pork, fresh, variety meats and by-products, spleen, cooked, braised	149	28	3	0	18.96	0.68
Pork, fresh, variety meats and by-products, spleen, raw	100	18	3	0	9.58	0.53
Pork, fresh, variety meats and by-products, stomach, cooked, simmered	157	21	7	0	12.88	0.61
Pork, fresh, variety meats and by-products, stomach, raw	159	17	10	0	9.69	0.57
Pork, fresh, variety meats and by-products, tail, cooked, simmered	396	17	36	0	6.40	0.38
Pork, fresh, variety meats and by-products, tail, raw	378	18	33	0	2.77	0.15
Pork, fresh, variety meats and by-products, tongue, cooked, braised	271	24	19	0	12.50	0.52

Pork Products

Food Description	Kcals	Protein	Fat	Carbs	PRAL	Acid Density
Pork, fresh, variety meats and by-products, tongue, raw	225	16	17	0	9.34	0.58
Pork, oriental style, dehydrated	615	12	62	1	7.18	0.60
Pork, pickled pork hocks	171	19	11	0	10.19	0.54
USDA Commodity, pork, cured, ham, boneless, cooked, heated	149	19	8	0	13.51	0.71
USDA Commodity, pork, cured, ham, boneless, cooked, unheated	133	17	6	1	12.50	0.74
USDA Commodity, pork, ground, fine/coarse, frozen, cooked	265	24	18	0	12.85	0.54
USDA Commodity, pork, ground, fine/coarse, frozen, raw	221	15	17	0	7.30	0.49

Breakfast Cereals

Food Description	Kcals	Protein	Fat	Carbs	PRAL	Alkali Density
AMARANTH FLAKES	353	16	7	71	11.57	0.16
Cereals ready-to-eat, bran flakes, single brand	320	9	2	80	4.17	0.05
Cereals ready-to-eat, bran, malted flour, single brand	287	13	2	78	8.20	0.11
Cereals ready-to-eat, corn flakes, low sodium	399	8	0	89	3.15	0.04
Cereals ready-to-eat, corn flakes, plain, single brand	360	7	0	87	2.29	0.03
Cereals ready-to-eat, granola, homemade	489	15	24	53	7.24	0.14
Cereals ready-to-eat, HEALTH VALLEY, FIBER 7 Flakes	353	14	1	78	4.84	0.06
Cereals ready-to-eat, HEALTHY CHOICE, KELLOGG'S Almond Crunch with Raisins	360	9	5	79	2.48	0.03
Cereals ready-to-eat, JUST RIGHT with Crunchy Nuggets	371	8	3	84	4.34	0.05
Cereals ready-to-eat, KASHI 7 Whole Grain Flakes by KELLOGG	350	11	2	82	6.27	0.08
Cereals ready-to-eat, KASHI GOLEAN by Kellogg	284	26	2	58	4.80	0.08
Cereals ready-to-eat, KASHI GOLEAN CRUNCH! by KELLOGG	377	17	6	68	1.28	0.02
Cereals ready-to-eat, KASHI Good Friends by Kellogg	316	9	4	82	-0.46	-0.01
Cereals ready-to-eat, KASHI HEART TO HEART Wild Blueberry by KELLOGG	369	11	5	76	1.37	0.02
Cereals ready-to-eat, KASHI Medley by Kellogg	354	11	13	67	-0.27	0
Cereals ready-to-eat, KASHI MIGHTY BITES Cinnamon Cereal	356	17	4	70	4.60	0.07
Cereals ready-to-eat, KASHI MIGHTY BITES, Honey Crunch Cereal	353	17	4	69	4.91	0.07
Cereals ready-to-eat, KASHI, CINNA-RAISIN CRUNCH by KELLOGG	330	8	3	82	-2.40	-0.03
Cereals ready-to-eat, KASHI, ORGANIC PROMISE Autumn Wheat by KELLOGG	335	10	2	83	3.13	0.04
Cereals ready-to-eat, KASHI, SEVEN IN THE MORNING by KELLOGG	356	12	3	81	4.88	0.06
Cereals ready-to-eat, MALT-O-MEAL, Corn Flakes	380	6	0	88	2.96	0.03
Cereals ready-to-eat, MALT-O-MEAL, Crispy Rice	381	6	1	86	4.24	0.05
Cereals ready-to-eat, MALT-O-MEAL, Frosted Flakes	387	5	0	91	2.09	0.02
Cereals ready-to-eat, MALT-O-MEAL, Frosted Whole Wheat Cereal	388	9	2	83	5.86	0.07
Cereals ready-to-eat, MALT-O-MEAL, Honey Nut TOASTY O'S Cereal	390	10	2	82	3.66	0.04
Cereals ready-to-eat, MALT-O-MEAL, MARSHMALLOW MATEYS	394	7	4	83	1.17	0.01
Cereals ready-to-eat, MALT-O-MEAL, Puffed Rice Cereal	401	8	1	90	5.06	0.06
Cereals ready-to-eat, MALT-O-MEAL, Puffed Wheat Cereal	396	16	2	79	9.63	0.12
Cereals ready-to-eat, MALT-O-MEAL, Raisin Bran Cereal	361	9	2	77	2.98	0.04
Cereals ready-to-eat, MALT-O-MEAL, TOOTIE FRUITIES	401	5	3	88	-2.32	-0.03
Cereals ready-to-eat, MUESLI, dried fruit and nuts	340	10	5	78	1.51	0.02
Cereals ready-to-eat, NATURE'S PATH, OPTIMUM	345	15	5	73	-3.45	-0.05

Breakfast Cereals

Food Description	Kcals	Protein	Fat	Carbs	PRAL	Alkali Density
Cereals ready-to-eat, NATURE'S PATH, OPTIMUM SLIM	327	16	5	69	-8.83	-0.13
Cereals ready-to-eat, OAT BRAN FLAKES, HEALTH VALLEY	353	11	1	79	12.39	0.16
Cereals ready-to-eat, oat, corn and wheat squares, presweetened, maple flavored	430	6	10	80	3.49	0.04
Cereals ready-to-eat, oats, corn puffed mixture, presweetened, single brand	405	8	4	83	5.36	0.06
Cereals ready-to-eat, oats, corn puffed mixture, presweetened, with marshmallows, single brand	398	6	3	87	4.42	0.05
Cereals ready-to-eat, Puffed KASHI by Kellogg	394	12	3	80	3.23	0.04
Cereals ready-to-eat, QUAKER, 100% Natural Granola Oats and Honey	455	10	13	73	3.05	0.04
Cereals ready-to-eat, QUAKER, Honey Graham bagged cereal	395	6	5	84	2.88	0.03
Cereals ready-to-eat, QUAKER, HONEY GRAHAM OH!S	411	4	7	84	3.74	0.04
Cereals ready-to-eat, QUAKER, Honey Nut Oats	385	6	4	85	6.28	0.07
Cereals ready-to-eat, QUAKER, KING VITAMAN	386	7	3	85	4.46	0.05
Cereals ready-to-eat, QUAKER, KRETSCHMER Honey Crunch Wheat Germ	372	27	8	58	22.45	0.39
Cereals ready-to-eat, QUAKER, KRETSCHMER Toasted Wheat Bran	200	18	5	60	13.64	0.23
Cereals ready-to-eat, QUAKER, KRETSCHMER Wheat Germ, Regular	366	31	10	49	25.38	0.52
Cereals ready-to-eat, QUAKER, Low Fat 100% Natural Granola with Raisins	390	8	6	81	2.23	0.03
Cereals ready-to-eat, QUAKER, MOTHER'S CINNAMON OAT CRUNCH	380	10	5	75	3.42	0.05
Cereals ready-to-eat, QUAKER, MOTHER'S COCOA BUMPERS	376	5	2	88	-11.22	-0.13
Cereals ready-to-eat, QUAKER, MOTHER'S GROOVY GRAHAMS	372	5	2	86	-10.47	-0.12
Cereals ready-to-eat, QUAKER, MOTHER'S HONEY ROUNDUP	382	5	2	88	3.01	0.03
Cereals ready-to-eat, QUAKER, MOTHER'S PEANUT BUTTER BUMPERS Cereal	403	8	7	78	-4.85	-0.06
Cereals ready-to-eat, QUAKER, MOTHER'S TOASTED OAT BRAN CEREAL, Brown Sugar Flavor	373	12	5	75	7.91	0.11
Cereals ready-to-eat, QUAKER, Oatmeal Cereal, Brown Sugar Bliss	384	9	6	80	2.52	0.03
Cereals ready-to-eat, QUAKER, QUAKER 100% Natural Cereal with oats, honey, and raisins	465	9	11	74	1.55	0.02
Cereals ready-to-eat, QUAKER, QUAKER Oat Bran Cereal	372	12	5	75	9.18	0.12
Cereals ready-to-eat, QUAKER, QUAKER OAT CINNAMON LIFE	375	9	4	79	6.33	0.08
Cereals ready-to-eat, QUAKER, QUAKER OAT LIFE, plain	375	10	4	78	7.18	0.09
Cereals ready-to-eat, QUAKER, QUAKER OATMEAL SQUARES	378	11	4	78	5.64	0.07
Cereals ready-to-eat, QUAKER, QUAKER Puffed Rice	383	7	1	88	4.46	0.05
Cereals ready-to-eat, QUAKER, QUAKER Puffed Wheat	366	16	2	76	8.80	0.12
Cereals ready-to-eat, QUAKER, QUAKER SWEET PUFFS	391	7	2	88	3.80	0.04
Cereals ready-to-eat, QUAKER, SUN COUNTRY Granola with Almonds	467	12	18	67	5.01	0.07

Breakfast Cereals

Food Description	Kcals	Protein	Fat	Carbs	PRAL	Alkali Density
Cereals ready-to-eat, QUAKER, SWEET CRUNCH/QUISP	405	5	6	85	2.85	0.03
Cereals ready-to-eat, QUAKER, Toasted Oats/OATMMM'S	380	9	5	78	9.66	0.12
Cereals ready-to-eat, Ralston Corn Biscuits	367	6	1	86	-2.93	-0.03
Cereals ready-to-eat, Ralston Corn Flakes	357	6	1	88	2.09	0.02
Cereals ready-to-eat, Ralston Crispy Hexagons	379	6	1	87	2.64	0.03
Cereals ready-to-eat, Ralston Crispy Rice	364	7	1	86	3.93	0.05
Cereals ready-to-eat, Ralston Enriched Bran flakes	310	10	3	83	5.96	0.07
Cereals ready-to-eat, Ralston TASTEEOS	398	12	6	84	10.86	0.13
Cereals ready-to-eat, rice, puffed, fortified	402	6	0	90	3.61	0.04
Cereals ready-to-eat, rice, puffed, presweetened, fruit flavored, single brand	401	4	4	88	1.04	0.01
Cereals ready-to-eat, rice, puffed, presweetened, with cocoa, single brand	398	4	4	88	0.52	0.01
Cereals ready-to-eat, UNCLE SAM CEREAL	431	16	12	66	5.71	0.09
Cereals ready-to-eat, USDA Commodity Corn and Rice (includes all commodity brands)	378	6	1	87	2.98	0.03
Cereals ready-to-eat, USDA Commodity Rice Crisps (includes all commodity brands)	381	6	1	86	3.75	0.04
Cereals ready-to-eat, WAFFELOS	405	6	4	86	30.14	0.35
Cereals ready-to-eat, WEETABIX WHOLE WHEAT CEREAL	373	11	3	77	-3.13	-0.04
Cereals ready-to-eat, wheat and bran, presweetened with nuts and fruits	385	7	6	76	1.37	0.02
Cereals ready-to-eat, wheat and malt barley flakes	365	10	3	82	5.74	0.07
Cereals ready-to-eat, wheat germ, toasted, plain	382	29	11	50	27.86	0.56
Cereals ready-to-eat, wheat, bran, shredded, plain, salt and sugar free, single brand	334	13	1	80	7.88	0.10
Cereals ready-to-eat, wheat, puffed, fortified	364	15	1	80	8.89	0.11
Cereals ready-to-eat, wheat, puffed, presweetened, single brand	398	5	1	91	3.32	0.04
Cereals ready-to-eat, wheat, shredded, plain, sugar and salt free, spoon size, single brand	340	10	1	83	5.96	0.07
Cereals ready-to-eat, wheat, shredded, plain, sugar and salt free	337	11	2	79	7.25	0.09
Cereals ready-to-eat, wheat, shredded, presweetened, single brand	352	8	2	84	4.58	0.05
Cereals ready-to-eat, whole wheat, rolled oats, presweetened, with nuts and fruit, single brand	377	8	8	73	1.77	0.02
Cereals ready-to-eat, whole wheat, rolled oats, presweetened, with pecans	408	9	12	71	3.44	0.05
Cereals ready-to-eat, whole wheat, rolled oats, presweetened, with walnuts and fruit, single brand	422	8	10	74	6.94	0.09
Cereals ready-to-eat, whole wheat, shredded, presweetened, single brand	385	10	4	81	5.60	0.07
Cereals, corn grits, white, regular and quick, enriched, cooked with water, without salt	59	1	0	13	0.49	0.04
Cereals, corn grits, white, regular and quick, enriched, dry	371	9	1	80	3.40	0.04
Cereals, corn grits, white, regular and quick, unenriched, cooked with water, without salt	59	1	0	13	0.49	0.04

Breakfast Cereals

Food Description	Kcals	Protein	Fat	Carbs	PRAL	Alkali Density
Cereals, corn grits, white, regular and quick, unenriched, dry	371	9	1	80	3.40	0.04
Cereals, corn grits, white, regular, quick, enriched, cooked with water, with salt	59	1	0	13	0.49	0.04
Cereals, corn grits, white, regular, quick, unenriched, cooked with water, with salt	60	1	0	13	0.56	0.04
Cereals, corn grits, yellow, regular and quick, enriched, cooked with water, without salt	59	1	0	13	0.49	0.04
Cereals, corn grits, yellow, regular and quick, enriched, dry	371	9	1	80	3.40	0.04
Cereals, corn grits, yellow, regular and quick, unenriched, cooked with water, without salt	59	1	0	13	0.49	0.04
Cereals, corn grits, yellow, regular and quick, unenriched, dry	371	9	1	80	3.40	0.04
Cereals, corn grits, yellow, regular, quick, enriched, cooked with water, with salt	59	1	0	13	0.49	0.04
Cereals, corn grits, yellow, regular, quick, unenriched, cooked with water, with salt	59	1	0	13	0.49	0.04
Cereals, CREAM OF RICE, cooked with water, with salt	52	1	0	11	0.53	0.05
Cereals, CREAM OF RICE, cooked with water, without salt	52	1	0	11	0.53	0.05
Cereals, CREAM OF RICE, dry	370	6	0	82	3.76	0.05
Cereals, CREAM OF WHEAT, instant, dry	366	11	1	76	1.06	0.01
Cereals, CREAM OF WHEAT, instant, prepared with water, with salt, (wheat)	62	2	0	13	0.16	0.01
Cereals, CREAM OF WHEAT, instant, prepared with water, without salt	62	2	0	13	0.16	0.01
Cereals, CREAM OF WHEAT, mix'n eat, apple, banana and maple flavored, prepared	88	2	0	19	-0.01	0
Cereals, CREAM OF WHEAT, mix'n eat, apple, banana and maple flavored, dry	373	7	1	82	0.09	0
Cereals, CREAM OF WHEAT, mix'n eat, plain, dry	361	10	1	76	2.92	0.04
Cereals, CREAM OF WHEAT, mix'n eat, plain, prepared with water	72	2	0	15	0.57	0.04
Cereals, CREAM OF WHEAT, quick, cooked with water, with salt	54	1	0	11	1.48	0.13
Cereals, CREAM OF WHEAT, quick, cooked with water, without salt	54	1	0	11	1.48	0.13
Cereals, CREAM OF WHEAT, quick, dry	361	10	1	75	7.90	0.11
Cereals, CREAM OF WHEAT, regular, cooked with water, with salt, (wheat)	52	2	0	11	0.31	0.03
Cereals, CREAM OF WHEAT, regular, cooked with water, without salt	52	2	0	11	0.31	0.03
Cereals, CREAM OF WHEAT, regular, dry	370	11	1	77	2.23	0.03
Cereals, farina, enriched, cooked with water, with salt	48	1	0	10	0.76	0.08
Cereals, farina, enriched, cooked with water, without salt	48	1	0	10	0.76	0.08
Cereals, farina, enriched, dry	369	11	0	78	5.95	0.08
Cereals, farina, unenriched, dry	369	11	0	78	5.95	0.08
Cereals, Oat Bran, QUAKER, QUAKER/MOTHER'S Oat Bran, prepared with water, salt	43	2	1	7	1.65	0.24
Cereals, oats, instant, fortified, plain, dry	369	13	6	68	4.88	0.07
Cereals, oats, instant, fortified, plain, prepared with water	55	2	1	13	0.69	0.05

Breakfast Cereals

Food Description	Kcals	Protein	Fat	Carbs	PRAL	Alkali Density
Cereals, oats, instant, fortified, with cinnamon and spice, dry	370	9	5	77	4.61	0.06
Cereals, oats, instant, fortified, with cinnamon and spice, prepared with water	107	2	1	22	1.26	0.06
Cereals, oats, instant, fortified, with raisins and spice, dry	360	8	4	76	0.72	0.01
Cereals, oats, instant, fortified, with raisins and spice, prepared with water	100	2	1	20	0.14	0.01
Cereals, oats, regular and quick and instant, not fortified, dry	384	13	7	69	13.50	0.20
Cereals, oats, regular and quick and instant, unenriched, cooked with water, with salt	62	3	2	14	2.18	0.16
Cereals, oats, regular and quick and instant, unenriched, cooked with water, without salt	63	3	2	14	2.18	0.16
Cereals, QUAKER Instant Oatmeal, NUTRITION FOR WOMEN, Vanilla Cinnamon, prepared with boiling water	104	3	1	20	-0.46	-0.02
Cereals, QUAKER, corn grits, instant, butter flavor, dry	366	8	6	75	-2.06	-0.03
Cereals, QUAKER, corn grits, instant, butter flavor, prepared with water	71	2	1	14	-0.43	-0.03
Cereals, QUAKER, corn grits, instant, cheddar cheese flavor, dry	366	8	6	73	4.11	0.06
Cereals, QUAKER, corn grits, instant, cheddar cheese flavor, prepared with water	72	2	1	14	0.73	0.05
Cereals, QUAKER, corn grits, instant, country bacon (imitation bacon bits), prepared with water	69	2	0	15	0.58	0.04
Cereals, QUAKER, corn grits, instant, plain, dry	342	8	1	79	3.92	0.05
Cereals, QUAKER, corn grits, instant, plain, prepared with water	68	2	0	15	0.71	0.05
Cereals, QUAKER, corn grits, instant, with imitation bacon bits, dry	349	10	2	77	3.37	0.04
Cereals, QUAKER, Creamy Wheat, farina, enriched, prepared with water, no salt	51	2	0	11	0.80	0.07
Cereals, QUAKER, Creamy Wheat, farina, enriched, prepared with water, salt	51	2	0	11	0.80	0.07
Cereals, QUAKER, farina, Creamy Wheat, enriched, dry	349	11	1	75	5.79	0.08
Cereals, QUAKER, farina, enriched cinnamon flavor, dry	346	12	1	75	6.21	0.08
Cereals, QUAKER, hominy grits, white, quick, dry	347	9	1	79	5.93	0.08
Cereals, QUAKER, hominy grits, white, regular, dry	347	9	1	79	5.93	0.08
Cereals, QUAKER, hominy grits, yellow, quick, dry	337	8	2	78	4.03	0.05
Cereals, QUAKER, Instant Grits Product with American Cheese Flavor, Dry	364	9	5	75	3.56	0.05
Cereals, QUAKER, Instant Grits Product with Imitation Bacon Bits and Cheddar Flavor, Dry	363	10	5	72	3.38	0.05
Cereals, QUAKER, Instant Grits Product with Redeye Gravy and Imitation Ham Bits, Dry	346	10	2	77	3.27	0.04
Cereals, QUAKER, Instant Grits Product--Ham 'n' Cheese	359	11	5	72	3.18	0.04
Cereals, QUAKER, Instant Oatmeal EXPRESS Cinnamon Roll, Dry	371	9	5	76	5.49	0.07
Cereals, QUAKER, Instant Oatmeal EXPRESS, Baked Apple, dry	367	8	5	77	3.46	0.04
Cereals, QUAKER, Instant Oatmeal EXPRESS, Golden Brown Sugar, dry	372	8	5	77	5.25	0.07

Breakfast Cereals

Food Description	Kcals	Protein	Fat	Carbs	PRAL	Alkali Density
Cereals, QUAKER, Instant Oatmeal, apples and cinnamon, dry	365	8	4	78	1.34	0.02
Cereals, QUAKER, Instant Oatmeal, Baked Apple, dry	363	8	4	77	-1.34	-0.02
Cereals, QUAKER, Instant Oatmeal, Baked Apple, prepared with boiling water	96	2	1	19	-0.39	-0.02
Cereals, QUAKER, Instant Oatmeal, Banana Bread, dry	368	4	2	31	3.86	0.12
Cereals, QUAKER, Instant Oatmeal, Cinnamon Spice, prepared with boiling water	107	2	1	22	1.26	0.06
Cereals, QUAKER, Instant Oatmeal, Cinnamon-Spice, dry	370	9	5	77	4.61	0.06
Cereals, QUAKER, Instant Oatmeal, DINOSAUR EGGS with DINOSAUR BONES, Brown Sugar Cinnamon, prepared with boiling water	119	2	2	23	1.16	0.05
Cereals, QUAKER, Instant Oatmeal, EXPRESS Baked Apple, prepared with boiling water	120	3	1	24	1.05	0.04
Cereals, QUAKER, Instant Oatmeal, EXPRESS Cinnamon Roll, prepared with boiling water	121	3	2	24	1.69	0.07
Cereals, QUAKER, Instant Oatmeal, EXPRESS, Golden Brown Sugar, prepared with boiling water	121	3	1	24	1.60	0.07
Cereals, QUAKER, Instant Oatmeal, French Vanilla Flavor, dry	369	9	5	76	4.89	0.06
Cereals, QUAKER, Instant Oatmeal, French Vanilla, prepared with boiling water	102	4	2	33	1.25	0.04
Cereals, QUAKER, Instant Oatmeal, fruit and cream variety, dry	386	8	8	75	2.83	0.04
Cereals, QUAKER, Instant Oatmeal, fruit and cream variety, prepared with boiling water	72	1	1	14	0.48	0.03
Cereals, QUAKER, Instant Oatmeal, Honey Nut, dry	389	9	8	73	4.81	0.07
Cereals, QUAKER, Instant Oatmeal, Honey Nut, prepared with boiling water	107	2	2	19	1.24	0.07
Cereals, QUAKER, Instant Oatmeal, low sodium, dry	365	13	7	67	6.62	0.10
Cereals, QUAKER, Instant Oatmeal, maple and brown sugar, dry	366	9	5	75	4.75	0.06
Cereals, QUAKER, Instant Oatmeal, maple and brown sugar, prepared with boiling water	101	2	1	20	1.22	0.06
Cereals, QUAKER, Instant Oatmeal, NUTRITION FOR WOMEN, Apple Spice, prepared with boiling water	107	3	1	21	-0.99	-0.05
Cereals, QUAKER, Instant Oatmeal, NUTRITION FOR WOMEN, Apple Spice, dry	360	11	4	74	-3.44	-0.05
Cereals, QUAKER, Instant Oatmeal, NUTRITION FOR WOMEN, Golden Brown Sugar, prepared with boiling water	105	3	1	20	-0.72	-0.04
Cereals, QUAKER, Instant Oatmeal, NUTRITION FOR WOMEN, Golden Brown Sugar, dry	363	12	5	72	-2.45	-0.03
Cereals, QUAKER, Instant Oatmeal, NUTRITION FOR WOMEN, Vanilla Cinnamon, dry	363	12	5	72	-1.50	-0.02
Cereals, QUAKER, Instant Oatmeal, Raisin and Spice, dry	360	8	4	76	0.72	0.01
Cereals, QUAKER, Instant Oatmeal, Raisin and Spice, prepared	100	2	1	20	0.14	0.01
Cereals, QUAKER, Instant Oatmeal, raisins, dates and walnuts, dry	365	8	5	74	1.82	0.02
Cereals, QUAKER, Instant Oatmeal, TREASURE HUNT, prepared with boiling water	108	2	1	22	1.04	0.05

Breakfast Cereals

Food Description	Kcals	Protein	Fat	Carbs	PRAL	Alkali Density
Cereals, QUAKER, Instant Oatmeal, TREASURE HUNT, dry	369	8	5	77	3.70	0.05
Cereals, QUAKER, Mother's Instant Oatmeal (Non-Fortified), Dry	359	14	7	66	11.45	0.17
Cereals, QUAKER, Oat Bran, QUAKER/MOTHER'S Oat Bran, dry	364	17	8	63	14.57	0.23
Cereals, QUAKER, Oat Bran, QUAKER/MOTHER'S Oat Bran, prepared with water, no salt	43	2	1	7	1.69	0.24
Cereals, QUAKER, oatmeal, instant, low sodium, prepared with water	93	4	2	17	1.81	0.11
Cereals, QUAKER, oatmeal, instant, raisins, dates and walnuts, prepared with water	116	3	2	24	0.55	0.02
Cereals, QUAKER, QUAKER MultiGrain Oatmeal, dry	333	11	3	73	6.27	0.09
Cereals, QUAKER, QUAKER MultiGrain Oatmeal, prepared with water, salt	61	2	0	13	1.09	0.08
Cereals, QUAKER, QUAKER MultiGrain Oatmeal, prepared with water, no salt	61	2	0	13	1.13	0.09
Cereals, QUAKER, Quick Oats, Dry	371	14	7	68	8.51	0.13
Cereals, QUAKER, Scotch Barley, regular and quick, dry	346	11	2	76	5.66	0.07
Cereals, QUAKER, Instant Oatmeal, apples and cinnamon, prepared with boiling water	87	2	1	18	0.23	0.01
Cereals, whole wheat hot natural cereal, cooked with water, with salt	66	2	0	14	1.34	0.10
Cereals, whole wheat hot natural cereal, cooked with water, without salt	66	2	0	14	1.34	0.10
Cereals, whole wheat hot natural cereal, dry	342	11	2	75	7.65	0.10
Millet, puffed	354	13	3	80	12.51	0.16

Sausage and Luncheon Meats

Food Description	Kcals	Protein	Fat	Carbs	PRAL	Acid Density
Bacon and beef sticks	517	29	44	1	10.80	0.37
Barbecue loaf, pork, beef	173	16	9	6	4.58	0.29
Beef sausage, fresh, cooked	332	18	28	0	8.21	0.46
Beef sausage, pre-cooked	405	15	38	0	8.99	0.60
Beef, bologna, reduced sodium	313	12	28	2	5.09	0.42
Beef, cured, corned beef, canned	250	27	15	0	14.01	0.52
Beef, cured, dried	153	31	2	3	15.74	0.51
Beef, cured, luncheon meat, jellied	111	19	3	0	5.41	0.28
Beef, cured, pastrami	146	22	6	0	11.59	0.53
Beef, cured, sausage, cooked, smoked	312	14	27	2	6.67	0.48
Beef, cured, smoked, chopped beef	133	20	4	2	8.02	0.40
Beef, cured, thin-sliced beef	176	28	4	6	10.34	0.37
Beerwurst, beer salami, pork	238	14	19	2	5.03	0.36
Beerwurst, beer salami, pork and beef	277	14	23	4	5.88	0.42
Beerwurst, pork and beef	276	14	23	4	5.88	0.42
Blood sausage	379	15	35	1	6.88	0.46
Bockwurst, pork, veal, raw	278	14	26	3	5.57	0.40
Bologna, beef	311	10	28	4	7.01	0.70
Bologna, beef and pork	308	15	25	5f	5.31	0.35
Bologna, beef and pork, low fat	230	11	19	3	8.60	0.78
Bologna, beef, low fat	204	12	15	5	8.85	0.74
Bologna, chicken, pork	336	10	31	4	6.93	0.69
Bologna, chicken, pork, beef	272	11	23	6	5.79	0.53
Bologna, chicken, turkey, pork	298	10	26	6	7.03	0.70
Bologna, pork	247	15	20	1	6.23	0.42
Bologna, pork and turkey, lite	211	13	16	3	5.91	0.45
Bologna, pork, turkey and beef	336	12	29	7	4.97	0.41
Bologna, turkey	209	11	16	5	4.96	0.45
Bratwurst, beef and pork, smoked	297	12	26	2	4.36	0.36
Bratwurst, chicken, cooked	176	19	10	0	10.27	0.54
Bratwurst, pork, beef and turkey, lite, smoked	186	14	14	2	6.25	0.45
Bratwurst, pork, cooked	333	14	29	3	8.69	0.62
Bratwurst, veal, cooked	341	14	32	0	6.99	0.50
Braunschweiger (a liver sausage), pork	327	15	28	3	8.73	0.58
Brotwurst, pork, beef, link	323	14	28	3	5.02	0.36
BUTCHER BOY MEATS, INC., Turkey Franks	239	13	18	5	9.43	0.73
Cheesefurter, cheese smokie, pork, beef	327	14	29	2	8.07	0.58
Chicken breast, fat-free, mesquite flavor, sliced	80	17	0	2	10.08	0.59
Chicken breast, oven-roasted, fat-free, sliced	79	17	0	2	8.72	0.51

Sausage and Luncheon Meats

Food Description	Kcals	Protein	Fat	Carbs	PRAL	Acid Density
Chicken roll, light meat	154	17	3	5	9.53	0.56
Chicken spread	158	18	18	4	9.37	0.52
Chorizo, pork and beef	455	24	38	2	8.42	0.35
Corned beef loaf, jellied	153	23	6	0	11.37	0.49
Dutch brand loaf, chicken, pork and beef	273	12	23	4	5.64	0.47
Frankfurter, beef	330	11	30	5	7.60	0.69
Frankfurter, beef and pork	305	12	28	2	4.92	0.41
Frankfurter, beef and pork, low fat	154	11	10	4	7.03	0.64
Frankfurter, beef, heated	326	12	29	5	8.37	0.70
Frankfurter, beef, low fat	233	12	20	2	9.84	0.82
Frankfurter, beef, pork, and turkey, fat free	109	13	2	11	5.32	0.41
Frankfurter, chicken	257	16	16	3	7.03	0.44
Frankfurter, low sodium	315	12	29	2	5.27	0.44
Frankfurter, meat	290	10	26	4	7.78	0.78
Frankfurter, meat and poultry, low fat	127	15	3	8	7.22	0.48
Frankfurter, meat, heated	278	10	24	5	7.95	0.80
Frankfurter, pork	269	13	24	0	3.19	0.25
Frankfurter, turkey	226	12	17	4	6.45	0.54
Ham and cheese loaf or roll	241	14	19	4	8.68	0.62
Ham and cheese spread	245	16	19	2	19.55	1.22
Ham salad spread	216	9	16	11	5.17	0.57
Ham, chopped, canned	239	15	19	0	6.61	0.44
Ham, chopped, not canned	180	17	10	4	6.61	0.39
Ham, honey, smoked, cooked	122	18	2	7	19.24	1.07
Ham, minced	263	16	21	2	6.70	0.42
Ham, sliced, extra lean	110	19	3	1	8.62	0.45
Ham, sliced, regular (approximately 11% fat)	163	17	9	4	6.88	0.40
Headcheese, pork	157	14	11	0	7.75	0.55
Honey loaf, pork, beef	125	11	4	10	5.15	0.47
Honey roll sausage, beef	182	19	11	2	7.52	0.40
Kielbasa, kolbassy, pork, beef, nonfat dry milk added	310	12	27	3	5.29	0.44
Knackwurst, knockwurst, pork, beef	307	11	28	3	4.45	0.40
Lebanon bologna, beef	184	19	10	0	8.71	0.46
Liver cheese, pork	304	15	26	2	9.94	0.66
Liver sausage, liverwurst, pork	326	14	28	2	11.19	0.80
Liverwurst spread	305	12	25	6	10.40	0.87
Luncheon meat, beef, loaved	308	14	26	3	6.58	0.47
Luncheon meat, beef, thin sliced	149	18	3	3	5.92	0.33

Sausage and Luncheon Meats

Food Description	Kcals	Protein	Fat	Carbs	PRAL	Acid Density
Luncheon meat, pork and chicken, minced, canned, includes SPAM Lite	196	15	14	1	0.84	0.06
Luncheon meat, pork with ham, minced, canned, includes SPAM (Hormel)	315	13	27	5	3.20	0.25
Luncheon meat, pork, beef	353	13	32	2	4.62	0.36
Luncheon meat, pork, canned	334	13	30	2	4.30	0.33
Luncheon meat, pork, ham, and chicken, minced, canned, reduced sodium, added ascorbic acid, includes SPAM, 25% less sodium	293	13	25	3	-2.05	-0.16
Luncheon sausage, pork and beef	260	15	21	2	6.37	0.42
Luxury loaf, pork	141	18	5	5	6.95	0.39
Macaroni and cheese loaf, chicken, pork and beef	228	12	15	12	3.30	0.28
Mortadella, beef, pork	311	16	25	3	7.66	0.48
Mother's loaf, pork	282	12	22	8	4.98	0.42
New England brand sausage, pork, beef	161	17	8	5	6.24	0.37
Olive loaf, pork	235	12	17	9	2.33	0.19
Oven-roasted chicken breast roll	134	15	8	2	4.30	0.29
Pastrami, beef, 98% fat-free	95	20	1	2	9.78	0.49
Pastrami, turkey	123	16	6	3	7.63	0.48
Pate, chicken liver, canned	201	13	13	7	10.60	0.82
Pate, goose liver, smoked, canned	462	11	44	5	8.84	0.80
Pate, liver, not specified, canned	319	14	28	1	10.21	0.73
Pate, truffle flavor	327	11	28	6	8.74	0.79
Peppered loaf, pork, beef	148	17	6	5	5.27	0.31
Pepperoni, pork, beef	466	23	44	0	9.12	0.40
Pickle and pimiento loaf, pork	225	11	16	10	2.19	0.20
Picnic loaf, pork, beef	232	15	17	5	5.32	0.35
Polish sausage, pork	326	14	29	2	6.44	0.46
Pork and beef sausage, fresh, cooked	396	14	36	3	6.31	0.45
Pork and turkey sausage, pre-cooked	342	12	31	4	4.49	0.37
Pork sausage rice links, brown and serve, cooked	407	14	38	2	5.99	0.43
Pork Sausage, Fresh, Cooked	339	19	28	0	8.76	0.46
Pork sausage, fresh, raw	304	15	27	0	6.70	0.45
Pork sausage, pre-cooked	378	14	35	0	8.70	0.62
Poultry salad sandwich spread	200	12	14	7	2.69	0.22
Roast beef spread	223	15	16	4	5.41	0.36
Salami, cooked, beef	261	13	22	2	9.39	0.72
Salami, cooked, beef and pork	250	22	26	2	6.35	0.29
Salami, cooked, turkey	152	19	9	1	11.71	0.62
Salami, dry or hard, pork	407	23	34	2	10.85	0.47
Salami, dry or hard, pork, beef	385	23	30	4	8.13	0.35
Salami, Italian, pork	425	22	37	1	11.26	0.51

Sausage and Luncheon Meats

Food Description	Kcals	Protein	Fat	Carbs	PRAL	Acid Density
Salami, Italian, pork and beef, dry, sliced, 50% less sodium	350	22	26	6	7.45	0.34
Salami, pork, beef, less sodium	396	15	30	15	-13.42	-0.89
Sandwich spread, pork, beef	235	8	17	12	3.26	0.41
Sausage, Berliner, pork, beef	230	15	17	3	5.80	0.39
Sausage, chicken and beef, smoked	296	18	24	0	9.74	0.54
Sausage, chicken, beef, pork, skinless, smoked	216	14	14	8	4.71	0.34
Sausage, Italian, pork, cooked	344	19	27	4	8.53	0.45
Sausage, Italian, pork, raw	346	14	31	1	6.32	0.45
Sausage, Italian, sweet, links	149	16	8	2	7	0.44
Sausage, Italian, turkey, smoked	158	15	9	5	9.16	0.61
Sausage, Polish, beef with chicken, hot	259	18	19	4	8.15	0.45
Sausage, Polish, pork and beef, smoked	301	12	27	2	5.50	0.46
Sausage, pork and beef, with cheddar cheese, smoked	296	13	26	2	7.49	0.58
Sausage, smoked link sausage, pork and beef	320	12	29	2	6.10	0.51
Sausage, summer, pork and beef, sticks, with cheddar cheese	426	19	38	2	10.39	0.55
Sausage, turkey, breakfast links, mild	235	15	18	2	9.19	0.61
Sausage, turkey, hot, smoked	158	15	9	5	9.16	0.61
Sausage, Vienna, canned, chicken, beef, pork	230	11	19	3	4.52	0.41
Scrapple, pork	213	8	14	14	3.01	0.38
Smoked link sausage, pork	389	12	28	1	8.93	0.74
Smoked link sausage, pork and beef, flour and nonfat dry milk added	268	14	21	4	6.46	0.46
Smoked link sausage, pork and beef, nonfat dry milk added	313	13	28	2	4.62	0.36
Swisswurst, pork and beef, with Swiss cheese, smoked	307	13	27	2	7.17	0.55
Thornier, cervelat, summer sausage, beef, pork	362	17	30	3	6.71	0.39
Turkey and pork sausage, fresh, bulk, patty or link, cooked	307	23	23	1	10.20	0.44
Turkey breast meat	104	17	2	4	7.36	0.43
Turkey ham, cured turkey thigh meat	126	17	5	2	12.75	0.75
Turkey ham, sliced, extra lean, prepackaged or deli-sliced	118	20	4	3	13.98	0.70
Turkey roll, light and dark meat	149	18	7	2	8.55	0.48
Turkey roll, light meat	147	15	2	5	9.72	0.65
Turkey sausage, fresh, cooked	196	24	10	0	12.09	0.50
Turkey sausage, fresh, raw	155	19	8	0	9.51	0.50
Turkey sausage, reduced fat, brown and serve, cooked (include BUTTERBALL breakfast links turkey sausage)	200	17	10	11	9.10	0.54
Turkey, pork, and beef sausage, low fat, smoked	101	8	3	11	1	0.13
Turkey, pork, and beef sausage, reduced fat, smoked	240	19	17	3	9.40	0.49
Turkey, white, rotisserie, deli cut	112	13	3	8	4.40	0.34

Sausage and Luncheon Meats

Food Description	Kcals	Protein	Fat	Carbs	PRAL	Acid Density
USDA Commodity, pork sausage, bulk/links/patties, frozen, raw	231	15	19	0	7.91	0.53
USDA Commodity, pork, sausage, bulk/links/patties, frozen, cooked	267	20	20	0	11.08	0.55

Dairy

Food Description	KCals	Protein	Fat	Carbs	PRAL	Acid Density
Beverage, instant breakfast powder, chocolate, not reconstituted	353	20	1	66	-3.97	-0.20
Beverage, instant breakfast powder, chocolate, sugar-free, not reconstituted	358	36	5	41	-16.9	-0.47
Beverage, milkshake mix, dry, not chocolate	328	2	3	53	-45.8	-22.89
Butter oil, anhydrous	876	0	0	99	0.09	!
Butter, salted	717	1	81	0	0.43	0.43
Butter, whipped, with salt	717	1	81	0	0.35	0.35
Butter, without salt	717	1	81	0	0.43	0.43
Cheese fondue	229	14	13	4	9.3	0.66
Cheese food, cold pack, american	331	20	24	8	9.56	0.48
Cheese food, imitation	141	22	1	9	14.29	0.65
Cheese food, pasteurized process, american, with di sodium phosphate	328	20	25	7	23.38	1.17
Cheese food, pasteurized process, american, without di sodium phosphate	330	18	25	8	10.93	0.61
Cheese food, pasteurized process, Swiss	323	22	24	5	14.11	0.64
Cheese product, pasteurized process, cheddar or american, reduced fat	240	18	14	11	24.63	1.37
Cheese sauce, prepared from recipe	197	10	15	5	6.01	0.60
Cheese spread, cream cheese base	295	7	29	4	3.41	0.49
Cheese spread, pasteurized process, american, with di sodium phosphate	290	16	21	9	27.27	1.70
Cheese spread, pasteurized process, american, without di sodium phosphate	290	16	21	9	21.24	1.33
Cheese substitute, mozzarella	248	11	12	24	8.64	0.79
Cheese, american cheddar, imitation	239	17	14	12	21.38	1.26
Cheese, blue	353	21	29	2	11.96	0.57
Cheese, brick	371	23	30	3	15.83	0.69
Cheese, brie	334	21	28	0	11.02	0.52
Cheese, camembert	300	20	24	0	13.05	0.65
Cheese, caraway	376	25	29	3	19.19	0.77
Cheese, cheddar	403	25	33	1	18.98	0.76
Cheese, Cheshire	387	23	31	5	17.71	0.77
Cheese, Colby	394	24	32	3	16.3	0.68
Cheese, cottage, creamed, large or small curd	103	11	4	3	8.33	0.76
Cheese, cottage, creamed, with fruit	97	11	4	5	6.65	0.60
Cheese, cottage, lowfat, 1% milkfat	72	12	1	3	8.3	0.69
Cheese, cottage, lowfat, 1% milkfat, lactose reduced	74	12	1	3	8.4	0.70
Cheese, cottage, lowfat, 1% milkfat, no sodium added	72	12	1	3	8.3	0.69
Cheese, cottage, lowfat, 1% milkfat, with vegetables	67	11	1	3	7.43	0.68
Cheese, cottage, lowfat, 2% milkfat	86	12	2	4	9.25	0.77
Cheese, cottage, nonfat, uncreamed, dry, large or small curd	72	10	0	7	11.11	1.11

Dairy

Food Description	KCals	Protein	Fat	Carbs	PRAL	Acid Density
Cheese, cottage, with vegetables	95	11	4	3	7.43	0.68
Cheese, cream	342	6	34	4	3.85	0.64
Cheese, cream, fat free	104	16	1	8	16.92	1.06
Cheese, cream, low fat	231	8	15	8	5.42	0.68
Cheese, edam	357	25	28	1	17.84	0.71
Cheese, feta	264	14	21	4	11.22	0.80
Cheese, fontina	389	26	31	2	16.48	0.63
Cheese, gjetost	466	10	30	43	-15.5	-1.55
Cheese, goat, hard type	452	31	36	2	27.88	0.90
Cheese, goat, semisoft type	364	22	30	3	16.5	0.75
Cheese, goat, soft type	268	19	21	1	15.76	0.83
Cheese, gouda	356	25	27	2	20.02	0.80
Cheese, gruyere	413	30	32	0	21.21	0.71
Cheese, limburger	327	20	27	0	14.67	0.73
Cheese, low fat, cheddar or Colby	173	24	7	2	22.64	0.94
Cheese, low-sodium, cheddar or Colby	398	24	33	2	17.64	0.74
Cheese, Mexican, queso anejo	373	21	30	5	15.53	0.74
Cheese, Mexican, queso asadero	356	23	28	3	16.39	0.71
Cheese, Mexican, queso chihuahua	374	22	30	6	16.76	0.76
Cheese, Monterey	373	24	30	0	16.32	0.68
Cheese, Monterey, low fat	313	28	22	1	18.67	0.67
Cheese, mozzarella, low sodium	280	27	17	3	20.68	0.77
Cheese, mozzarella, nonfat	149	32	0	4	24.22	0.76
Cheese, mozzarella, part skim milk	254	24	16	3	16.49	0.69
Cheese, mozzarella, part skim milk, low moisture	302	26	20	4	19.93	0.77
Cheese, mozzarella, whole milk	300	22	22	2	15.28	0.69
Cheese, mozzarella, whole milk, low moisture	318	22	25	2	16.23	0.74
Cheese, muenster	368	23	30	1	15.95	0.69
Cheese, muenster, low fat	274	25	18	4	19.02	0.76
Cheese, Neufchatel	260	9	23	4	6.33	0.70
Cheese, parmesan, grated	431	38	29	4	27.78	0.73
Cheese, parmesan, hard	392	36	26	0	24.72	0.69
Cheese, parmesan, low sodium	456	42	30	4	28.78	0.69
Cheese, parmesan, shredded	415	38	27	3	26.09	0.69
Cheese, pasteurized process, american, low fat	180	25	7	4	29.35	1.17
Cheese, pasteurized process, american, with di sodium phosphate	375	22	31	2	18.4	0.84
Cheese, pasteurized process, american, without di sodium phosphate	375	22	31	2	15.3	0.70
Cheese, pasteurized process, cheddar or american, fat-free	148	22	1	13	29.71	1.35

Dairy

Food Description	KCals	Protein	Fat	Carbs	PRAL	Acid Density
Cheese, pasteurized process, cheddar or american, low sodium	375	22	31	2	26.46	1.20
Cheese, pasteurized process, pimento	375	22	31	2	26.41	1.20
Cheese, pasteurized process, Swiss, low fat	170	26	5	4	29.79	1.15
Cheese, pasteurized process, Swiss, with di sodium phosphate	334	25	25	2	24.98	1
Cheese, pasteurized process, Swiss, without di sodium phosphate	334	25	25	2	16.77	0.67
Cheese, port de salut	352	24	28	1	13.04	0.54
Cheese, provolone	351	26	27	2	17.43	0.67
Cheese, ricotta, part skim milk	138	11	8	5	5.8	0.53
Cheese, ricotta, whole milk	174	11	13	3	6.18	0.56
Cheese, Romano	387	32	27	4	26.99	0.84
Cheese, Roquefort	369	22	31	2	13.76	0.63
Cheese, Swiss	380	27	28	5	21.28	0.79
Cheese, Swiss, low fat	179	28	5	3	20.54	0.73
Cheese, Swiss, low sodium	376	28	27	3	20.54	0.73
Cheese, titlist	340	24	26	2	19.65	0.82
Cream substitute, liquid, light	69	1	4	s	-0.56	-0.56
Cream substitute, liquid, with hydrogenated vegetable oil and soy protein	136	1	10	11	-1.27	-1.27
Cream substitute, liquid, with lauric acid oil and sodium caseinate	136	1	10	11	-1.27	-1.27
Cream substitute, powdered	545	5	35	55	0.51	0.10
Cream substitute, powdered, light	431	2	16	73	-13	-6.50
Cream, fluid, half and half	130	3	11	4	0.61	0.20
Cream, fluid, heavy whipping	345	2	37	3	0.69	0.35
Cream, fluid, light (coffee cream or table cream)	195	3	19	4	0.23	0.08
Cream, fluid, light whipping	292	2	31	3	0.2	0.10
Cream, half and half, fat free	59	3	1	9	0.87	0.29
Cream, sour, cultured	214	2	20	4	-0.12	-0.06
Cream, sour, reduced fat, cultured	135	3	12	4	0.63	0.21
Cream, whipped, cream topping, pressurized	257	3	22	12	0.17	0.06
Dessert topping, powdered	577	5	40	53	1.25	0.25
Dessert topping, powdered, 1.5 ounce prepared with 1/2 cup milk	189	4	12	17	0.34	0.09
Dessert topping, pressurized	264	1	22	16	0.65	0.65
Dessert topping, semi solid, frozen	318	1	25	23	0.4	0.40
Egg substitute, frozen	160	11	11	3	2.38	0.22
Egg substitute, liquid	84	12	3	1	2.5	0.21
Egg substitute, powder	444	56	13	22	23.32	0.42
Egg, duck, whole, fresh, raw	185	14	13	1	8.48	0.61
Egg, goose, whole, fresh, raw	185	14	13	1	8.88	0.63

Dairy

Food Description	KCals	Protein	Fat	Carbs	PRAL	Acid Density
Egg, quail, whole, fresh, raw	158	13	11	0	10.81	0.83
Egg, turkey, whole, fresh, raw	171	14	12	1	8.38	0.60
Egg, white, dried	382	81	0	8	17.12	0.21
Egg, white, dried, flakes, glucose reduced	351	77	0	4	16.05	0.21
Egg, white, dried, powder, glucose reduced	376	82	0	4	17.2	0.21
Egg, white, raw, fresh	52	11	0	1	2.09	0.19
Egg, white, raw, frozen	47	10	0	1	2.07	0.21
Egg, whole, cooked, fried	196	14	15	1	10.18	0.73
Egg, whole, cooked, hard-boiled	155	13	11	1	8.97	0.69
Egg, whole, cooked, omelet	157	11	12	1	7.93	0.72
Egg, whole, cooked, poached	142	13	10	1	9.37	0.72
Egg, whole, cooked, scrambled	167	11	12	2	7.59	0.69
Egg, whole, dried	594	47	41	5	39.5	0.84
Egg, whole, dried, stabilized, glucose reduced	615	48	44	2	35.08	0.73
Egg, whole, raw, fresh	143	13	10	1	9.41	0.72
Egg, whole, raw, frozen	148	12	10	1	9.54	0.80
Egg, yolk, dried	666	34	56	4	41.66	1.23
Egg, yolk, raw, fresh	322	16	27	4	18.1	1.13
Egg, yolk, raw, frozen	303	15	26	1	18.51	1.23
Egg, yolk, raw, frozen, salted	274	14	23	2	18.6	1.33
Egg, yolk, raw, frozen, sugared	307	14	23	11	16.94	1.21
Eggnog	135	4	7	14	0.25	0.06
Eggs, scrambled, frozen mixture	131	13	6	8	3.96	0.30
Ensure plus, liquid nutrition	141	13	11	20	-0.29	-0.02
Imitation cheese, american or cheddar, low cholesterol	390	25	32	1	20.76	0.83
Milk shakes, thick chocolate	119	3	3	21	-0.68	-0.23
Milk shakes, thick vanilla	112	4	3	18	0.09	0.02
Milk substitutes, fluid with hydrogenated vegetable oils	61	2	3	6	0.61	0.31
Milk substitutes, fluid, with lauric acid oil	61	2	3	6	0.61	0.31
Milk, buttermilk, dried	387	34	6	49	-0.35	-0.01
Milk, buttermilk, fluid, cultured, lowfat	40	3	1	5	-0.05	-0.02
Milk, buttermilk, fluid, cultured, reduced fat	56	4	2	5	-0.93	-0.23
Milk, canned, condensed, sweetened	321	8	9	54	1.07	0.13
Milk, canned, evaporated, nonfat	78	8	0	11	-0.53	-0.07
Milk, canned, evaporated, with added vitamin A	134	7	8	10	0.46	0.07
Milk, canned, evaporated, without added vitamin A	134	7	8	10	0.46	0.07
Milk, chocolate beverage, hot cocoa, homemade	77	4	2	11	-0.49	-0.12
Milk, chocolate, fluid, commercial, lowfat	63	3	1	10	-0	0

Dairy

Food Description	KCals	Protein	Fat	Carbs	PRAL	Acid Density
Milk, chocolate, fluid, commercial, reduced fat	76	3	2	12	-0.09	-0.03
Milk, chocolate, fluid, commercial, reduced fat, with added calcium	78	3	2	12	-1.19	-0.40
Milk, chocolate, fluid, commercial, whole	83	3	3	10	-0.01	0
Milk, dry, nonfat, calcium reduced	354	36	0	52	35.32	0.98
Milk, dry, nonfat, instant, with added vitamin A	358	35	1	52	-1.2	-0.03
Milk, dry, nonfat, instant, without added vitamin A	358	35	1	52	-1.2	-0.03
Milk, dry, nonfat, regular, with added vitamin A	362	36	1	52	-3.34	-0.09
Milk, dry, nonfat, regular, without added vitamin A	362	36	1	52	-3.34	-0.09
Milk, dry, whole	496	26	27	0	-0.38	-0.01
Milk, filled, fluid, with blend of hydrogenated vegetable oils	63	3	3	5	0.3	0.10
Milk, filled, fluid, with lauric acid oil	63	3	3	5	0.3	0.10
Milk, fluid, nonfat, calcium fortified (fat free or skim)	35	3	0	5	-1.02	-0.34
Milk, goat, fluid	69	4	4	4	-0.53	-0.13
Milk, human, mature, fluid	70	1	4	7	-0.54	-0.54
Milk, imitation, non-soy	46	2	2	5	0.24	0.12
Milk, Indian buffalo, fluid	97	4	7	5	-0.57	-0.14
Milk, low sodium, fluid	61	3	3	4	-2.05	-0.68
Milk, lowfat, fluid, 1% milkfat, protein fortified, with added vitamin A	48	4	1	6	-0.01	0
Milk, lowfat, fluid, 1% milkfat, with added nonfat milk solids and vitamin A	43	3	1	5	-0.02	-0.01
Milk, lowfat, fluid, 1% milkfat, with added vitamin A	42	3	1	5	0.18	0.06
Milk, nonfat, fluid, protein fortified, with added vitamin A (fat free and skim)	41	4	0	6	-0.01	0
Milk, nonfat, fluid, with added nonfat milk solids and vitamin A (fat free or skim)	37	4	0	5	-0.06	-0.02
Milk, nonfat, fluid, with added vitamin A (fat free or skim)	34	3	0	5	0.2	0.07
Milk, nonfat, fluid, without added vitamin A (fat free or skim)	34	3	0	5	0.03	0.01
Milk, producer, fluid, 3.7% milkfat	64	3	4	5	-0.01	0
Milk, reduced fat, fluid, 2% milkfat, protein fortified, with added vitamin A	56	4	2	5	-0.01	0
Milk, reduced fat, fluid, 2% milkfat, with added nonfat milk solids and vitamin A	51	3	2	5	-0.02	-0.01
Milk, reduced fat, fluid, 2% milkfat, with added nonfat milk solids, without added vitamin A	56	4	2	5	08	0
Milk, reduced fat, fluid, 2% milkfat, with added vitamin A	50	3	2	5	0.13	0.04
Milk, sheep, fluid	108	6	7	5	2.92	0.49
Milk, whole, 3.25% milkfat	60	3	3	5	0.21	0.07
Parmesan cheese topping, fat free	370	40	5	40	21.46	0.54
Reddi Wip Fat Free Whipped Topping	149	3	5	25	0.1	0.03
Sour cream, fat free	74	3	0	16	0.44	0.15

Dairy

Food Description	KCals	Protein	Fat	Carbs	PRAL	Acid Density
Sour cream, imitation, cultured	208	2	20	7	-0.73	-0.37
Sour cream, light	136	4	11	7	-2.2	-0.55
Sour cream, reduced fat	181	7	14	7	0.02	0
Sour dressing, non-butterfat, cultured, filled cream-type	178	3	17	5	-0.32	-0.11
USDA Commodity, cheese, cheddar, reduced fat	282	27	18	2	20.27	0.75
Whey, acid, dried	339	12	1	73	-24.3	-2.02
Whey, acid, fluid	24	1	0	5	-1.34	-1.34
Whey, sweet, dried	353	13	1	74	-17.8	-1.37
Whey, sweet, fluid	27	1	0	5	-2.08	-2.08
Whipped cream substitute, dietetic, made from powdered mix	100	1	6	11	0.94	0.94
Whipped topping, frozen, low fat	220	3	13	s	0.98	0.33
Yogurt, chocolate, nonfat milk	108	4	0	24	-1.43	-0.36
Yogurt, fruit variety, nonfat	94	4	0	19	0.11	0.03
Yogurt, fruit, low fat, 10 grams protein per 8 ounce	102	4	1	19	0.08	0.02
Yogurt, fruit, low fat, 11 grams protein per 8 ounce	105	5	1	19	0.15	0.03
Yogurt, fruit, low fat, 9 grams protein per 8 ounce	99	4	1	19	0.13	0.03
Yogurt, fruit, lowfat, with low calorie sweetener	105	5	1	19	0.83	0.17
Yogurt, plain, low fat, 12 grams protein per 8 ounce	63	5	2	7	0.16	0.03
Yogurt, plain, skim milk, 13 grams protein per 8 ounce	56	6	0	8	0.18	0.03
Yogurt, plain, whole milk, 8 grams protein per 8 ounce	61	3	3	5	0.07	0.02
Yogurt, vanilla or lemon flavor, nonfat milk, sweetened with low-calorie sweetener	47	4	0	8	0.01	0
Yogurt, vanilla, low fat, 11 grams protein per 8 ounce	85	5	1	14	0.17	0.03

Soups, Sauces, and Gravies

Food Description	Kcals	Protein	Fat	Carbs	PRAL	Alkali Density
Adobo fresco	226	2	21	19	-3.73	-0.20
Fish broth	16	5	1	1	-0.13	-0.13
Gravy, au jus, canned	16	1	0	3	-0.10	-0.03
Gravy, au jus, dry	313	9	10	47	1.03	0.02
Gravy, beef, canned	53	4	2	5	1.11	0.22
Gravy, brown instant, dry	380	9	12	60	1.97	0.03
Gravy, brown, dry	367	11	10	59	4.67	0.08
Gravy, chicken, canned	79	2	5	6	-0.58	-0.10
Gravy, chicken, dry	381	11	10	62	3.31	0.05
Gravy, HEINZ Home Style Savory Beef Gravy	39	1	1	6	0.28	0.05
Gravy, instant beef, dry	369	10	9	61	1.29	0.02
Gravy, instant turkey, dry	409	12	15	58	4.55	0.08
Gravy, meat or poultry, prepared, low sodium	53	4	2	6	1.14	0.19
Gravy, mushroom, canned	50	1	2	5	-1.19	-0.24
Gravy, mushroom, dehydrated, dry	328	10	4	65	3.03	0.05
Gravy, onion, dehydrated, dry	322	9	3	68	1.89	0.03
Gravy, pork, dry	367	9	9	64	3.63	0.06
Gravy, turkey, canned	51	6	5	12	-0.04	0
Gravy, turkey, dry	367	3	2	5	2.47	0.49
Gravy, unspecified type, dry	344	13	8	58	5.25	0.09
Peppers, hot, chili, immature green, canned, chili sauce	20	1	0	5	-11.36	-2.27
Peppers, hot, chili, mature red, canned, chili sauce	21	1	1	4	-11.24	-2.81
Potato soup, instant, dry mix	343	9	3	76	-15.22	-0.20
Sauce, alfredo mix, dry	535	15	36	37	10.62	0.29
Sauce, barbecue sauce	150	0	0	36	-4.20	-0.12
Sauce, barbecue, low sodium	150	0	0	36	-4.20	-0.12
Sauce, cheese sauce mix, dry	438	8	18	61	1.65	0.03
Sauce, cheese, dehydrated, dry	448	23	25	34	10.82	0.32
Sauce, cheese, ready-to-serve	174	7	13	7	5.84	0.83
Sauce, fish, ready-to-serve	35	5	0	4	-8.41	-2.10
Sauce, hoisin, ready-to-serve	220	3	3	44	-0.51	-0.01
Sauce, hollandaise, with butter fat, dehydrated, dry	554	11	46	32	5.89	0.18
Sauce, hollandaise, with vegetable oil, dehydrated, dry	374	14	9	62	2.61	0.04
Sauce, homemade, white, medium	147	4	11	9	0.33	0.04
Sauce, homemade, white, thick	186	4	14	12	0.57	0.05
Sauce, homemade, white, thin	105	4	7	7	0.13	0.02
Sauce, mole poblano, dry mix, single brand	571	7	42	42	-6.80	-0.16
Sauce, oyster, ready-to-serve	51	1	0	11	-0.17	-0.02

Soups, Sauces, and Gravies

Food Description	Kcals	Protein	Fat	Carbs	PRAL	Alkali Density
Sauce, pasta, spaghetti/marinara, ready-to-serve	74	2	3	14	-6.50	-0.46
Sauce, pizza, canned, ready-to-serve	54	2	1	9	-5.76	-0.64
Sauce, plum, ready-to-serve	184	1	1	43	-4.65	-0.11
Sauce, ready-to-serve, pepper or hot	11	1	0	2	-2.60	-1.30
Sauce, ready-to-serve, pepper, TABASCO	12	1	1	1	-1.67	-1.67
Sauce, ready-to-serve, salsa	27	2	0	6	-5.07	-0.85
Sauce, sofrito, prepared from recipe	237	13	18	5	2.08	0.42
Sauce, spaghetti, low sodium	109	2	3	14s	-6.83	#VALUE!
Sauce, sweet and sour, prepared-from-recipe	79	2	1	17	-2.58	-0.15
Sauce, teriyaki, dehydrated, dry	283	9	2	60	3.83	0.06
Sauce, teriyaki, ready-to-serve	84	6	0	16	1.96	0.12
Sauce, teriyaki, ready-to-serve, reduced sodium	84	6	0	16	1.96	0.12
Sauce, tomato chili sauce, bottled, no salt, low sodium	104	3	0	20	-5.19	-0.26
Sauce, tomato chili sauce, bottled, with salt	104	3	0	20	-5.19	-0.26
Sauce, white, dehydrated, dry	463	11	27	51	-3.12	-0.06
Sauce, white, thin, prepared-from-recipe, with butter	72	4	3	8	0.48	0.06
Sauce, worcestershire	67	0	19	0	-16.30	!
Soup, bean & ham, canned, reduced sodium, prepared with water or ready-to-serve	74	4	1	14	-1.77	-0.13
Soup, bean with bacon, dehydrated, dry mix	370	19	8	58	-8.26	-0.14
Soup, bean with bacon, dehydrated, prepared with water	40	2	1	6	-0.87	-0.15
Soup, bean with frankfurters, canned, condensed, commercial	142	8	5	17	-1.05	-0.06
Soup, bean with frankfurters, canned, prepared with equal volume water, commercial	75	4	3	9	-0.56	-0.06
Soup, bean with ham, canned, chunky, ready-to-serve, commercial	95	5	4	11	0.14	0.01
Soup, bean with pork, canned, condensed, commercial	129	6	4	17	-1.43	-0.08
Soup, bean with pork, canned, prepared with equal volume water, commercial	68	3	2	8	-0.77	-0.10
Soup, beef and mushroom, low sodium, chunk style	69	4	2	10	0.79	0.08
Soup, beef broth bouillon and consomme, canned, condensed, commercial	24	3	0	1	0.38	0.38
Soup, beef broth or bouillon canned, ready-to-serve	7	1	0	0	-0.22	!
Soup, beef broth or bouillon, powder, dry	238	16	9	24	8.19	0.34
Soup, beef broth or bouillon, powder, prepared with water	8	0	0	0	0.18	!
Soup, beef broth, cubed, dry	170	17	4	16	6.25	0.39
Soup, beef broth, cubed, prepared with water	3	0	0	0	0.15	!
Soup, beef mushroom, canned, condensed, commercial	61	5	2	5	0.44	0.09
Soup, beef mushroom, canned, prepared with equal volume water, commercial	30	2	1	3	0.22	0.07
Soup, beef noodle, canned, condensed, commercial	67	4	2	7	1.31	0.19

Soups, Sauces, and Gravies

Food Description	Kcals	Protein	Fat	Carbs	PRAL	Alkali Density
Soup, beef noodle, canned, prepared with equal volume water, commercial	34	2	1	4	0.68	0.17
Soup, beef stroganoff, canned, chunky style, ready-to-serve	98	5	5	9	1.09	0.12
Soup, beef, canned, chunky, ready-to-serve	71	4	1	10	1.08	0.11
Soup, black bean, canned, condensed, commercial	91	5	1	15	-1.42	-0.09
Soup, black bean, canned, prepared with equal volume water, commercial	47	2	1	8	-0.29	-0.04
Soup, bouillon cubes and granules, low sodium, dry	438	17	14	65	3.94	0.06
Soup, broccoli cheese, canned, condensed, commercial	87	2	5	8	-2.63	-0.33
Soup, CAMPBELL'S HEALTHY REQUEST Chicken with Rice, canned, condensed	49	2	58	7	-1.14	-0.16
Soup, cheese, canned, condensed, commercial	121	4	8	8	1.94	0.24
Soup, cheese, canned, prepared with equal volume milk, commercial	92	4	6	6	0.98	0.16
Soup, cheese, canned, prepared with equal volume water, commercial	63	2	4	4	1.01	0.25
Soup, chicken broth cubes, dehydrated, dry	198	15	5	24	2.44	0.10
Soup, chicken broth or bouillon, dehydrated, dry	267	17	14	18	3.92	0.22
Soup, chicken broth or bouillon, dehydrated, prepared with water	9	0	0	0	0.11	!
Soup, chicken broth, canned, condensed, commercial	31	4	1	1	0.68	0.68
Soup, chicken broth, canned, less/reduced sodium	7	1	0	0	-0.58	!
Soup, chicken broth, canned, prepared with equal volume water, commercial	16	2	1	0	0.21	!
Soup, chicken broth, low sodium, canned	16	2	1	1	0.20	0.20
Soup, chicken gumbo, canned, condensed, commercial	45	2	1	7	0.18	0.03
Soup, chicken gumbo, canned, prepared with equal volume water, commercial	23	1	1	3	0.06	0.02
Soup, chicken mushroom, canned, condensed, commercial	109	4	7	8	-0.59	-0.07
Soup, chicken mushroom, canned, prepared with equal volume water, commercial	54	2	4	4	-0.29	-0.07
Soup, chicken noodle mix, dehydrated, dry form	377	15	7	62	6.64	0.11
Soup, chicken noodle, canned, chunky, ready-to-serve	37	3	1	4	2.52	0.63
Soup, chicken noodle, canned, condensed, commercial	53	3	2	6	1.31	0.22
Soup, chicken noodle, canned, prepared with equal volume water, commercial	31	1	1	3	0.75	0.25
Soup, chicken noodle, dehydrated, prepared with water	23	1	1	4	0.47	0.12
Soup, chicken noodle, low sodium	31	1	1	3	-0.03	-0.01
Soup, chicken rice, canned, chunky, ready-to-serve	53	5	1	5	2.38	0.48
Soup, chicken rice, dehydrated, prepared with water	24	1	1	24	0.50	0.02
Soup, chicken vegetable with potato and cheese, chunky, ready-to-serve	65	1	4	5	-0.58	-0.12
Soup, chicken vegetable, canned, chunky, ready-to-serve	69	5	2	8	0.68	0.09

Soups, Sauces, and Gravies

Food Description	Kcals	Protein	Fat	Carbs	PRAL	Alkali Density
Soup, chicken vegetable, canned, condensed, commercial	61	2	2	7	-0.29	-0.04
Soup, chicken vegetable, canned, prepared with equal volume water, commercial	31	1	1	4	-0.14	-0.04
Soup, chicken with dumplings, canned, condensed, commercial	79	5	5	5	1.86	0.37
Soup, chicken with dumplings, canned, prepared with equal volume water, commercial	40	2	2	3	0.92	0.31
Soup, chicken with rice, canned, condensed, commercial	49	3	2	6	0.14	0.02
Soup, chicken with rice, canned, prepared with equal volume water, commercial	25	1	1	3	0.08	0.03
Soup, chicken, canned, chunky, ready-to-serve, commercial	71	5	3	7	2.46	0.35
Soup, chili beef, canned, condensed, commercial	129	5	3	19	-2.75	-0.14
Soup, chili beef, canned, prepared with equal volume water, commercial	68	2	1	9	-1.44	-0.16
Soup, clam chowder, Manhattan style, canned, chunky, ready-to-serve	56	3	1	8	-1.15	-0.14
Soup, clam chowder, Manhattan style, dehydrated, dry	345	2	2	10	-11.32	-1.13
Soup, clam chowder, Manhattan, canned, condensed, commercial	61	2	2	10	-1.53	-0.15
Soup, clam chowder, Manhattan, canned, prepared with equal volume water	32	1	1	5	-0.82	-0.16
Soup, clam chowder, new England, canned, condensed, commercial	70	3	2	10	0.88	0.09
Soup, clam chowder, new England, canned, prepared with equal volume water, commercial	39	2	1	5	0.20	0.04
Soup, clam chowder, new England, canned, prepared with equal volume milk, commercial	61	3	2	7	0.45	0.06
Soup, consomme with gelatin, dehydrated, prepared with water	7	1	0	1	0.41	0.41
Soup, crab, canned, ready-to-serve	31	2	1	4	-0.88	-0.22
Soup, cream of asparagus, canned, condensed, commercial	69	2	3	9	-1.23	-0.14
Soup, cream of asparagus, canned, prepared with equal volume milk, commercial	65	3	3	7	-0.62	-0.09
Soup, cream of asparagus, canned, prepared with equal volume water, commercial	35	1	2	4	-0.64	-0.16
Soup, cream of celery, canned, condensed, commercial	72	1	4	7	-0.84	-0.12
Soup, cream of celery, canned, prepared with equal volume milk, commercial	66	2	4	6	-0.45	-0.08
Soup, cream of celery, canned, prepared with equal volume water, commercial	37	1	2	4	-0.44	-0.11
Soup, cream of chicken, canned, condensed, commercial	89	2	6	7	0.99	0.14
Soup, cream of chicken, canned, condensed, reduced sodium	58	2	1	9	-4.17	-0.46
Soup, cream of chicken, canned, prepared with equal volume water, commercial	48	1	3	4	0.28	0.07
Soup, cream of chicken, dehydrated, prepared with water	41	1	2	5	-0.44	-0.09
Soup, cream of chicken, prepared with equal volume milk, commercial	77	3	5	6	0.29	0.05
Soup, cream of mushroom, canned, condensed, commercial	85	2	6	7	0.18	0.03
Soup, cream of mushroom, canned, condensed, reduced sodium	52	1	2	8	-5.67	-0.71

Soups, Sauces, and Gravies

Food Description	Kcals	Protein	Fat	Carbs	PRAL	Alkali Density
Soup, cream of mushroom, canned, prepared with equal volume milk, commercial	67	2	4	6	0.09	0.02
Soup, cream of mushroom, canned, prepared with equal volume water, commercial	42	1	3	3	0.04	0.01
Soup, cream of mushroom, low sodium, ready-to-serve, canned	53	1	4	5	0.07	0.01
Soup, cream of onion, canned, condensed, commercial	88	2	4	10	-0.35	-0.04
Soup, cream of onion, canned, prepared with equal volume milk, commercial	75	3	4	7	-0.15	-0.02
Soup, cream of onion, canned, prepared with equal volume water, commercial	44	1	2	5	-0.15	-0.03
Soup, cream of potato, canned, condensed	59	1	2	9	-0.47	-0.05
Soup, cream of potato, canned, prepared with equal volume milk, commercial	60	2	3	7	-0.23	-0.03
Soup, cream of potato, canned, prepared with equal volume water, commercial	30	1	1	5	-0.25	-0.05
Soup, cream of shrimp, canned, condensed	72	2	4	7	0.69	0.10
Soup, cream of shrimp, canned, prepared with equal volume milk, commercial	66	3	3	6	0.33	0.06
Soup, cream of shrimp, canned, prepared with equal volume water, commercial	37	1	2	3	0.34	0.11
Soup, cream of vegetable, dehydrated, dry	446	8	24	52	0.79	0.02
Soup, escarole, canned, ready-to-serve	11	1	1	1	-0.98	-0.98
Soup, gazpacho, canned, ready-to-serve	19	3	0	2	-0.16	-0.08
Soup, lentil with ham, canned, ready-to-serve	56	4	1	8	1.09	0.14
Soup, minestrone, canned, chunky, ready-to-serve	53	2	1	9	-3.09	-0.34
Soup, minestrone, canned, condensed, commercial	68	3	2	9	-2.46	-0.27
Soup, minestrone, canned, prepared with equal volume water, commercial	34	2	1	5	-1.27	-0.25
Soup, minestrone, canned, reduced sodium, ready-to-serve	50	2	1	9	-2.26	-0.25
Soup, mushroom barley, canned, condensed, commercial	61	1	2	10	0.67	0.07
Soup, mushroom barley, canned, prepared with equal volume water, commercial	30	1	1	5	0.33	0.07
Soup, mushroom with beef stock, canned, condensed, commercial	68	3	3	7	-0.62	-0.09
Soup, mushroom with beef stock, canned, prepared with equal volume water, commercial	35	1	2	4	-0.33	-0.08
Soup, mushroom, dehydrated, prepared with water	38	1	2	4	-0.50	-0.13
Soup, onion, canned, condensed, commercial	46	3	1	7	0.31	0.04
Soup, onion, canned, prepared with equal volume water, commercial	24	1	1	3	0.19	0.06
Soup, onion, dehydrated, prepared with water	11	0	0	3	0	0
Soup, oxtail, dehydrated, prepared with water	28	1	1	4	0.58	0.15
Soup, oyster stew, canned, condensed, commercial	48	2	3	3	1.10	0.37
Soup, oyster stew, canned, prepared with equal volume milk, commercial	55	1	2	2	0.56	0.28
Soup, oyster stew, canned, prepared with equal volume water, commercial	24	1	2	2	0.57	0.29
Soup, pea, green, canned, condensed, commercial	125	7	2	20	2.62	0.13

Soups, Sauces, and Gravies

Food Description	Kcals	Protein	Fat	Carbs	PRAL	Alkali Density
Soup, pea, green, canned, prepared with equal volume milk, commercial	94	5	3	13	1.34	0.10
Soup, pea, green, canned, prepared with equal volume water, commercial	66	3	1	10	1.38	0.14
Soup, pea, low sodium, with water	66	3	1	10	1.36	0.14
Soup, pea, split with ham, canned, chunky, ready-to-serve	77	5	2	11	1.73	0.16
Soup, pea, split with ham, canned, condensed, commercial	141	8	3	21	2.26	0.11
Soup, pea, split with ham, canned, prepared with equal volume water, commercial	75	4	2	11	1.17	0.11
Soup, pepperpot, canned, condensed, commercial	84	5	4	8	0.84	0.11
Soup, pepperpot, canned, prepared with equal volume water, commercial	43	3	2	4	0.41	0.10
Soup, ramen noodle, any flavor, dehydrated, dry	453	9	17	66	5.20	0.08
Soup, ramen noodle, beef flavor, dehydrated, dry	436	10	16	63	4.62	0.07
Soup, ramen noodle, chicken flavor, dehydrated, dry	437	11	16	64	5.03	0.08
Soup, scotch broth, canned, condensed, commercial	66	4	2	8	0.68	0.09
Soup, scotch broth, canned, prepared with equal volume water, commercial	33	2	1	4	0.34	0.09
Soup, shark fin, restaurant-prepared	46	3	2	4	0.92	0.23
Soup, stock, beef, home-prepared	13	2	0	1	-2.05	-2.05
Soup, stock, chicken, home-prepared	36	3	1	4	-0.11	-0.03
Soup, stock, fish, home-prepared	17	2	1	0	-0.06	!
Soup, stockpot, canned, condensed, commercial	78	4	3	9	-0.77	-0.09
Soup, stockpot, canned, prepared with equal volume water, commercial	40	2	2	5	-0.40	-0.08
Soup, SWANSON Chicken Broth 99% Fat Free	4	1	0	0	-0.03	!
Soup, tomato beef with noodle, canned, condensed, commercial	112	4	3	17	-0.63	-0.04
Soup, tomato beef with noodle, canned, prepared with equal volume water, commercial	57	2	2	8	-0.31	-0.04
Soup, tomato bisque, canned, condensed, commercial	96	2	2	18	-4.80	-0.27
Soup, tomato bisque, canned, prepared with equal volume milk, commercial	79	3	3	12	-2.50	-0.21
Soup, tomato bisque, canned, prepared with equal volume water, commercial	50	1	1	10	-2.52	-0.25
Soup, tomato rice, canned, condensed, commercial	93	2	2	17	-3.96	-0.23
Soup, tomato rice, canned, prepared with equal volume water, commercial	48	1	1	9	-2.04	-0.23
Soup, tomato vegetable mix, dehydrated, dry form	325	12	5	60	-4.14	-0.07
Soup, tomato vegetable, dehydrated, prepared with water	22	1	0	4	-0.27	-0.07
Soup, tomato, canned, condensed, commercial	60	2	1	13	-3.48	-0.27
Soup, tomato, canned, condensed, reduced sodium	65	2	1	13	-1.50	-0.12
Soup, tomato, canned, prepared with equal volume milk, commercial	65	3	3	12	-1.44	-0.12
Soup, tomato, canned, prepared with equal volume water, commercial	35	1	0	7	-1.48	-0.21

Soups, Sauces, and Gravies

Food Description	Kcals	Protein	Fat	Carbs	PRAL	Alkali Density
Soup, tomato, dehydrated, prepared with water	39	1	1	7	-1.34	-0.19
Soup, tomato, low sodium, with water	35	1	0	7	-1.50	-0.21
Soup, turkey noodle, canned, condensed, commercial	55	3	2	7	1.44	0.21
Soup, turkey noodle, canned, prepared with equal volume water, commercial	28	2	1	4	0.75	0.19
Soup, turkey vegetable, canned, condensed, commercial	60	3	2	7	-0.80	-0.11
Soup, turkey vegetable, canned, prepared with equal volume water, commercial	30	1	1	4	-0.42	-0.11
Soup, turkey, chunky, ready-to-serve	57	4	2	6	0	0
Soup, vegetable beef, canned, condensed, commercial	63	4	2	8	0.16	0.02
Soup, vegetable beef, dehydrated, dry	344	4	2	6	2.83	0.47
Soup, vegetable beef, dehydrated, prepared with water	21	1	0	3	0.15	0.05
Soup, vegetable beef, prepared with equal volume water, commercial	32	2	1	4	0.11	0.03
Soup, vegetable chicken, low sodium	69	5	2	9	0.66	0.07
Soup, vegetable with beef broth, canned, condensed, commercial	66	2	2	11	-1.23	-0.11
Soup, vegetable with beef broth, canned, prepared with equal volume water, commercial	34	1	1	5	-0.65	-0.13
Soup, vegetable, canned, chunky, ready-to-serve, commercial	51	1	2	8	-2.01	-0.25
Soup, vegetable, canned, low sodium, condensed	65	2	1	12	-7.26	-0.61
Soup, vegetarian vegetable, canned, condensed, commercial	59	2	2	10	-2.08	-0.21
Soup, vegetarian vegetable, canned, prepared with equal volume water, commercial	30	1	1	5	-1.07	-0.21
USDA Commodity, salsa	36	1	0	7	-4.39	-0.63
USDA Commodity, spaghetti sauce, meatless, canned	48	1	1	9	-5.21	-0.58
Vegetable soup, low sodium, with water	22	5	2	9	-2.83	-0.31

Poultry Products

Food Description	Kcals	Protein	Fat	Carbs	PRAL	Acid Density
Chicken, broilers or fryers, back, meat and skin, cooked, fried, batter	331	22	22	10	11.22	0.51
Chicken, broilers or fryers, back, meat and skin, cooked, fried, flour	331	22	22	10	14.10	0.64
Chicken, broilers or fryers, back, meat and skin, cooked, roasted	300	26	21	0	13.21	0.51
Chicken, broilers or fryers, back, meat and skin, cooked, stewed	258	22	18	0	11.61	0.53
Chicken, broilers or fryers, back, meat and skin, raw	319	14	29	0	7.48	0.53
Chicken, broilers or fryers, back, meat only, cooked, fried	288	30	15	6	14.94	0.50
Chicken, broilers or fryers, back, meat only, cooked, roasted	239	28	13	0	14.05	0.50
Chicken, broilers or fryers, back, meat only, cooked, stewed	209	25	11	0	13.17	0.53
Chicken, broilers or fryers, back, meat only, raw	137	20	6	0	10.09	0.50
Chicken, broilers or fryers, breast, meat and skin, cooked, fried, flour	222	32	9	2	17.79	0.56
Chicken, broilers or fryers, breast, meat and skin, cooked, fried, batter	260	25	13	9	13.91	0.56
Chicken, broilers or fryers, breast, meat and skin, cooked, roasted	197	30	8	0	16.49	0.55
Chicken, broilers or fryers, breast, meat and skin, cooked, stewed	184	27	7	0	14.71	0.54
Chicken, broilers or fryers, breast, meat and skin, raw	172	21	9	0	11.24	0.54
Chicken, broilers or fryers, breast, meat only, cooked, fried	187	33	5	1	18.67	0.57
Chicken, broilers or fryers, breast, meat only, cooked, roasted	165	31	4	0	17.31	0.56
Chicken, broilers or fryers, breast, meat only, cooked, stewed	151	29	3	0	15.58	0.54
Chicken, broilers or fryers, breast, meat only, raw	110	23	1	0	12.34	0.54
Chicken, broilers or fryers, dark meat, meat and skin, cooked, fried, batter	298	22	19	9	11.39	0.52
Chicken, broilers or fryers, dark meat, meat and skin, cooked, fried, flour	285	27	7	4	14.17	0.52
Chicken, broilers or fryers, dark meat, meat and skin, cooked, roasted	253	26	16	0	13.55	0.52
Chicken, broilers or fryers, dark meat, meat and skin, cooked, stewed	233	24	15	0	12.30	0.51
Chicken, broilers or fryers, dark meat, meat and skin, raw	237	17	18	0	8.83	0.52
Chicken, broilers or fryers, dark meat, meat only, cooked, fried	239	29	12	3	14.92	0.51
Chicken, broilers or fryers, dark meat, meat only, cooked, roasted	205	27	10	0	14.20	0.53
Chicken, broilers or fryers, dark meat, meat only, cooked, stewed	192	26	9	0	13.51	0.52
Chicken, broilers or fryers, dark meat, meat only, raw	125	20	4	0	10.41	0.52
Chicken, broilers or fryers, drumstick, meat and skin, cooked, fried, flour	245	27	14	2	14.15	0.52
Chicken, broilers or fryers, drumstick, meat and skin, cooked, fried, batter	268	22	16	8	11.54	0.52
Chicken, broilers or fryers, drumstick, meat and skin, cooked, roasted	216	27	11	0	14.15	0.52
Chicken, broilers or fryers, drumstick, meat and skin, cooked, stewed	204	25	11	0	13.09	0.52

Poultry Products

Food Description	Kcals	Protein	Fat	Carbs	PRAL	Acid Density
Chicken, broilers or fryers, drumstick, meat and skin, raw	161	19	9	0	10.12	0.53
Chicken, broilers or fryers, drumstick, meat only, cooked, fried	195	29	8	0	14.89	0.51
Chicken, broilers or fryers, drumstick, meat only, cooked, roasted	172	28	6	0	14.72	0.53
Chicken, broilers or fryers, drumstick, meat only, cooked, stewed	169	27	6	0	14.15	0.52
Chicken, broilers or fryers, drumstick, meat only, raw	119	21	3	0	10.74	0.51
Chicken, broilers or fryers, giblets, cooked, fried	277	33	13	4	18.71	0.57
Chicken, broilers or fryers, giblets, cooked, simmered	158	27	5	0	18.74	0.69
Chicken, broilers or fryers, giblets, raw	124	18	4	2	10.66	0.59
Chicken, broilers or fryers, leg, meat and skin, cooked, fried, batter	273	22	16	9	11.56	0.53
Chicken, broilers or fryers, leg, meat and skin, cooked, fried, flour	254	27	14	3	14.20	0.53
Chicken, broilers or fryers, leg, meat and skin, cooked, roasted	232	26	13	0	13.67	0.53
Chicken, broilers or fryers, leg, meat and skin, cooked, stewed	220	24	13	0	12.62	0.53
Chicken, broilers or fryers, leg, meat and skin, raw	187	18	12	0	9.57	0.53
Chicken, broilers or fryers, leg, meat only, cooked, fried	208	28	9	1	14.89	0.53
Chicken, broilers or fryers, leg, meat only, cooked, roasted	191	27	8	0	14.15	0.52
Chicken, broilers or fryers, leg, meat only, cooked, stewed	185	26	8	0	13.70	0.53
Chicken, broilers or fryers, leg, meat only, raw	120	20	4	0	10.49	0.52
Chicken, broilers or fryers, light meat, meat and skin, cooked, fried, batter	277	24	15	9	13.03	0.54
Chicken, broilers or fryers, light meat, meat and skin, cooked, fried, flour	246	30	12	2	16.87	0.56
Chicken, broilers or fryers, light meat, meat and skin, cooked, roasted	222	29	11	0	16	0.55
Chicken, broilers or fryers, light meat, meat and skin, cooked, stewed	201	26	10	0	14.01	0.54
Chicken, broilers or fryers, light meat, meat and skin, raw	186	20	11	0	10.93	0.55
Chicken, broilers or fryers, light meat, meat only, cooked, fried	192	33	6	0	18.14	0.55
Chicken, broilers or fryers, light meat, meat only, cooked, roasted	173	31	5	0	17.05	0.55
Chicken, broilers or fryers, light meat, meat only, cooked, stewed	159	29	4	0	15.51	0.53
Chicken, broilers or fryers, light meat, meat only, raw	114	23	2	0	12.41	0.54
Chicken, broilers or fryers, meat and skin and giblets and neck, cooked, fried, flour	272	29	15	3	15.32	0.53
Chicken, broilers or fryers, meat and skin and giblets and neck, cooked, fried, batter	291	23	18	9	12.22	0.53
Chicken, broilers or fryers, meat and skin and giblets and neck, roasted	234	27	13	0	14.61	0.54
Chicken, broilers or fryers, meat and skin and giblets and neck, raw	213	18	15	0	9.86	0.55
Chicken, broilers or fryers, meat and skin and giblets and neck, stewed	216	24	12	0	13.22	0.55

Poultry Products

Food Description	Kcals	Protein	Fat	Carbs	PRAL	Acid Density
Chicken, broilers or fryers, meat and skin, cooked, fried, batter	289	23	17	9	12.07	0.52
Chicken, broilers or fryers, meat and skin, cooked, fried, flour	269	29	15	3	15.27	0.53
Chicken, broilers or fryers, meat and skin, cooked, roasted	239	27	14	0	14.63	0.54
Chicken, broilers or fryers, meat and skin, cooked, stewed	219	25	13	0	13.08	0.52
Chicken, broilers or fryers, meat and skin, raw	215	19	15	0	9.92	0.52
Chicken, broilers or fryers, meat only, cooked, fried	219	31	9	2	16.24	0.52
Chicken, broilers or fryers, meat only, raw	119	21	3	0	11.26	0.54
Chicken, broilers or fryers, meat only, roasted	190	29	7	0	15.44	0.53
Chicken, broilers or fryers, meat only, stewed	177	27	7	0	14.41	0.53
Chicken, broilers or fryers, neck, meat and skin, cooked simmered	247	20	18	0	11.16	0.56
Chicken, broilers or fryers, neck, meat and skin, cooked, fried, batter	330	20	24	9	9.97	0.50
Chicken, broilers or fryers, neck, meat and skin, cooked, fried, flour	332	24	24	4	11.97	0.50
Chicken, broilers or fryers, neck, meat and skin, raw	297	14	26	0	7.58	0.54
Chicken, broilers or fryers, neck, meat only, cooked, fried	229	27	12	2	12.63	0.47
Chicken, broilers or fryers, neck, meat only, cooked, simmered	179	25	8	0	12.84	0.51
Chicken, broilers or fryers, neck, meat only, raw	154	18	9	0	8.31	0.46
Chicken, broilers or fryers, separable fat, raw	629	4	68	0	2.23	0.56
Chicken, broilers or fryers, skin only, cooked, fried, batter	394	10	29	23	5.79	0.58
Chicken, broilers or fryers, skin only, cooked, fried, flour	502	19	43	9	10.76	0.57
Chicken, broilers or fryers, skin only, cooked, roasted	454	20	41	0	11.17	0.56
Chicken, broilers or fryers, skin only, cooked, stewed	363	7	15	0	8.17	1.17
Chicken, broilers or fryers, skin only, raw	349	13	32	0	7.58	0.58
Chicken, broilers or fryers, thigh, meat and skin, cooked, fried, batter	277	22	17	9	11.51	0.52
Chicken, broilers or fryers, thigh, meat and skin, cooked, fried, flour	262	27	15	3	14.21	0.53
Chicken, broilers or fryers, thigh, meat and skin, cooked, roasted	247	25	15	0	13.32	0.53
Chicken, broilers or fryers, thigh, meat and skin, cooked, stewed	232	23	15	0	12.33	0.54
Chicken, broilers or fryers, thigh, meat and skin, raw	211	17	15	0	9.14	0.54
Chicken, broilers or fryers, thigh, meat only, cooked, fried	218	28	10	1	14.88	0.53
Chicken, broilers or fryers, thigh, meat only, cooked, roasted	209	26	11	0	13.70	0.53
Chicken, broilers or fryers, thigh, meat only, cooked, stewed	195	25	10	0	13.23	0.53
Chicken, broilers or fryers, thigh, meat only, raw	119	20	4	0	10.24	0.51
Chicken, broilers or fryers, wing, meat and skin, cooked, fried, batter	324	20	22	11	10.63	0.53

Poultry Products

Food Description	Kcals	Protein	Fat	Carbs	PRAL	Acid Density
Chicken, broilers or fryers, wing, meat and skin, cooked, fried, flour	321	5	4	0	13.93	2.79
Chicken, broilers or fryers, wing, meat and skin, cooked, roasted	290	27	18	0	14.19	0.53
Chicken, broilers or fryers, wing, meat and skin, cooked, stewed	249	32	24	0	12.14	0.38
Chicken, broilers or fryers, wing, meat and skin, raw	222	18	16	0	9.96	0.55
Chicken, broilers or fryers, wing, meat only, cooked, fried	211	30	9	0	15.73	0.52
Chicken, broilers or fryers, wing, meat only, cooked, roasted	203	30	8	0	15.90	0.53
Chicken, broilers or fryers, wing, meat only, cooked, stewed	181	27	7	0	14.42	0.53
Chicken, broilers or fryers, wing, meat only, raw	126	22	4	0	11.68	0.53
Chicken, canned, meat only, with broth	165	22	8	0	11.38	0.52
Chicken, canned, no broth	184	25	8	1	14.16	0.57
Chicken, capons, giblets, cooked, simmered	164	26	5	1	17.72	0.68
Chicken, capons, giblets, raw	130	18	5	1	11.27	0.63
Chicken, capons, meat and skin and giblets and neck, cooked, roasted	226	28	12	0	16.83	0.60
Chicken, capons, meat and skin and giblets and neck, raw	232	19	17	0	10.60	0.56
Chicken, capons, meat and skin, cooked, roasted	229	29	12	0	17.13	0.59
Chicken, capons, meat and skin, raw	234	18	17	0	10.72	0.60
Chicken, cornish game hens, meat and skin, cooked, roasted	260	22	18	0	10.53	0.48
Chicken, cornish game hens, meat and skin, raw	200	17	14	0	8.01	0.47
Chicken, cornish game hens, meat only, cooked, roasted	134	23	4	0	11.01	0.48
Chicken, cornish game hens, meat only, raw	116	20	3	0	9.38	0.47
Chicken, feet, boiled	215	19	15	0	10.65	0.56
Chicken, gizzard, all classes, cooked, simmered	146	30	3	0	17.82	0.59
Chicken, gizzard, all classes, raw	94	18	2	0	8.61	0.48
Chicken, heart, all classes, cooked, simmered	185	26	8	0	16.76	0.64
Chicken, heart, all classes, raw	153	16	9	1	9.92	0.62
Chicken, liver, all classes, cooked, pan-fried	172	26	6	1	21.53	0.83
Chicken, liver, all classes, cooked, simmered	167	24	7	1	20.65	0.86
Chicken, liver, all classes, raw	116	17	5	0	13.85	0.81
Chicken, roasting, dark meat, meat only, cooked, roasted	178	23	9	0	12.35	0.54
Chicken, roasting, dark meat, meat only, raw	113	19	4	0	10.33	0.54
Chicken, roasting, giblets, cooked, simmered	165	27	5	1	16.96	0.63
Chicken, roasting, giblets, raw	127	18	5	1	10.35	0.58
Chicken, roasting, light meat, meat only, cooked, roasted	153	27	4	0	15.60	0.58
Chicken, roasting, light meat, meat only, raw	109	22	2	0	13.04	0.59
Chicken, roasting, meat and skin and giblets and neck, cooked, roasted	220	24	13	0	13.39	0.56

Poultry Products

Food Description	Kcals	Protein	Fat	Carbs	PRAL	Acid Density
Chicken, roasting, meat and skin and giblets and neck, raw	213	17	15	0	9.73	0.57
Chicken, roasting, meat and skin, cooked, roasted	223	24	13	0	13.26	0.55
Chicken, roasting, meat and skin, raw	216	17	16	0	9.80	0.58
Chicken, roasting, meat only, cooked, roasted	167	25	7	0	13.84	0.55
Chicken, roasting, meat only, raw	111	20	3	0	11.56	0.58
Chicken, stewing, dark meat, meat only, cooked, stewed	258	26	9	0	15.69	0.60
Chicken, stewing, dark meat, meat only, raw	157	20	8	0	10.87	0.54
Chicken, stewing, giblets, cooked, simmered	194	26	9	0	16.93	0.65
Chicken, stewing, giblets, raw	168	18	9	2	10.74	0.60
Chicken, stewing, light meat, meat only, cooked, stewed	213	22	8	0	19.55	0.89
Chicken, stewing, light meat, meat only, raw	137	23	4	0	13.56	0.59
Chicken, stewing, meat and skin, and giblets and neck, cooked, stewed	214	25	12	0	13.52	0.54
Chicken, stewing, meat and skin, and giblets and neck, raw	251	17	20	0	10.03	0.59
Chicken, stewing, meat and skin, cooked, stewed	285	27	19	0	15.32	0.57
Chicken, stewing, meat and skin, raw	258	18	20	0	10.03	0.56
Chicken, stewing, meat only, cooked, stewed	237	30	12	0	17.47	0.58
Chicken, stewing, meat only, raw	148	21	6	0	12.12	0.58
Chicken, wing, frozen, glazed, barbecue flavored	211	20	13	3	12.34	0.62
Chicken, wing, frozen, glazed, barbecue flavored, heated (conventional oven)	242	22	15	3	14.03	0.64
Chicken, wing, frozen, glazed, barbecue flavored, heated (microwave)	248	25	14	0	15.95	0.64
Dove, cooked (includes squab)	219	24	13	0	17.72	0.74
Duck, domesticated, liver, raw	136	19	5	4	13.53	0.71
Duck, domesticated, meat and skin, cooked, roasted	337	19	28	0	10.23	0.54
Duck, domesticated, meat and skin, raw	404	11	39	0	5.85	0.53
Duck, domesticated, meat only, cooked, roasted	201	23	11	0	13.04	0.57
Duck, domesticated, meat only, raw	132	18	6	0	10.14	0.56
Duck, wild, breast, meat only, raw	123	20	4	0	10.37	0.52
Duck, wild, meat and skin, raw	211	17	0	15	8.93	0.53
Emu, fan fillet, cooked, broiled	154	31	2	0	16.19	0.52
Emu, fan fillet, raw	103	22	1	0	12.32	0.56
Emu, flat fillet, raw	102	22	1	0	13.49	0.61
Emu, full rump, cooked, broiled	168	34	3	0	20.67	0.61
Emu, full rump, raw	112	23	2	0	11.89	0.52
Emu, ground, cooked, pan-broiled	163	28	5	0	15.15	0.54
Emu, ground, raw	134	23	4	0	11.93	0.52
Emu, inside drum, raw	108	22	1	0	11.95	0.54
Emu, inside drums, cooked, broiled	156	32	2	0	19.73	0.62

Poultry Products

Food Description	Kcals	Protein	Fat	Carbs	PRAL	Acid Density
Emu, outside drum, raw	103	23	0	0	12.12	0.53
Emu, oyster, raw	141	23	5	0	13.12	0.57
Emu, top loin, cooked, broiled	152	29	3	0	15.63	0.54
Goose, domesticated, meat and skin, cooked, roasted	305	25	22	0	14.66	0.59
Goose, domesticated, meat and skin, raw	371	16	34	0	9.33	0.58
Goose, domesticated, meat only, cooked, roasted	238	29	13	0	16.64	0.57
Goose, domesticated, meat only, raw	161	23	7	0	13.07	0.57
Goose, liver, raw	133	16	4	6	11.66	0.73
Guinea hen, meat and skin, raw	158	23	6	0	12.35	0.54
Guinea hen, meat only, raw	110	21	2	0	10.98	0.52
Ostrich, fan, raw	117	22	3	0	11.37	0.52
Ostrich, ground, cooked, pan-broiled	175	26	7	0	13.61	0.52
Ostrich, ground, raw	165	20	9	0	10.54	0.53
Ostrich, inside leg, cooked	141	29	2	0	15.12	0.52
Ostrich, inside leg, raw	111	22	2	0	11.75	0.53
Ostrich, inside strip, cooked	164	29	4	0	15.32	0.53
Ostrich, inside strip, raw	127	24	3	0	12.37	0.52
Ostrich, outside leg, raw	115	23	2	0	11.95	0.52
Ostrich, outside strip, cooked	156	29	4	0	14.94	0.52
Ostrich, outside strip, raw	120	23	2	0	12.26	0.53
Ostrich, oyster, cooked	159	29	4	0	15.09	0.52
Ostrich, oyster, raw	125	22	4	0	11.24	0.51
Ostrich, round, raw	116	22	2	0	11.51	0.52
Ostrich, tenderloin, raw	123	22	3	0	11.58	0.53
Ostrich, tip trimmed, cooked	145	28	3	0	14.91	0.53
Ostrich, tip trimmed, raw	114	22	2	0	11.44	0.52
Ostrich, top loin, cooked	155	28	4	0	14.70	0.53
Ostrich, top loin, raw	119	22	3	0	11.33	0.52
Pate de foie gras, canned (goose liver pate), smoked	462	11	44	5	8.84	0.80
Pheasant, breast, meat only, raw	133	24	3	0	13.67	0.57
Pheasant, cooked, total edible	247	32	12	0	18.35	0.57
Pheasant, leg, meat only, raw	134	22	4	0	14.12	0.64
Pheasant, raw, meat and skin	181	23	9	0	13.26	0.58
Pheasant, raw, meat only	133	24	4	0	13.86	0.58
Poultry food products, ground turkey, cooked	235	27	13	0	14.03	0.52
Poultry food products, ground turkey, raw	149	17	8	0	8.77	0.52
Poultry, mechanically deboned, from backs and necks with skin, raw	272	11	25	0	6.17	0.56
Poultry, mechanically deboned, from backs and necks without skin, raw	199	14	15	0	7.83	0.56

Poultry Products

Food Description	Kcals	Protein	Fat	Carbs	PRAL	Acid Density
Poultry, mechanically deboned, from mature hens, raw	243	15	20	0	7.17	0.48
Quail, breast, meat only, raw	123	23	3	0	13.18	0.57
Quail, cooked, total edible	234	25	14	0	17.31	0.69
Quail, meat and skin, raw	192	20	12	0	14.49	0.72
Quail, meat only, raw	134	22	5	0	16.22	0.74
Squab, (pigeon), light meat without skin, raw	134	22	5	0	12.78	0.58
Squab, (pigeon), meat and skin, raw	294	18	24	0	13.31	0.74
Squab, (pigeon), meat only, raw	142	17	8	0	14.13	0.83
Turkey and gravy, frozen	67	6	3	5	4.20	0.70
Turkey bacon, cooked	382	30	28	3	22.35	0.75
Turkey breast, pre-basted, meat and skin, cooked, roasted	126	22	3	0	12.90	0.59
Turkey patties, breaded, battered, fried	283	14	18	16	10.50	0.75
Turkey roast, boneless, frozen, seasoned, light and dark meat, raw	120	18	2	6	6.37	0.35
Turkey roast, boneless, frozen, seasoned, light and dark meat, roasted	155	21	6	3	12.58	0.60
Turkey sticks, breaded, battered, fried	279	14	17	17	9.58	0.68
Turkey thigh, pre-basted, meat and skin, cooked, roasted	157	19	9	0	9.93	0.52
Turkey, all classes, back, meat and skin, cooked, roasted	243	27	14	0	13.56	0.50
Turkey, all classes, back, meat and skin, raw	196	18	13	0	9.03	0.50
Turkey, all classes, breast, meat and skin, cooked, roasted	189	28	7	0	14.81	0.53
Turkey, all classes, breast, meat and skin, raw	157	32	10	0	11.04	0.35
Turkey, all classes, dark meat, cooked, roasted	187	29	7	0	14.41	0.50
Turkey, all classes, dark meat, meat and skin, cooked, roasted	221	27	12	0	13.94	0.52
Turkey, all classes, dark meat, meat and skin, raw	160	19	9	0	9.33	0.49
Turkey, all classes, dark meat, raw	125	20	4	0	9.84	0.49
Turkey, all classes, giblets, cooked, simmered, some giblet fat	199	21	12	0	12.56	0.60
Turkey, all classes, giblets, raw	129	19	4	2	10.39	0.55
Turkey, all classes, leg, meat and skin, cooked, roasted	208	28	10	0	14.12	0.50
Turkey, all classes, leg, meat and skin, raw	144	20	7	0	9.62	0.48
Turkey, all classes, light meat, cooked, roasted	157	30	3	0	15.37	0.51
Turkey, all classes, light meat, meat and skin, cooked, roasted	197	29	8	0	14.76	0.51
Turkey, all classes, light meat, meat and skin, raw	159	22	7	0	10.92	0.50
Turkey, all classes, light meat, raw	115	24	2	0	11.82	0.49
Turkey, all classes, meat and skin and giblets and neck, cooked, roasted	205	28	8	0	14.43	0.52
Turkey, all classes, meat and skin and giblets and neck, raw	157	20	8	0	10.22	0.51
Turkey, all classes, meat and skin, cooked, roasted	208	28	10	0	14.41	0.51

Poultry Products

Food Description	Kcals	Protein	Fat	Carbs	PRAL	Acid Density
Turkey, all classes, meat and skin, raw	160	20	12	0	10.23	0.51
Turkey, all classes, meat only, cooked, roasted	170	29	5	0	14.98	0.52
Turkey, all classes, meat only, raw	119	22	3	0s	10.83	0.49
Turkey, all classes, neck, meat only, cooked, simmered	180	27	7	0	13.66	0.51
Turkey, all classes, neck, meat only, raw	135	20	5	0	9.47	0.47
Turkey, all classes, skin only, cooked, roasted	442	20	40	0	10.49	0.52
Turkey, all classes, skin only, raw	387	13	37	0	6.67	0.51
Turkey, all classes, wing, meat and skin, cooked, roasted	229	27	12	0	14.15	0.52
Turkey, all classes, wing, meat and skin, raw	197	20	12	0	10.24	0.51
Turkey, canned, meat only, with broth	163	24	7	0	12.21	0.51
Turkey, diced, light and dark meat, seasoned	138	18	6	1	11.07	0.62
Turkey, drumstick, smoked, cooked, with skin, bone removed	208	28	10	0	14.14	0.51
Turkey, fryer-roasters, back, meat and skin, cooked, roasted	204	26	10	0	13.74	0.53
Turkey, fryer-roasters, back, meat and skin, raw	151	20	7	0	10.45	0.52
Turkey, fryer-roasters, back, meat only, cooked, roasted	170	28	6	0	14.68	0.52
Turkey, fryer-roasters, back, meat only, raw	120	21	4	0	10.88	0.52
Turkey, fryer-roasters, breast, meat and skin, cooked, roasted	153	29	3	0	15.45	0.53
Turkey, fryer-roasters, breast, meat and skin, raw	125	24	3	0	12.24	0.51
Turkey, fryer-roasters, breast, meat only, cooked, roasted	135	30	1	0	15.97	0.53
Turkey, fryer-roasters, breast, meat only, raw	111	25	1	0	12.66	0.51
Turkey, fryer-roasters, dark meat, meat and skin, cooked, roasted	182	28	7	0	14.67	0.52
Turkey, fryer-roasters, dark meat, meat and skin, raw	129	20	5	0	10.28	0.51
Turkey, fryer-roasters, dark meat, meat only, cooked, roasted	162	19	4	0	15.25	0.80
Turkey, fryer-roasters, dark meat, meat only, raw	111	20	3	0	10.48	0.52
Turkey, fryer-roasters, leg, meat and skin, cooked, roasted	170	28	5	0	15.14	0.54
Turkey, fryer-roasters, leg, meat and skin, raw	118	20	4	0	10.22	0.51
Turkey, fryer-roasters, leg, meat only, cooked, roasted	159	29	4	0	15.49	0.53
Turkey, fryer-roasters, leg, meat only, raw	108	19	2	0	10.30	0.54
Turkey, fryer-roasters, light meat, meat and skin, cooked, roasted	164	29	5	0	15.27	0.53
Turkey, fryer-roasters, light meat, meat and skin, raw	133	23	4	0	11.95	0.52
Turkey, fryer-roasters, light meat, meat only, cooked, roasted	140	30	1	0	16.04	0.53
Turkey, fryer-roasters, light meat, meat only, raw	108	24	0	0	12.49	0.52
Turkey, fryer-roasters, meat and skin and giblets and neck, cooked, roasted	171	28	6	0	15	0.54
Turkey, fryer-roasters, meat and skin and giblets and neck, raw	133	22	4	0	11.42	0.52

Poultry Products

Food Description	Kcals	Protein	Fat	Carbs	PRAL	Acid Density
Turkey, fryer-roasters, meat and skin, cooked, roasted	172	28	6	0	14.98	0.54
Turkey, fryer-roasters, meat and skin, raw	134	20	4	0	11.51	0.58
Turkey, fryer-roasters, meat only, cooked, roasted	150	30	3	0	15.68	0.52
Turkey, fryer-roasters, meat only, raw	110	22	2	0	11.50	0.52
Turkey, fryer-roasters, skin only, cooked, roasted	299	21	23	0	11.11	0.53
Turkey, fryer-roasters, skin only, raw	283	17	24	0	8.67	0.51
Turkey, fryer-roasters, wing, meat and skin, cooked, roasted	207	28	10	0	14.67	0.52
Turkey, fryer-roasters, wing, meat and skin, raw	159	21	8	0	10.96	0.52
Turkey, fryer-roasters, wing, meat only, cooked, roasted	163	31	3	0	16.36	0.53
Turkey, fryer-roasters, wing, meat only, raw	106	22	1	0	11.86	0.54
Turkey, gizzard, all classes, cooked, simmered	123	22	4	0	8.83	0.40
Turkey, gizzard, all classes, raw	118	19	5	0	7.30	0.38
Turkey, heart, all classes, cooked, simmered	130	21	5	1	13.22	0.63
Turkey, heart, all classes, raw	113	17	5	0	9.76	0.57
Turkey, light or dark meat, smoked, cooked, skin and bone removed	170	29	5	0	14.97	0.52
Turkey, light or dark meat, smoked, cooked, with skin, bone removed	208	28	10	0	14.41	0.51
Turkey, liver, all classes, cooked, simmered	273	20	21	1	15.75	0.79
Turkey, liver, all classes, raw	228	18	16	2s	13.25	0.74
Turkey, mechanically deboned, from turkey frames, raw	201	13	16	0	4.91	0.38
Turkey, wing, smoked, cooked, with skin, bone removed	229	27	12	0	14.16	0.52
Turkey, young hen, back, meat and skin, cooked, roasted	254	26	16	0	13.41	0.52
Turkey, young hen, back, meat and skin, raw	218	18	16	0	8.68	0.48
Turkey, young hen, breast, meat and skin, cooked, roasted	194	29	8	0	14.85	0.51
Turkey, young hen, breast, meat and skin, raw	167	22	8	0	10.83	0.49
Turkey, young hen, dark meat, meat and skin, cooked, roasted	232	27	13	0	13.86	0.51
Turkey, young hen, dark meat, meat and skin, raw	172	19	10	0	9.23	0.49
Turkey, young hen, dark meat, meat only, cooked, roasted	192	28	8	0	14.30	0.51
Turkey, young hen, dark meat, meat only, raw	130	20	5	0	9.82	0.49
Turkey, young hen, leg, meat and skin, cooked, roasted	213	28	11	0	13.97	0.50
Turkey, young hen, leg, meat and skin, raw	151	19	8	0	9.58	0.50
Turkey, young hen, light meat, meat and skin, cooked, roasted	207	29	9	0	14.74	0.51
Turkey, young hen, light meat, meat and skin, raw	165	22	8	0	10.80	0.49
Turkey, young hen, light meat, meat only, cooked, roasted	161	30	4	0	15.32	0.51
Turkey, young hen, light meat, meat only, raw	116	24	2	0	11.81	0.49

Poultry Products

Food Description	Kcals	Protein	Fat	Carbs	PRAL	Acid Density
Turkey, young hen, meat and skin and giblets and neck, cooked, roasted	215	28	11	0	14.40	0.51
Turkey, young hen, meat and skin and giblets and neck, raw	166	20	9	0	10.07	0.50
Turkey, young hen, meat and skin, cooked, roasted	218	28	11	0	14.36	0.51
Turkey, young hen, meat and skin, raw	168	20	9	0	10.07	0.50
Turkey, young hen, meat only, cooked, roasted	175	29	6	0	14.89	0.51
Turkey, young hen, meat only, raw	122	22	3	0	10.80	0.49
Turkey, young hen, skin only, cooked, roasted	482	19	44	0	10.18	0.54
Turkey, young hen, skin only, raw	417	12	41	0	6.07	0.51
Turkey, young hen, wing, meat and skin, cooked, roasted	238	27	14	0	14.11	0.52
Turkey, young hen, wing, meat and skin, raw	210	20	14	0	10.03	0.50
Turkey, young tom, back, meat and skin, cooked, roasted	238	27	14	0	13.62	0.50
Turkey, young tom, back, meat and skin, raw	179	18	11	0	9.17	0.51
Turkey, young tom, breast, meat and skin, cooked, roasted	189	29	7	0	14.74	0.51
Turkey, young tom, breast, meat and skin, raw	151	22	2	0	11.11	0.51
Turkey, young tom, dark meat, meat and skin, cooked, roasted	216	28	11	0	13.95	0.50
Turkey, young tom, dark meat, meat and skin, raw	152	19	8	0	9.39	0.49
Turkey, young tom, dark meat, meat only, cooked, roasted	185	29	7	0	14.43	0.50
Turkey, young tom, dark meat, meat only, raw	123	20	4	0	9.80	0.49
Turkey, young tom, leg, meat and skin, cooked, roasted	206	28	10	0	14.13	0.50
Turkey, young tom, leg, meat and skin, raw	141	20	6	0	9.60	0.48
Turkey, young tom, light meat, meat and skin, cooked, roasted	191	28	8	0	14.68	0.52
Turkey, young tom, light meat, meat and skin, raw	156	22	7	0	10.94	0.50
Turkey, young tom, light meat, meat only, cooked, roasted	154	30	3	0	15.35	0.51
Turkey, young tom, light meat, meat only, raw	114	23	2	0	11.76	0.51
Turkey, young tom, meat and skin and giblets and neck, cooked, roasted	199	28	9	0	14.38	0.51
Turkey, young tom, meat and skin and giblets and neck, raw	152	20	7	0	10.20	0.51
Turkey, young tom, meat and skin, cooked, roasted	202	27	14	0	14.35	0.53
Turkey, young tom, meat and skin, raw	154	20	7	0	10.22	0.51
Turkey, young tom, meat only, cooked, roasted	168	29	7	0	14.98	0.52
Turkey, young tom, meat only, raw	117	22	3	0	10.82	0.49
Turkey, young tom, skin only, cooked, roasted	422	20	37	0	10.74	0.54
Turkey, young tom, skin only, raw	368	13	35	0	7.06	0.54
Turkey, young tom, wing, meat and skin, cooked, roasted	221	27	11	0	14.21	0.53
Turkey, young tom, wing, meat and skin, raw	188	20	11	0	10.42	0.52

Poultry Products

Food Description	Kcals	Protein	Fat	Carbs	PRAL	Acid Density
USDA Commodity, turkey ham, dark meat, smoked, frozen	118	16	4	3	12.86	0.80

Fats and Oils

Food Description	Kcals	Protein	Fat	Carbs	PRAL	Alkali Density
Animal fat, bacon grease	900	0	100	0	0	
Butter replacement, without fat, powder	373	2	1	89	0.93	0.01
Butter, light, stick, with salt	499	3	55	0	0.63	
Butter, light, stick, without salt	499	3	55	0	0.63	
Butter-margarine blend, stick, unsalted	718	1	81	1	0.09	0.09
Creamy dressing, made with sour cream and/or buttermilk and oil, reduced calorie, fat-free	107	1	3	20	0.14	0.01
Creamy dressing, made with sour cream and/or buttermilk and oil, reduced calorie	160	1	14	7	0.10	0.01
Creamy dressing, made with sour cream and/or buttermilk and oil, reduced calorie, cholesterol-free	140	1	8	16	2.56	0.16
Fat, beef tallow	900	0	100	0	0	
Fat, chicken	900	0	100	0	0	
Fat, duck	900	0	100	0	0	
Fat, goose	900	0	100	0	0	
Fat, mutton tallow	900	0	100	0	0	
Fat, turkey	900	0	100	0	0	
Fish oil, cod liver	900	0	100	0	0	
Fish oil, herring	900	0	100	0	0	
Fish oil, menhaden	900	0	100	0	0	
Fish oil, menhaden, fully hydrogenated	900	0	100	0	0	
Fish oil, salmon	900	0	100	0	0	
Fish oil, sardine	900	0	100	0	0	
Flaxseed oil	900	0	100	0	0	
Lard	900	0	100	0	0	
Margarine Spread, approximately 48% fat, tub	424	0	48	1	-0.58	-0.58
Margarine spread, fat-free, tub	44	0	3	4	-0.76	-0.19
Margarine, 70% vegetable oil spread, soybean and soybean(hydrogenated)	619	0	70	2	-0.63	-0.32
Margarine, 80% fat, stick, includes regular and hydrogenated corn and soybean oils	705	0	81	0	-0.17	
Margarine, industrial, non-dairy, cottonseed, soy oil (partially hydrogenated), for flaky pastries	714	0	80	1	-0.17	-0.17
Margarine, industrial, soy and partially hydrogenated soy oil, use for baking, sauces and candy	714	0	80	1	-0.17	-0.17
Margarine, regular, hard, corn (hydrogenated and regular)	719	1	81	1	-0.05	-0.05
Margarine, regular, hard, corn (hydrogenated)	719	1	81	1	-0.05	-0.05
Margarine, regular, hard, corn and soybean (hydrogenated) and cottonseed (hydrogenated), without salt	714	0	80	1	-0.07	-0.07
Margarine, regular, hard, corn and soybean (hydrogenated) and cottonseed (hydrogenated), with salt	719	1	81	1	-0.05	-0.05
Margarine, regular, hard, safflower and soybean (hydrogenated and regular) and cottonseed (hydrogenated)	719	1	81	1	-0.05	-0.05

Fats and Oils

Food Description	Kcals	Protein	Fat	Carbs	PRAL	Alkali Density
Margarine, regular, hard, safflower and soybean (hydrogenated)	719	1	81	1	-0.05	-0.05
Margarine, regular, hard, safflower and soybean (hydrogenated) and cottonseed (hydrogenated)	719	1	81	1	-0.05	-0.05
Margarine, regular, hard, soybean (hydrogenated and regular)	719	1	81	1	-0.05	-0.05
Margarine, regular, hard, soybean (hydrogenated)	719	1	81	1	-0.05	-0.05
Margarine, regular, hard, soybean (hydrogenated) and corn and cottonseed (hydrogenated)	719	1	81	1	-0.05	-0.05
Margarine, regular, hard, soybean (hydrogenated) and cottonseed	719	1	81	1	-0.05	-0.05
Margarine, regular, hard, soybean (hydrogenated) and cottonseed (hydrogenated)	719	1	81	1	-0.05	-0.05
Margarine, regular, hard, soybean (hydrogenated) and palm (hydrogenated and regular)	719	1	81	1	-0.05	-0.05
Margarine, regular, hard, soybean (hydrogenated) and palm (hydrogenated)	719	1	81	1	-0.05	-0.05
Margarine, regular, hard, soybean (hydrogenated), cottonseed (hydrogenated), and soybean	719	1	81	1	-0.05	-0.05
Margarine, regular, hard, soybean, soybean (hydrogenated), and cottonseed (hydrogenated)	719	1	81	1	-0.05	-0.05
Margarine, regular, hard, sunflower and soybean (hydrogenated) and cottonseed (hydrogenated)	719	1	81	1	-0.05	-0.05
Margarine, regular, liquid, soybean (hydrogenated and regular) and cottonseed	721	2	81	0	-0.17	
Margarine, regular, stick, composite, 80% fat, with salt	705	0	81	1	-0.17	-0.17
Margarine, regular, stick, unsalted, composite, 80% fat	719	1	81	1	0.12	0.12
Margarine, regular, tub, composite, 80% fat, with salt	716	0	80	1	-0.05	-0.05
Margarine, regular, tub, unsalted, composite, 80% fat	716	0	80	1	-0.05	-0.05
Margarine, regular, unspecified oils, with salt added	719	1	81	1	-0.05	-0.05
Margarine, regular, unspecified oils, without added salt	714	0	80	1	-0.07	-0.07
Margarine, vegetable oil spread, 20% fat	175	0	20	0	-0.03	
Margarine, vegetable oil spread, 20% fat, without salt	175	0	20	0	-0.03	
Margarine, vegetable oil spread, 60% fat, stick	518	0	60	1	-0.06	-0.06
Margarine, vegetable oil spread, 60% fat, stick, no salt	519	0	60	1	-0.06	-0.06
Margarine, vegetable oil spread, 60% fat, tub/bottle	531	0	60	1	-0.06	-0.06
Margarine, vegetable oil spread, 60% fat, tub/bottle, unsalted	531	0	60	1	-0.06	-0.06
Margarine, vegetable oil spread, stick/tub/bottle, 60% fat	526	0	60	1	-0.06	-0.06
Margarine-butter blend, soybean oil and butter	714	0	80	1	-0.09	-0.09
Margarine-like shortening, industrial, soy (partially hydrogenated), cottonseed, and soy, principal use flaky pastries	628	0	71	0	0	
Margarine-like spread, 70% fat, liquid, with salt	621	0	70	0	-0.22	

Fats and Oils

Food Description	Kcals	Protein	Fat	Carbs	PRAL	Alkali Density
Margarine-like spread, fat free, liquid, salted	43	1	3	3	0.19	0.06
Margarine-like spread, made with yogurt, stick, salted	630	0	70	0	-0.09	
Margarine-like spread, reduced calorie, 40% fat, stick, with salt	356	1	40	0	-0.06	
Margarine-like spread, reduced calorie, about 40% fat, made with yogurt, tub, salted	330	2	35	2	0.29	0.15
Margarine-like spread, stick or tub, sweetened	534	0	52	17	-0.03	0
Mayonnaise dressing, no cholesterol	688	0	78	0	0.51	
Mayonnaise, low sodium, low calorie or diet	231	0	19	16	-0.06	0
Mayonnaise, made with tofu	322	6	32	3	1.24	0.41
Mayonnaise, reduced-calorie or diet, cholesterol-free	333	1	33	7	-0.96	-0.14
Meat drippings (lard, beef tallow, mutton tallow)	900	0	100	0	0	
Oil, canola and soybean	900	0	100	0	0	
Oil, corn and canola	900	0	100	0	0	
Oil, corn, peanut, and olive	900	0	100	0	0	
Oil, industrial, canola with antifoaming agent, principal uses salads, woks and light frying	900	0	100	0	0	
Oil, industrial, coconut (hydrogenated), used for whipped toppings and coffee whiteners	900	0	100	0	-0.05	
Oil, industrial, coconut, principal uses candy coatings, oil sprays, roasting nuts	900	0	100	0	0	
Oil, industrial, palm kernel (hydrogenated), filling fat	900	0	100	0	-0.04	
Oil, industrial, soy (partially hydrogenated) and cottonseed, principal use as a tortilla shortening	900	0	100	0	0	
Oil, olive, salad or cooking	900	0	100	0	-0.03	
Oil, peanut, salad or cooking	900	0	100	0	0	
Oil, sesame, salad or cooking	900	0	100	0	0	
Oil, soybean, salad or cooking	900	0	100	0	0	
Oil, soybean, salad or cooking, (hydrogenated)	900	0	100	0	0	
Oil, soybean, salad or cooking, (hydrogenated) and cottonseed	900	0	100	0	0	
Oil, vegetable safflower, salad or cooking, linoleic, (over 70%)	900	0	100	0	0	
Oil, vegetable safflower, salad or cooking, oleic, over 70% (primary safflower oil of commerce)	900	0	100	0	0	
Oil, vegetable, almond	900	0	100	0	0	
Oil, vegetable, apricot kernel	900	0	100	0	0	
Oil, vegetable, babassu	900	0	100	0	0	
Oil, vegetable, cocoa butter	900	0	100	0	0	
Oil, vegetable, corn, industrial and retail, all purpose salad or cooking	900	0	100	0	0	
Oil, vegetable, cottonseed, salad or cooking	900	0	100	0	0	
Oil, vegetable, cupu assu	900	0	100	0	0	
Oil, vegetable, grapeseed	900	0	100	0	0	
Oil, vegetable, hazelnut	900	0	100	0	0	

Fats and Oils

Food Description	Kcals	Protein	Fat	Carbs	PRAL	Alkali Density
Oil, vegetable, industrial, canola (partially hydrogenated) oil for deep fat frying	900	0	100	0	0	
Oil, vegetable, industrial, canola for salads, woks and light frying	900	0	100	0	0	
Oil, vegetable, industrial, coconut, confection fat, typical basis for ice cream coatings	900	0	100	0	-0.06	
Oil, vegetable, industrial, mid-oleic, sunflower, principal uses frying and salad dressings	900	0	100	0	0	
Oil, vegetable, industrial, palm and palm kernel, filling fat	900	0	100	0	-0.09	
Oil, vegetable, industrial, palm kernel (hydrogenated), used for whipped toppings, non-dairy	900	0	100	0	-0.05	
Oil, vegetable, industrial, palm kernel (hydrogenated), confection fat, intermediate grade product	900	0	100	0	-0.03	
Oil, vegetable, industrial, palm kernel (hydrogenated), confection fat, uses similar to 95 degree hard butter	900	0	100	0	-0.03	
Oil, vegetable, industrial, palm kernel, confection fat, uses similar to high quality cocoa butter	900	0	100	0	-0.05	
Oil, vegetable, industrial, soy (partially hydrogenated), all purpose	900	0	100	0	0	
Oil, vegetable, industrial, soy (partially hydrogenated) and soy (winterized), pourable clear fry	900	0	100	0	0	
Oil, vegetable, industrial, soy (partially hydrogenated), palm, principal uses icings and fillings	900	0	100	0	0	
Oil, vegetable, industrial, soy (partially hydrogenated), multiuse for non-dairy butter flavor	900	0	100	0	0	
Oil, vegetable, industrial, soy (partially hydrogenated), principal uses popcorn and flavoring vegetables	900	0	100	0	0	
Oil, vegetable, industrial, soy, refined, for woks and light frying	900	0	100	0	0	
Oil, vegetable, nutmeg butter	900	0	100	0	0	
Oil, vegetable, palm	900	0	100	0	0	
Oil, vegetable, poppyseed	900	0	100	0	0	
Oil, vegetable, rice bran	900	0	100	0	0	
Oil, vegetable, sheanut	900	0	100	0	0	
Oil, vegetable, sunflower, high oleic (70% and over)	900	0	100	0	0	
Oil, vegetable, sunflower, linoleic (less than 60%)	900	0	100	0	0	
Oil, vegetable, sunflower, linoleic, (approx. 65%)	900	0	100	0	0	
Oil, vegetable, sunflower, linoleic, (hydrogenated)	900	0	100	0	0	
Oil, vegetable, teaseed	900	0	100	0	0	
Oil, vegetable, tomatoseed	900	0	100	0	0	
Oil, vegetable, ucuhuba butter	900	0	100	0	0	
Oil, vegetable, walnut	900	0	100	0	0	
Oil, wheat germ	900	0	100	0	0	

Fats and Oils

Food Description	Kcals	Protein	Fat	Carbs	PRAL	Alkali Density
Salad dressing, bacon and tomato	326	2	35	2	-0.66	-0.33
Salad dressing, blue or Roquefort cheese dressing, commercial, regular	504	5	52	7	3.26	0.47
Salad dressing, blue or Roquefort cheese dressing, fat-free	115	2	1	26	-0.25	-0.01
Salad dressing, blue or Roquefort cheese dressing, reduced calorie	86	2	3	13	0.70	0.05
Salad dressing, blue or Roquefort cheese, low calorie	99	5	7	3	4.12	1.37
Salad dressing, buttermilk, lite	225	1	17	16	3.09	0.19
Salad dressing, caesar dressing, regular	528	1	58	3	0.31	0.10
Salad dressing, caesar, low calorie	110	0	4	19	-0.12	-0.01
Salad dressing, coleslaw	390	1	33	24	0.98	0.04
Salad Dressing, coleslaw dressing, reduced fat	329	0	20	4	-0.53	-0.13
Salad dressing, french dressing, commercial, regular	457	1	45	16	-0.76	-0.05
Salad dressing, french dressing, commercial, regular, without salt	459	1	45	16	-0.76	-0.05
Salad dressing, french dressing, fat-free	132	0	0	33	-1.80	-0.05
Salad dressing, french dressing, reduced calorie	200	0	13	27	-1.08	-0.04
Salad dressing, french dressing, reduced fat	232	1	13	30	-1.72	-0.06
Salad dressing, french dressing, reduced fat, without salt	233	1	13	30	-1.72	-0.06
Salad dressing, french, home recipe	631	0	70	3	-0.42	-0.14
Salad dressing, green goddess, regular	427	2	43	7	0.23	0.03
Salad dressing, home recipe, cooked	157	4	9	15	1.43	0.10
Salad dressing, home recipe, vinegar and oil	449	0	50	3	-0.16	-0.05
Salad dressing, Italian dressing, commercial, regular	291	0	28	10	-0.65	-0.07
Salad dressing, Italian dressing, commercial, regular, without salt	292	0	28	10	-0.65	-0.07
Salad dressing, Italian dressing, fat-free	47	1	1	9	1.84	0.20
Salad dressing, Italian dressing, reduced calorie	200	0	20	7	-0.41	-0.06
Salad dressing, Italian dressing, reduced fat	75	0	6	5	-1.36	-0.27
Salad dressing, Italian dressing, reduced fat, without salt	76	0	6	5	-1.36	-0.27
Salad dressing, mayonnaise and mayonnaise-type, low calorie	263	1	19	24	0.81	0.03
Salad dressing, Mayonnaise dressing, diet, no cholesterol	390	1	33	24	0.98	0.04
Salad dressing, mayonnaise type, regular, with salt	390	1	33	24	0.98	0.04
Salad dressing, mayonnaise, imitation, milk cream	97	2	5	11	-0.01	0
Salad dressing, mayonnaise, imitation, soybean	232	0	19	16	-0.06	0
Salad dressing, mayonnaise, imitation, soybean without cholesterol	482	0	48	16	-0.16	-0.01
Salad dressing, mayonnaise, light	324	1	33	8	0.73	0.09
Salad dressing, mayonnaise, soybean and safflower oil, with salt	717	1	79	3	0.60	0.20

Fats and Oils

Food Description	Kcals	Protein	Fat	Carbs	PRAL	Alkali Density
Salad dressing, mayonnaise, soybean oil, with salt	717	1	79	3	0.60	0.20
Salad Dressing, mayonnaise-like, fat-free	84	0	3	15	-0.87	-0.06
Salad dressing, peppercorn dressing, commercial, regular	564	1	61	4	-2.48	-0.62
Salad dressing, ranch dressing, commercial, regular	484	1	51	7	4.62	0.66
Salad dressing, ranch dressing, fat-free	119	0	2	27	1.11	0.04
Salad dressing, ranch dressing, reduced fat	219	1	17	16	3.09	0.19
Salad dressing, Russian dressing	355	2	28	31	-2.61	-0.08
Salad dressing, Russian dressing, low calorie	141	0	4	28	-1.93	-0.07
Salad dressing, sesame seed dressing, regular	443	3	45	9	-0.65	-0.07
Salad dressing, sweet and sour	15	0	0	4	-0.66	-0.17
Salad dressing, thousand island dressing, fat-free	132	1	1	32	-2.50	-0.08
Salad dressing, thousand island dressing, reduced fat	204	1	13	24	-3.68	-0.15
Salad dressing, thousand island, commercial, regular	370	1	35	16	-1.14	-0.07
Sandwich spread, with chopped pickle, regular, unspecified oils	389	1	34	22	0.43	0.02
Shortening bread, soybean (hydrogenated) and cottonseed	900	0	100	0	0	
Shortening cake mix, soybean (hydrogenated) and cottonseed (hydrogenated)	900	0	100	0	0	
Shortening confectionery, coconut (hydrogenated) and or palm kernel (hydrogenated)	900	0	100	0	0	
Shortening frying (heavy duty), beef tallow and cottonseed	900	0	100	0	0	
Shortening frying (heavy duty), palm (hydrogenated)	900	0	100	0	0	
Shortening frying (heavy duty), soybean (hydrogenated), linoleic (30%) stabilizers with silicon	900	0	100	0	0	
Shortening frying (heavy duty), soybean (hydrogenated), linoleic (less than 1%)	900	0	100	0	0	
Shortening frying (regular), soybean (hydrogenated) and cottonseed (hydrogenated)	900	0	100	0	0	
Shortening household soybean (hydrogenated) and palm	900	0	100	0	0	
Shortening industrial, lard and vegetable oil	900	0	100	0	0	
Shortening industrial, soybean (hydrogenated) and cottonseed	900	0	100	0	0	
Shortening, confectionery, fractionated palm	900	0	100	0	0	
Shortening, CRISCO 0 Grams Trans Fat Per Serving All-Vegetable, can	900	0	100	0	-0.01	
Shortening, CRISCO 0 Grams Trans Fat Per Serving All-Vegetable, sticks	900	0	100	0	-0.01	
Shortening, household, lard and vegetable oil	900	0	100	0	0	
Shortening, household, soybean (hydrogenated)-cottonseed (hydrogenated)	900	0	100	0	0	
Shortening, industrial, soy (partially hydrogenated) and corn for frying	900	0	100	0	0	
Shortening, industrial, soy (partially hydrogenated) for baking and confections	900	0	100	0	0	

Fats and Oils

Food Description	Kcals	Protein	Fat	Carbs	PRAL	Alkali Density
Shortening, industrial, soy (partially hydrogenated), pourable liquid fry shortening	900	0	100	0	0	
Shortening, institutional, composite	900	0	100	0	0	
Shortening, multipurpose, soybean (hydrogenated) and palm (hydrogenated)	900	0	100	0	0	
Shortening, special purpose for baking, soybean (hydrogenated) palm and cottonseed	900	0	100	0	0	
Shortening, special purpose for cakes and frostings, soybean (hydrogenated)	900	0	100	0	0	
Shortening, vegetable, household, composite	900	0	100	0	-0.01	
USDA Commodity Food, oil, vegetable, low saturated fat	900	0	100	0	0	
USDA Commodity Food, oil, vegetable, soybean, refined	900	0	100	0	0	
USDA Commodity Food, shortening, all purpose, soybean (partially hydrogenated) and cottonseed	900	0	100	0	0	
USDA Commodity Food, shortening, type III, creamy liquid, soybean and soybean (partially hydrogenated)	900	0	100	0	0	
Vegetable oil, avocado	900	0	100	0	0	
Vegetable oil, canola	900	0	100	0	0	
Vegetable oil, coconut	900	0	100	0	0	
Vegetable oil, mustard	900	0	100	0	0	
Vegetable oil, oat	900	0	100	0	0	
Vegetable oil, palm kernel	900	0	100	0	0	
Vegetable oil, soybean lecithin	900	0	100	0	0	
Vegetable oil-butter spread, reduced calorie	465	0	53	0	0.16	
Vegetable oil-butter spread, reduced calorie, tub, salted	450	1	50	1	0.14	0.14
Vegetable oil-butter spread, tub, salted	362	1	40	1	0.11	0.11

Spices and Herbs

Food Description	Kcals	Protein	Fat	Carbs	PRAL	Alkali Density
Basil, fresh	27	3	1	3	-10.01	-3.34
Capers, canned	23	2	1	5	-0.69	-0.14
Dill weed, fresh	43	3	1	7	-15.49	-2.21
Horseradish, prepared	48	1	11	1	-4.87	-4.87
Mustard, prepared, yellow	67	4	4	5	1.13	0.23
Peppermint, fresh	70	4	1	15	-12.65	-0.84
Rosemary, fresh	131	3	6	21	-16.45	-0.78
Salt, table	0	0	0	0	-0.50	
Spearmint, dried	285	20	7	52	-55.42	-1.07
Spearmint, fresh	44	3	1	8	-10.01	-1.25
Spices, allspice, ground	263	6	9	72	-26.86	-0.37
Spices, anise seed	337	18	16	50	-18.17	-0.36
Spices, basil, dried	251	14	4	61	-85.36	-1.40
Spices, bay leaf	313	8	8	75	-17.16	-0.23
Spices, caraway seed	333	20	15	50	-13.33	-0.27
Spices, cardamom	311	11	7	68	-22.57	-0.33
Spices, celery seed	392	18	25	41	-34.71	-0.85
Spices, chervil, dried	237	23	4	49	-92.40	-1.89
Spices, chili powder	314	3	5	15	-31.05	-2.07
Spices, cinnamon, ground	261	0	0	6	-23.75	-3.96
Spices, cloves, ground	323	0	1	4	-31.58	-7.90
Spices, coriander leaf, dried	279	22	5	52	-99.48	-1.91
Spices, coriander seed	298	12	18	55	-23.21	-0.42
Spices, cumin seed	375	18	22	44	-31.97	-0.73
Spices, curry powder	325	13	14	58	-26.10	-0.45
Spices, dill seed	305	4	15	4	-33.19	-8.30
Spices, dill weed, dried	253	20	4	16	-74.51	-4.66
Spices, fennel seed	345	16	15	42	-35.37	-0.84
Spices, fenugreek seed	323	23	6	58	-1.20	-0.02
Spices, garlic powder	332	17	1	73	-2	-0.03
Spices, ginger, ground	347	9	6	71	-24.55	-0.35
Spices, mace, ground	475	7	32	50	-9.87	-0.20
Spices, marjoram, dried	271	13	7	61	-49.30	-0.81
Spices, mustard seed, yellow	469	25	29	35	14.49	0.41
Spices, nutmeg, ground	525	6	36	49	-3.75	-0.08
Spices, onion powder	347	10	1	81	-10.15	-0.13
Spices, oregano, dried	306	11	10	64	-49.76	-0.78
Spices, paprika	289	15	13	56	-36.33	-0.65
Spices, parsley, dried	276	22	4	52	-81.49	-1.57
Spices, pepper, black	255	11	3	65	-25.39	-0.39

Spices and Herbs

Food Description	Kcals	Protein	Fat	Carbs	PRAL	Alkali Density
Spices, pepper, red or cayenne	318	12	17	57	-31.44	-0.55
Spices, pepper, white	296	10	2	69	4.29	0.06
Spices, poppy seed	533	18	45	24	-1.87	-0.08
Spices, poultry seasoning	307	10	8	66	-22.11	-0.34
Spices, pumpkin pie spice	342	6	13	69	-19.13	-0.28
Spices, rosemary, dried	331	5	15	64	-37.43	-0.58
Spices, saffron	310	11	6	65	-29.58	-0.46
Spices, sage, ground	315	11	13	61	-46.49	-0.76
Spices, savory, ground	272	7	6	69	-51.11	-0.74
Spices, tarragon, dried	295	23	7	50	-64.51	-1.29
Spices, thyme, dried	276	9	7	64	-35.48	-0.55
Spices, turmeric, ground	354	8	10	65	-46.66	-0.72
Thyme, fresh	101	6	2	24	-15.56	-0.65
Vanilla extract	288	0	0	13	-3.31	-0.25
Vanilla extract, imitation, alcohol	237	0	0	2	-1.35	-0.68
Vanilla extract, imitation, no alcohol	56	0	0	14	-0.05	0
Vinegar, balsamic	88	0	17	0	-2.07	
Vinegar, cider	21	0	0	1	-1.45	-1.45
Vinegar, distilled	18	0	0	1	0	0
Vinegar, red wine	19	0	0	1	-0.68	-0.68

Appendix B: Hormone Screens

Appendix B: Hormone Screens

The questionnaires are not designed to diagnose a medical condition or health-related condition. If you suspect an underlying hormonal dysfunction unrelated to acidity, consult with your healthcare professional for further evaluation.

Appendix B: Hormone Screens

Growth Hormone

Growth hormone (GH) is a hormone that is synthesized and secreted by the anterior pituitary gland. It is a major participant in the control of several processes including growth and metabolism.

The following are signs and symptoms of a growth hormone deficiency.

Check all of the following that apply.

- Reduced muscle mass
- Increased abdominal fat
- Reduced strength
- Insulin resistance
- Balding
- Reduced bone mass and/or osteoporosis
- Reduced energy
- Elevated cholesterol (LDL)

Appendix B: Hormone Screens

Thyroid Hormone

Thyroid hormones increase metabolic rate, control the body's response to the stress hormone adrenaline, and regulates the overall metabolism of protein, fats, and carbohydrates

The following are signs and symptoms of hypothyroidism.

Check all of the following that apply.

- Fatigue
- Weakness
- Weight gain or increased difficulty losing weight
- Coarse, dry hair
- Dry, rough pale skin
- Hair loss
- Intolerance to cold
- Muscle cramps and frequent muscle aches
- Constipation
- Depression
- Irritability
- Memory loss
- Abnormal menstrual cycles
- Decreased libido

Appendix B: Hormone Screens

Cortisol

Cortisol, or the stress hormone as it is commonly known, is produced by the adrenal glands. This hormone is involved in the metabolism of glucose, possesses anti-inflammatory properties, and affects your body's ability to burn fat.

The following are signs and symptoms of elevated cortisol levels.

Check all of the following that apply.

- Depression
- Memory issues
- Anxiety
- Fatigue
- Stomach ulcers
- High blood pressure
- Increased levels of cholesterol
- Weight gain/loss
- Alcohol craving
- Insulin resistance
- Heart disease
- Osteoporosis
- Frequent illnesses

Appendix B: Hormone Screens

Insulin

The release of insulin causes an increased uptake of nutrients into the cells, and as the blood concentrations of these substances drop, insulin secretion is suppressed.

The following are signs and symptoms of insulin resistance.

Check all of the following that apply.

- Abdominal weight gain
- Fatigue
- Cardiovascular disease
- Elevated blood pressure
- Intestinal swelling and bloating
- Depression
- Inability to focus
- Vision problems

Appendix C: Biomarker Assessment Tables

Appendix C: Biomarker Assessment Tables
Lean Body Mass (LBM)

Lean Body Mass consists of muscle, bone and other vital organ tissues of the body, in short, everything that is not fat. LBM is one of the most crucial components of the body to preserve and build. Protein provides the building blocks for the maintenance and growth of LBM, which determines approximately 90 percent of the Basal Metabolic Rate (BMR) of the body. Lean Body Mass is also known as Fat Free Mass (FFM).

Body Mass Index

Classification	BMI	Risk of Co-morbidities
Underweight	< 18.50	Low (but risk of other clinical problems)
Normal range	18.50-24.99	Average
Overweight	>=25	Increased
Pre-obese	25-29.99	Increased
Obese class I	30-34.99	Moderate
Obese class II	35-39.99	Severe
Obese class III	>=40	Very severe

Body Mass Index is a ratio between a person's body weight and height. It is a mathematical formula that correlates somewhat with body fat. In general, if your BMI is high, you may have an increased risk of developing certain disease including hypertension, cardiovascular disease and others. BMI is a better predictor of disease risk than body weight alone. Competitive athletes, body builders, women who are pregnant or lactating, growing children or frail and sedentary elderly individuals should not use BMI as the basis for estimating their body fat content.

Appendix C: Biomarker Assessment Tables
Percent Body Fat

Males

Age	RISKY	EXCELLENT	GOOD	FAIR	POOR	VERY POOR
19-24	<6%	10.8%	14.9%	19.0%	23.3%	>23.3%
25-29		12.8%	16.5%	20.3%	24.4%	
30-34		14.5%	18.0%	21.5%	25.2%	
35-39		16.1%	19.4%	22.6%	26.1%	
40-44		17.5%	20.5%	23.6%	26.9%	
45-49		18.6%	21.5%	24.5%	27.6%	
50-54		19.8%	22.7%	25.6%	28.7%	

Females

Age	RISKY	EXCELLENT	GOOD	FAIR	POOR	VERY POOR
19-24	<9%	18.9%	22.1%	25.0%	29.6%	>29.6%
25-29		18.9%	22.0%	25.4%	29.8%	
30-34		19.7%	22.7%	26.4%	30.5%	
35-39		21.0%	24.0%	27.7%	31.5%	
40-44		22.6%	25.6%	29.3%	32.8%	
45-49		24.3%	27.3%	30.9%	34.1%	
50-54		26.6%	29.7%	33.1%	36.2%	
55-59		27.4%	30.7%	34.0%	37.3%	
60+		27.6%	31.0%	34.4%	38.0%	

Body Fat Mass is the body's less metabolically active storage tissue, technically known as "adipose tissue." With advancing age, even if our body weight doesn't change much, most of us tend to gain fat and lose heavier muscle tissue.

Appendix C: Biomarker Assessment Tables
Waist to Hip Ratio

	Ideal	Excessive Abdominal Body Fat
Males	0.9	>0.9
Females	0.8	>0.8

Your *Waist to Hip Ratio* is a measure of how fat is distributed throughout your body. Abdominal fat is related to an increased risk of many conditions, such as cardiovascular disease and diabetes.

Glossary

Glossary

Ammomia

Ammonia is a chemical and buffer that contains hydrogen and nitrogen (NH3) and combines with extra hydrogen ions, forming ammomium, eliminating is the hydrogen from the body.

Anabollsm

Anabolism is the process by which various building blocks are put together to form other structures, such as protein and fat.

Anterior Pituitary Gland

The anterior pituitary gland, which sits below the brain, is a major organ of the hormonal or endocrine system that regulates the majority of the body's processes, including growth, sex, and reproduction.

Ash Analysis

Ash analysis involves the combustion of a food, and the subsequent analysis of the ash to see how much of the food was acidic and how much was alkaline.

Basal Metabolic Rate (BMR)

Our basal metabolic rate (BMR), that is, the amount of calories we burn at rest, accounts for the largest portion of energy expenditure, and muscle (and bone) is the only part of BMR that is variable.

Bioavailability

Bioavailability refers to the amount of a nutrient, such as protein, that when entering the body actually gets into the circulation.

Bicarbonate

Bicarbonate is a chemical and powerful base with the chemical formula (HCO3). It is produced in red blood cells from the reaction between water (H20) and carbon dioxide (C02).

Glossary

Body Mass Index (BMI)

Body Mass Index is a ratio between a person's body weight and height. It is a mathematical formula that correlates somewhat with body fat. In general, if your BMI is high, you may have an increased risk of developing certain disease including hypertension, cardiovascular disease and others. BMI is a better predictor of disease risk than body weight alone. Competitive athletes, body builders, women who are pregnant or lactating, growing children or frail and sedentary elderly individuals should not use BMI as the basis for estimating their body fat content.

Buffering

Buffering is the process by which a chemical reduces the change in pH of a solution by soaking up (or donating) extra hydrogen molecules. When a solution is too acidic a buffer is like a sponge soaking up water, or in this case, extra hydrogen molecules. If the solution is too alkaline, the buffer can be squeezed out to release hydrogen.

Catabolism

Catabolism is the process of breaking down substances, usually from food, into smaller, more usable substances with the aim of producing energy

Degenerative Disease

Unlike an infectious or congenital disease, a degenerative disease is a disease in which the function or structure of the body will progressively deteriorate over time, due to normal aging or poor lifestyle choices.

DNA

DNA is the molecule that houses all of genetic information, determining skin and eye colour, height, and other outwardly physical characteristics

Empty calorie

Empty calories, such as alcohol and refined foods, do not contain the nutrients required to break itself down into useable energy.

Glossary

Enzymes

Enzymes are proteins that speed up a reaction, but are not consumed by the reaction

Essential amino acids

Essential amino acids cannot be produced by the body and must be provided by diet.

Glomerular filtration rat (GFR)

GFR is the volume of blood filtered at the kidney per unit time.

Glucocorticoid

Glucocorticoids are chemicals that control sugar concentration in the body. The main one is cortisol.

Glycemic index

The glycemic index is a measure of how quickly one's blood sugar level increases in response to carbohydrate dominant foods.

Glycogen

Glycogen is the storage form of sugar or glucose, and is produced primarily in the liver and muscle, where it is also stored. Your body stores approximately 500g of glycogen to be used when dietary sources are inadequate, as in extreme starvation, stress, of exercise.

Gluconeogenesis

Gluconeogenesis is the production of glucose from non-carbohydrate sources, such as fat stores and skeletal muscle. This is an important process as the brain and nervous system require glucose to function.

Glossary

Hormones

Hormones are chemicals produced by the body and travel in the blood and control all of your body's metabolic processes. Common hormones include cortisol, insulin, and thyroid hormone.

Hydrogenated Fats (Trans Fats, Hydrogenation)

The process of hydrogenation takes a healthy, unsaturated fat and adds hydrogen molecules to it, thereby, saturating it, increasing its shelf life. This renders these fats more harmful than saturated fats because the hydrogen is placed in an unnatural *trans-* position. Your body cannot metabolize it, leading to accumulation in blood vessels and cell membranes.

Hyperplasia

Hyperplasia is the process by which the body increases the number of fat cells. Once these fat cells are formed, they cannot be destroyed.

Insulin sensitivity or Insulin Resistance

Insulin sensitivity can be best described by explaining insulin resistance. Insulin resistance occurs when your cells become less sensitive to the effects of insulin, causing your pancreas to produce more insulin.

Insulinemic index (II)

The insulinemic index specifically refers to the rise in insulin that occurs after a meal. It takes into account the effect of dietary protein and fat, as well as carbohydrates. The II is somewhat of an intermediary between dietary intake and the glycemic index.

Ketones

Ketones or ketone bodies are a group of chemicals produced by the body when fat and protein are used for energy instead of carbohydrates, as in extreme fasting. They are an important source of fuel for the brain, if glucose is not available.

Glossary

Metabolic Acidosis

Metabolic acidosis is a state where the body's pH is below its optimal range.. Essentially, metabolic acidosis is a pH imbalance in which the body has accumulated too much acid and cannot, for various reasons, neutralize this acid.

Net Acid Excretion

The NAE is determined by measuring the acid and the ammonium appearing in the urine and then subtracting out the measured urinary bicarbonate. This method reflects total acid and base load of a mixed diet.

Nitrogen Balance

Nitrogen is a substance unique to protein and therefore provides a good indicator as to whether your building (or losing) muscle. Nitrogen balance compares nitrogen input (through diet) to nitrogen loss (urine).

PRAL – formula

The PRAL provides an estimation of the body's acid production over alkali production (or vice versa) for a given amount of food ingested daily. The PRAL is physiologically based and takes into account different absorption rates of individualized minerals (calcium, potassium, phosphorus, and magnesium) and sulphur containing protein, as well as sulphur produced from metabolized proteins.

$$PRAL = 0.49*protein\,(g) + 0.037*phosphorous(mg) - 0.021*potassium(mg) - 0.026*magnesium(mg) - 0.013*calcium(mg)$$

PRAL Density

The PRAL density is a measure of the alkalinity per gram of carbohydrate of carbohydrate-dominant foods. Similarly, the PRAL density measures the acidity per gram of protein of protein-dominant foods.

Glossary
Ratio of Omega 3 and Omega 6 Fatty Acids

The ideal ratio of omega 6: omega 3 fatty acids should range from 2:1 to 4:1, but the typical Western diet has a ratio of 14:1 to 15:1. It has been shown that this ratio is a cause of inflammation, as well as atherosclerosis, insulin resistance, and arthritis.

Thermic effect of food (TEF)

The thermic effect of food is the caloric expenditure (above your BMR) required to digest food. The TEF is highest for dietary protein.

Waist Hip Ratio (WHR)

Your waist to hip ratio is a measure of how fat is distributed throughout your body.

References

References

Introduction

1. Centers for Disease Control and Prevention. National Center for Health Statistics Prevalence of Overweight and Obesity Among Adults: United States, 1999, accessed 2/22/y002.
2. Katzmarzyk PT, Janssen I. The economic costs associated with physical inactivity and obesity in Canada: an update. Can J Appl Physiol. 2004 Feb 29(1):90-115
3. McCrory MA, Hajduk CL, Roberts SB, Mayer J. Food group associations with BMI: Influence of energy reporting accuracy. (abstract) FASEB J. 2001; 15 (5): A951.
4. U.S. Department of Health and Human Services. Overweight and obesity: a major public health issue. Prevention Report 2001;16.
5. Epstein LH, Gordy CC, Raynor HA, Beddome M, Kilanowski CK, Paluch R. Increasing fruit and vegetable intake and decreasing fat and sugar intake in families at risk for childhood obesity. Obesity Res.
6. Manz, F. (2001) History of nutrition and acid-base physiology. European Journal of Nutrition. 40:189-199.
7. Robergs, RA., Ghiasvand, F, Parker, D. Biochemistry of exercise-induced metabolic acidosis. American Journal of Physiol Regul Integr Comp Physiol, 2004. 287(3): R502-16
8. Edge, J. Bishop, Goodman, C. (2006) Effects of chronic $NaHCO_3$ ingestion during interval training on changes on muscle buffer capacity, metabolism, and short-term endurance performance. 101(3): 918-25.
9. Induced metabolic alkalosis affects muscle metabolism and repeated-sprint ability. Medicine and Science in Sports and Exercise. May 36(5): 807-13
10. Toldeo et al. Effects of Physical Activity and Weight Loss on Skeletal Muscle Mitochondria and Relationship With Glucose Control in Type 2 Diabetes Diabetes 2007; 56:2142-2147, 2007
11. Alexy,U, Remer, T, Manz, F, Neu, C, Schoemau, E. (2005) Long-term protein intake and dietary potential renal acid load are associated with bone modeling and remodeling at the proximal radius in healthy children. American Journal of Clinical Nutrition. 82: 1107-1114.
12. Barzel, US, Massey, LK. (1998). Excess Dietary Protein Can Adversely Affect Bone. Journal of Nutrition. 128: 1051-1053.
13. Frassetto, L, Morris, RC, Sebastien, A. (1997). Potassium Bicarbonate Reduces Urinary Nitrogen Excretion in Postmenopausal Women. Journal of Endocrinology and Metabolism.82: 254-259.
14. Macdonald, HM, New, SA, Fraser, WD, Campbell, MK, Reid, DM. (2005) Low dietary potassium intakes and high dietary estimates of net endogenous acid production are associated with low bone mineral density in premenopausal women and increased markers of bone resorption in postmenopausal women. American Journal of Clinical Nutrition. 81:923-933

15. Massey, LK. Dietary Animal and Plant Protein and Human Bone Health: A

References

Whole Foods Approach. (2003) Journal of Nutrition. 133: 862S-865S.

16. Maurer, M, Riesen, W, Muser, J, Hulter, HN, Krapt, R. (2003) Neutralization of Western diets inhibits boen resorption independently of potassium intake and reduces cortisol secretion in humans. *American Journal of Physiology: Renal Physiology.* 284: F32-F40.
17. Remer, T, Dimitriou, T, Manz, F. (2003). Dietary potential renal acid load and renal net acid excretion in healthy, free-living children and adolescents. *American Journal of Clinical Nutrition.* 77: 1255-1260.
18. Remer,T, Manz, F. (1995). Potential renal acid load of foods and its influence on urine pH. *Journal of the American Dietetic Association.* 95: 791-797.
19. Sebastien, A, Frassetto, LA, Sellmeyer, DE, Merriam, RL, Morris, RC. (2002). Estimation of the net acid load of the diet of ancestral preagricultural Homo sapiens and their hominid ancestors. *American Journal of Clinical Nutrition.* 76:1308-1316.
20. Trichchieri, A, Zanetti, G, Curro, A, Lizzano, R. (2001). Effect of potential renal acid load of foods on calcium metabolism of renal calcium formers. *European Urology.* 39(2): 33-36.
21. Zwart, SR, Davis, JE, Paddon-James, D, Ferrando, AA, Wolfe, RR, Smith, SM. (2005). Amino acid supplementation alters bone metabolism during simulated weightlessness. *Journal of Applied Physiology* 99: 134-140.

Growth Hormone

1. McSherry, E. Morris, RC, Jr. Attainment and maintenance of norm stature of alkali therapy in infancnts and children with cliassic renal tubular acidosis. *J. Clinic Invest.* 1978; 61:509-27.
2. Challa, A, Krieg, RJ, Thabet, MA, Velduis, JD, Chan, JCM,. Meabolic acidiosis inhibits growth homreone secretion in rates: mechanismsm of growth retardation. *Am. J. Physiology.* 1993; 265: E547-53.
3. Challa, A, Chan, W, Krieg, RH, Thabet, MA, Liu, F, Hintz, RL, Chan, JCM. Effect of metabolic acidosis on the expression of insulin-like growth factor and growth hormone receptor. *Kidney International.* 1993; 44: 1224-7.
4. Brungger, M, Hulter, HN, Krapf, R. Effect of chronic metabolic acidosis on the growth hormone and IGF-1 endocrine axis: New cause of growth hormone insensitivity in humans. *Kidney International.* 1997; 51: 216-21.
5. Sicuro, A, Mahlbacher, K, Hulter, HN, Krapf, R. Effect of growth hormone on renal and systemic acid-base homestasis in humans. *Am J Physiol* 1998. Renal Physiol 43: F650-7.
6. Mahlbacher, K, Sicuro, A, Gerber, H, Hulter, HN, Krapf, R, Growth Hormone corrects acidosis induced negative niroogen balance and renal phosphate depletion and attenuates reanl magenisum wasting in humans. *Metabolism.* 1999; 48: 763-70.
7. Haffner, D, Schaefer, F, Girard, J, Ritz, E, Mels, O. Metabolic clearance of recombinant human growth hormone in health and chronic renal failure. *J*

References

Clin Invest. 1994; 93: 1163-1171.

8. Fouque, D, Peng, SC, Kopple, JD. Impaired metabolic response to recombinant insulin-like growth factor-1 in dialysis patients. Kidney Int. 1995: 47: 876-883.
9. Wiederkehr, M, Krapf, R. Metabolic and endocrine effects of metabolic acidosis in humans. Swiss Med Wkly 2001; 131: 127-132.
10. Wiederkehr, M, Kalogiris, J. Krapf, R. Correction of metabolic acidosis improves thyroid and growth hormone axes in haemodialysis patients. Nephrology Dialysis Transplantation. 2004; 19: 1190-1197.
11. Sicuro, A, Mahlbacher, K, Hulter, HN, Krapf, R. Effect of growth hormone on renal and systemic acid-base homeostasis in humans. 1998; 274(4): F650-F657
12. Salomon F, Cuneo RC, Hesp R, et al. The Effects of Treatment with Recombinant HGH on Body Composition and Metabolism in Adults with Growth Hormone Deficiency. New Eng JMed1989;321:1797-03.
13. Bengtsson BA. The Consequences of Growth Hormone Deficiency in Adults. Acta Endocrin 1993;128:2-5.
14. Cuneo RC, Salomon F, Wiles CM et al. HGH Treatment in GH Deficient Adults. II. Effects on Exercise Performance. J Appl Physiol 1991;70:695-700.
15. O'Halloran DJ, Tsatsoulis A, Whitehouse RW et al. Increased Bone Density after Growth Hormone (HGH) Therapy in Adults with Isolated HGH Deficiency. J Clin Endo Metab 1993;76:1344-48.
16. McGauley GA, Cuneo RC, Salomon F et al. Psychological Well-Being Before and After Growth Hormone Treatment in Adults with HGH Deficiency. Hormone Research 1990;33(Suppl 4):52-54.
17. Bengtsson BA, Eden S, Lonn L et al. Treatment of Adults with Growth Hormone (HGH) Deficiency with Recombinant (HGH).J Clin EndoMetab1993;76:309-17.
18. Johnston DG, Bengtsson BA. The Effects of GH and GH Deficiency on Lipids and the Cardiovascular System.Acta Endocrinologica 1993;128(Suppl 2):69-70.
19. Amato G, Carella C, Fazio S et al. Body Composition, Bone Metabolism, and Heart Structure and Function in Growth Hormone (HGH)-Deficient Adults Before and After HGH Replacement Therapy at Low Doses. J. of Clinical Endocrinology & Metabolism. 1993;77:1671-76.
20. Fazio S, Sabatini D, Capaldo B, et.al. A preliminary study of GH in the treatment of dilated cardiomyopathy. New Engl J Medicine.1996;334:809-14.
21. Borst SE and Lowenthal DT: Role of IGF-1 in muscular atrophy of aging. Endocrine 7:61-63, 1997.
22. Cummings DE and Merriam GR: Growth hormone therapy in adults. Annu Rev Med 54:513-533, 2003.
23. Holloway L, Butterfield G, Hintz RL, et al.: Effect of recombinant human growth hormone on metabolic indices, body composition, and bone turnover in healthy elderly women. J Clin Endocrinol Metab 79:470-479, 1994.
24. Marcus R and Hoffman AR: Growth hormone as therapy for older men and women. Annu Rev Pharmacol Toxicol 38:45-61, 1998.

References

25. Papadakis MA, Grady D, Black D, et al.: Growth hormone replacement in healthy older men improves body composition but not functional ability. Ann Int Med 124:708-716, 1996.

26. Rudman D, Feller AG, Nagraj HS, et al.: Effects of human growth hormone in men over 60 years old. New Eng J Med 323:1-6, 1990.
27. Taaffe DR, Pruitt L, Reim J, et al.: Effects of recombinant human growth hormone on the muscle strength response to resistance exercise in elderly men. J Clin Endocrinol Metab 79:1361-1366, 1994.
28. Takala J, Ruokonen E, Webster NR, et al.: Increased mortality associated with growth hormone treatment in critically ill adults. New Eng J Med 341:785-792, 1999.
29. Vance ML and Mauras N: Drug therapy: Growth hormone therapy in adults and children. New Eng J Med 341:1206-1216, 1999.
30. Cohen, Pinchas, et al. "Insulin-like growth factors (IGFs), IGF receptors, and IGF-binding proteins in primary cultures of prostate epithelial". Journal of Clinical Endocrinology and Metabolism, Vol. 73, No. 2, 1991, pp. 401-07

Insulin

1. Mak, RH. Effect of metabolic acidosis on insulin action and secretion in uremia. Kidney Int. 1998; 54: 603-607.
2. Bigner, Dr, Goff, JP, Faust, MA, Burton, JL, Tyler, HD, Horst, RL. Acidosis Effects on Insulin Response During Glucose Tolerance Tests in Jersey Cows. J Dairy Scie. 79: 2182-2188.

Thyroid Hormone

1. Michael, UFR, Chavez, SL, Cookson, SL, Vaamonde, CA. Impaired urinary acidification in the hypothyroid rat. Pfluegers Arch. 1976; 61: 215-20.
2. Brungger, M, Hulter, HN, Krapf, R. Effect of chronic metabolic acidosis on thyroid hormone homeostasis in humans. Am J Physiol 1997; 272: F648-F653
3. Lim VS, Fang, VS, Katz, AI, Refetoff, S. Thyroid Dysfunction in chronic renal failure. J. Clin Invest 1977; 60: 522-534.
4. Wiederkehr, M, Krapf, R. Metabolic and endocrine effects of metabolic acidosis in humans. Swiss Med Wkly 2001; 131: 127-132.
5. Wiederkehr, M, Kalogiris, J. Krapf, R. Correction of metabolic acidosis improves thyroid and growth hormone axes in haemodialysis patients. Nephrology Dialysis Transplantation. 2004; 19: 1190-1197.
6. Balch JF, Balch PA. Prescription for Natural Healing. Garden City Park, NY, 1990, Avery.
7. Werbach MR. Nutritional Influences on Illness, ed. 2. Tarzana, CA, 1996, Third Line Press.

References

8. Grabowski RJ. *Current Nutritional Therapy: A Clinical Reference.* San Antonio, 1993, Image Press.
9. Schaff L, et al. Screening for thyroid disorders in a working population, Clin Investig 71:126-31, 1993.

Muscle Loss

1. Bailey, JL. Metabolic Acidosis and Protein Catabolism: Mechanisms and Clinical Implications. Protein Metabolism in Renal Diseases. 1998; 24: 13-19.
2. Schambelan, M, Sebastien, A, Katuna, BA, Arteaga, E. Adrenocortical hormone secretory response to chronic NH4CL-induced metabolic acidosis. Am J Physiol Endocrin Metab 252: E454-E460.
3. Cynober, L, Harris, RA. Branched-Chain Amino Acids: Metabolism, Physiological Function, and Application. The Journal of Nutrition. 2006; 136: 333S-336S.
4. May, RC, Kelly, RA, Mitch, WF. Metabolic acidosis stimulates protein breakdown from skeletal muscle. J. Clin. Invest 1986; 77: 614-21.
5. Kahlhoff, H, MAnz, F, Dickman, L. Decreased growth rate of low birth-weight infants whith prolonged maximum renal acid simtuatlation. Acta Pediatr 1993: 82: 522-37.
6. McSherry, E. Morris, RC, Jr. Attainment and maintenance of norm stature of alkalki therapy in infancnts and children with cliassic renal tubular acidosis. J. Clinic Invest. 1978; 61:509-27.
7. May, RC, Hara, Y, Kelly, B, RA, Block, KP, Buse, MG, Mitche, WE. Branched-chain amino acid metabolism in rate muscle: abnormal regulation by acidosis: Am J Physiology 1987; 252: E712-8.
8. Ballmer, PE, McNurlan, MA. Hulter, Hn, Anderson, SE, Garlick, PJ, Krapf, R. Chronic metabolic acidosis decreases albumin synthesis and induces negative nitrogen balance in humans. J. Clin Invest 1995; 95: 39-43.
9. Maniar, S. Laouari, D, Dechaux, M, Motel, V Uyvert, JP, Mathian, B, Kleinknecht, C. I n vivo unaltered muscle protein sysntehsis in experimental chronic metabolic acidosis. Kidney Int. 1994; 46: 1705-12.
10. Papadoyannakis, NJ, Stefanidis, CJ, McGeown, M. The effect of correction of metabolic acidosis on nitrogen and potassium balance of patients with chronic renal failure. Am J Clin Nutr 1984; 40: 623-7.
11. Kotler, DP, Tierney, AR, Wang, J, Peterson, RN. Magnitude of body-cell mass depletion and the timing of death. Am J Clin Nutr 1989; 50: 444-7.
12. Mahlbacher, K, Sicuro, A, Gerber, H, Hulter, HN, Krapf, R, Growth Hormone corrects acidosis induced negative niroogen balance and renal phosphate depletion and attenuates reanl magenisum wasting in humans. Metabolism. 1999; 48: 763-70.
13. Brungger, M, Hulter, HN, Krapf, R. Effect of chronic metabolic acidosis on the growth hormone and IGF-1 endocrine axis: New cause of growth hormone

References

insensitivity in humans. Kidney International. 1997; 51: 216-21.

14. Wiederkehr, M, Krapf, R. Metabolic and endocrine effects of metabolic acidosis in humans. Swiss Med Wkly 2001; 131: 127-132.

General

1. Tilkian S, et al: Clinical Implications of Laboratory Tests, ed 3, St. Louis, 1993, C.V. Mosby Co.
2. Berkow R, Fletcher AJ, editors. The Merck Manual, ed 16, Rahway, NJ, 1992, Merck & Co.
3. Guyton AC, Hall JE. Textbook of Medical Physiology, ed 9, Philadelphia, 1996, W. B. Saunders.
4. Tierney LM, et al, editors: Current Medical Diagnosis & Treatment, ed. 35, Stamford, CT, 1996, Appleton & Lange.
5. Fischbach F. A Manual of Laboratory & Diagnostic Tests, ed 5, Philadelphia, 1996, J. B. Lippincott Co.

Bone Loss

1. Kiberistis P, et al: Bone health in the balance. Science 289:1497, 2000.
2. Dacy P, et al: The osteoblast: a sophisticated fibroblast under central surveillance. Science 289:1501-1504, 2000.
3. Teitelbaum S: Bone resorption by osteoclasts. Science 289:1505-1508, 2000.
4. Wachman A, et al: Diet and osteoporosis. The Lancet 1:958-959, 1968.
5. Lemann J Jr, Lennon EJ: Role of diet, gastrointestinal tract, and bone in acid-base homeostasis. Kidney Int 1:275-279, 1972.
6. Barzel US, Massey LK: Excess dietary protein can adversely affect bone. J Nutr 128:1051-1053, 1998.
7. Anand C, Linkswiler H: Effect of protein intake on calcium balance of young men given 500mg of calcium daily. J Nutr 104:695-700, 1974.
8. Chu J, et al: Studies in calcium metabolism II. Effects of low calcium and variable protein intake on human calcium metabolism. Am J Clin Nutr 28:1028-1035, 1975.
9. Johnson NE, et al: Effect of protein intake on urinary and fecal calcium and calcium retention of young adult males. J Nutr 100:1425-1430, 1970.
10. Margen S, et al: The calciuretic effect of dietary protein. Am J Clin Nutr 27:548-588, 1974.
11. Schwartz R, et al: Effect of magnesium and protein level on calcium balance. Am JClin Nutr 26:519-523, 1973.
12. Walker Rm, Linkswiler HM: Calcium retention in the adult human male as affected by protein intake. J Nutr 102:1297-1302, 1972.
13. Heaney RP, Recker RR: Effects of nitrogen, phosphorus, and caffeine on calcium balance in women. J Lab Clin Med 99:46-55, 1982.

References

14. Bushinsky DA: Metabolic alkalosis decreases bone calcium efflux by suppressing osteoclasts and stimulating osteoblasts. Am J Physiol 271:F216-F22, 1996.
15. Heaney RP: Excess dietary protein may not adversely affect bone. J Nutr. 128:1054-1057, 1998.
16. Kleinman JG, Lemann J Jr: Acid production. In: Maxwell MH, et al (eds): Clinical Disorders of Fluid and Electrolyte Metabolism, 4th Edition. New York: McGraw Hill, 1987, pp. 159-173.
17. Green J, Kleeman CR: The role of bone in the regulation of systemic acid base balance. Contrib Nephrol 91:61-76, 1991.
18. Remer T, Manz F: Estimation of the renal net acid excretion by adults consuming diets containing variable amounts of protein. Am J Clin Nutr 59:1356-1361, 1994.
19. Frassetto L, Sebastian A: Age and systemic acid-base equilibrium: analysis of published data. J Gerontol 51:B91-B99, 1996.
20. Lennon EJ, et al: The effect of diet and stool composition on the net external acid balance of normal subjects. J Clin Invest 45:1601-1607, 1966.
21. Kurtz I, et al: Effect of diet on plasma acid-base composition in normal humans.Kidney Int 24:670-680, 1983.
22. Schwarz WB, Relman AS: A critique of the parameters used in the evaluation of acid-base disorders. New Engl J Med 268:1382, 1963.
23. Szent-Gyrogy A: Quantum Biochemistry. New York: Blackwell, 1957.
24. Jaffe R: Autoimmunity: clinical relevance of biological response modifiers in diagnosis, treatment, and testing. Int J Integr Med 2(2):7-14, March/April 2000.
25. Sebastian A: Improved mineral balance and skeletal metabolism in post-menopausal women treated with potassium bicarbonate. N Engl J Med 330:1776-1781, 1994.
26. Frassetto L, et al: Potassium bicarbonate reduces urinary nitrogen excretion in postmenopausal women. J Clin Endocrinol Metab 82:254-259, 1997.
27. Halperin ML, Goldstein MB: Fluid, Electrolyte, and Acid-Base Physiology: A Problem-Based Approach, 3rd Edition. Philadelphia: WB Saunders Company, 1999.
28. 40. Cohn SH, et al: Body elemental composition: comparison between black and white adults. Am J Physiol 232:E419-E422, 1977.
29. 41. Armstrong WD, Singer L: Composition and constitution of the mineral phase of bone. Clin Orthop 38:179-190, 1965.
30. 42. Flynn MA, et al: Total body potassium in aging humans: a longitudinal study. Am J Clin Nutr 50:713-717, 1989.
31. 43. Poyart CF, et al: The bone CO_2 compartment: evidence for a bicarbonate pool. Respir Physiol 25:89-99, 1975.
32. Vatassery GT, et al: Determination of hydroxyl content of calcified tissue mineral. Calcif Tissue Res 5:183-188, 1970.
33. 46. Triffitt JT, et al: A comparative study of the exchange in vivo of major constituents of bone mineral. Calcif Tissue Res 2:165-176, 1968.

References

34. 54. Schweitzer C, et al: Dietary intake of carotenoids, fruits, and vegetables in the US: CSFII 1994-1996, a national survey. Proceedings from the 12th International Carotenoid Symposium, July 18-23, 1999, Cairns, Australia.
35. 55. Krebs-Smith SM, et al: Fruit and vegetable intakes of children and adolescents in the United States. Arch Pediatr Adolesc Med 150:81-86, 1996.
36. 56. Breslau NA, et al: Relationship of animal protein-rich diet to kidney stone formation and calcium metabolism. J Clin Endocrinol Metab 66:140-146,1988.
37. 57. Licata AA, et al: Acute effects of dietary protein on calcium metabolism in patients with osteoporosis. J Gerontol 36:14-19, 1981.
38. 59. Beyene Y: Cultural significance and physiological manifestation of menopause: a biocultural analysis. Cult Med Psychiatry 10:47-71, 1986.
39. 60. Luyken R, Luyken-Koning R: Studies on the physiology of nutrition in Surinam VIII. Metabolism of calcium. Trop Geogr Med 13:46-54, 1961.
40. 61. Chalmers J, Ho K: Geographical variations in senile osteoporosis. J Bone and Joint Surgery 52B:667-675, 1970.
41. 63. Melton L, Riggs B: Epidemiology of age-related fractures. In: The Osteoporotic Syndrome: Detection, Prevention and Treatment. New York: Grune and Stratton, 1983.
42. 64. Krieger NS, et al: Acidosis inhibits osteoblastic and stimulates osteoclastic activity in vitro. Am J Physiol 31:F442-F448, 1992.
43. 65. Arnett TR, Spowage M: Modulation of the resorptive activity of rat osteoclasts by small changes in extracellular pH near the physiological range. Bone 18:277-279, 1996.
44. 66. Arnett TR, Dempster DW: Effect of pH on bone resorption by rat osteoclasts in vitro. Endocrinology 119:119-124, 1986.
45. 67. Grinspoon SK, et al: Decreased bone formation and increased mineral dissolution during acute fasting in young women. J Clin Endocrinol Metab 80:3628-3633, 1995.
46. 68. Marsh A, et al: Cortical bone density of adult lactovegetarian women and omnivorous women. J Amer Diet Assoc 76:148-151, 1980.

Nutrition

1. Terry P, Terry JB, Wolk A. Fruit and vegetable consumption in the prevention of cancer: an update. J Int Med. 2001;250:280-290.
2. Feskanich D, Ziegler RG, Michaud DS, et al. Prospective study of fruit and vegetable consumption and risk of lung cancer among men and women. J Natl Cancer Inst. 2000;92(22):1812-1823.
3. Voorips LE, Goldbohm RA, Verhoeven DT, van Poppel G, Sturmans F, Hermus RJJ. Vegetable and fruit consumption and lung cancer risk in the Netherlands Cohort Study on diet and cancer. Cancer Causes and Control. 2000;11:101-115.

References

4. Michaud DS, Feskanich D, Rimm EB, et al. Intake of specific carotenoids and risk of lung cancer in two prospective U.S. cohorts. Am J Clin Nutr. 2000;72:900-997.
5. Marchand LL, Murphy SP, Hankin JH, Wilkens LR, Kolonel LN. Intake of flavonoids and lung cancer. J Natl Cancer Inst. 2000;92:154-160.
6. Jansen MC, Bueno-de-Mesquita HB, Rasanen L, et al. Cohort analysis of fruit and vegetable consumption and lung cancer mortality in European men. Int J Cancer. 2001;92:913-918.
7. Smith-Warner SA, Spiegelman D, Yaun S-S, et al. Intake of fruits and vegetables and risk of breast cancer. JAMA. 2001;285:769-776.
8. Terry P, Wolk A, Magnusson C. Brassica vegetables and breast cancer risk. JAMA. 2001.
9. Fowke JH, Longcope C, Hebert JR. Brassica vegetable consumption shifts estrogen metabolism in healthy postmenopausal women. Cancer Epidem, Bio & Prev. 2000;9:773-779.
10. Cohen JH, Kristal AR, Stanford JL. Fruit and vegetable intakes and prostate cancer risk. J Natl Cancer Inst. 2000;92:61-68.
11. Steinmetz KA, Potter JD. Vegetables, fruit and cancer prevention: A review. JADA. 1996;96:1027-1093.
12. Terry P, Giovannucci E, Michels KB, et al. Fruit, vegetables, dietary fiber, and risk of colorectal cancer. J Natl Cancer Inst. 2001;93:525-533.
13. Michels KB, Giovannucci E, Joshipura KJ, et al. Prospective study of ruit and vegetable consumption and incidence of colon and rectal cancers. J Natl Cancer Inst. 2000;92:1740-1752.
14. Voorips LE, Goldbohm RA, van Poppel G, Sturmans F, Hermus RJJ, van den Brandt PA. Vegetable and fruit consumption and risks of colon and rectal cancer in a prospective cohort study. Am J Epidemiol. 2000;152:1081-1092.
15. Flood A, Schatzkin A. Colorectal cancer: Does it matter if you eat your fruits and vegetables. J Natl Cancer Inst. 2000;92(21):1706-1707.
16. Zhang SM, Hunter DJ, Rosner BA, et al. Intakes of fruits, vegetables, and related nutrients and the risk of Non-Hodgkins Lymphoma among women. Cancer Epidem, Bio & Prev. 2000;9:477-485.
17. McCann SE, Moysich KB, Mettlin C. Intakes of selected nutrients and food groups and risk of ovarian cancer. Nutr and Cancer. 2001;39(1):19-28.
18. Cramer DW, Kuper H, Harlow BL, Titus-Ernstoff L. Carotenoids, antioxidants and ovarian cancer risk in pre-and postmenopausal women. Int J Cancer. 2001;94:128-134.
19. Gallus S, Bosetti C, Franceschi S, et al. Oesophageal cancer in women: tobacco, alcohol, nutritional and hormonal factors. Brit J Cancer. 2001;85(3):341-345.
20. Castellsague X, Munoz N, De Stefani E, Victoria CG, Castelletto R, Rolon PA. Influence of mate drinking, hot beverages and diet on esophageal cancer risk in South America. Int J Cancer. 2000;88:658-664.
21. De Stefani E, Brennan P, Boffetta P, Ronco AL, Mendilaharsu M, Deneo-Pellegrini H. Vegetables, fruits, related dietary antioxidants, and risk of

References

squamous cell carcinoma of the esophagus: A case control study in Uruguay. Nutr and Cancer. 2000;38(1):23-29.

22. Bosetti C, Vecchia CL, Talamini R, et al. Food groups and risk of squamous cell esophageal cancer in northern Italy. Int J Cancer. 2000;87:289-294.

23. De Stefani E, Boffetta P, Oreggia F, et al. Plant foods and risk of laryngeal cancer: A case-control study in Uruguay. Int J Cancer. 2000;87:129-132.

24. Nagano J, Kono S, Preston DL, et al. Bladder-cancer incidence in relation to vegetable and fruit consumption: A prospective study of atomic-bomb survivors. Int J Cancer. 2000;86:132-138.

25. Steinmaus CM, Nunex S, Smith A. Diet and bladder cancer: a metaanalysis of six dietary variables. Am J Epidemiol. 2000;151:693-702.

26. Michaud DS, Spiegelman D, Clinton S, Rimm EB, Willett WC, Giovannucci E. Fruit and vegetable intake and incidence of bladder cancer in a male prospective cohort. J Natl Cancer Inst. 1999;91:605-613.

27. Littman AJ, Beresford SA, White E. The association of dietary fat and plant foods with endometrial cancer (United States). Cancer Causes and Control. 2001;12:691-702.

28. McCann SE, Freudenheim JL, Marshall J, Brasure RR, Swanson MK, Graham S. Diet in the epidemiology of endometrial cancer in western New York (United States). Cancer Causes and Control. 2000;11:965-974.

29. Jain MG, Howe GR, Rohan TE. Nutritional factors and endometrial cancer in Ontario, Canada. Cancer Causes and Control. 2000;7:288-296.

30. McCullough ML, Robertson A, Jacobs EJ, Chao A, Calle EE, Thun MJ. A prospective study of diet and stomach cancer mortality in United States men and women. Cancer

31. Epidem, Bio & Prev. 2001;10(11):1201-1205.

32. Fung TT, Willett WC, Stampfer MJ, Manson JE, Hu FB. Dietary patterns and the risk of coronary heart disease in women. Arch Intern Med. 2001;161:1857-1862.

33. Joshipura KJ, Hu FB, Manson JE, et al. The effect of fruit and vegetable intake on risk

34. for coronary heart disease. Ann Int Med. 2001;134:1106-1114.

35. Liu S, Lee I, Ajani U, Cole S, Buring J, Manson J. Intake of vegetables rich in carotenoids and risk of coronary heart disease in men: the Physician's Health Study. Int J Epidemiol. 2000.

36. Liu S, Manson JE, Lee M-I, et al. Fruit and vegetable intake and risk of cardiovascular disease: The Women's Healthy Study. Am J Clin Nutr. 2000;72:922-928.

37. Eichholzer M, Luthy J, Gutzwiller F, Stahelin HB. The role of folate, antioxidant vitamins and other constituents in fruit and vegetables in the prevention of cardiovascular disease: The epidemiological evidence. Int J Vitam Nutr Res. 2001;71(1):5-17.

38. Brouwer IA, van Dusseldorp M, West CE, et al. Dietary folate from vegetables and citrus fruits decreases plasma homocysteine concentrations in humans in a dietary controlled trial. J Nutr. 1999;129:1135-1139.

References

39. Broekmans WMR, Klopping-Ketelaars WAA, Schuurman CRW, et al. Fruits and vegetables increase plasma carotenoids and vitamins and decrease homocysteine in humans. J Nutr. 2000;130:1578-1583.
40. Rock C, Moskowitz A, Huizar B, et al. High vegetable and fruit diet intervention in premenopausal women with cervical intraepithelial neoplasia. JADA. 2001;101:1167-1174.
41. Jenkins DJA, Kendall CWC, Popovich DG, et al. Effect of a very-high fiber vegetable, fruit, and nut dish on serum lipids, and colonic function. Metabolism. 2001;50(4):494-503.
42. Obarzanek E, Sacks FM, Vollmer WM, et al. Effects on blood lipids of a blood pressure-lowering diet: the Dietary Approaches to Stop Hypertension (DASH) Trial. Am J Clin Nutr. 2001;74:80-89.
43. Appel LJ, Moore TJ, Obarzanek E, et al. A clinical trial of the effects of dietary patterns on blood pressure. N Engl J Med. 1997;136:1117-1124.
44. Cao G, Russell RM, Lischner N, Prior RL. Serum antioxidant capacity is increased by consumption of strawberries, spinach, red wine or vitamin C in elderly women. J Nutr. 1998;128:2383-2390.
45. Pederson CB, Kyle J, Jenkinson AM, Gardner PT, McPhail DB, Duthie GG. Effects of blueberry and cranberry juice consumption on the plasma antioxidant capacity of healthy female volunteers. Eur J Clin Nutrition. 2000;54:405-408.
46. Strain JJ, Elwood PC, Davis A, et al. Frequency of fruit and vegetable consumption and blood antioxidants in the Caerphilly cohort of older men. Eur J Clin Nutr. 2000;54:828-833.
47. Maskarinee G, Chan CLY, Meng L, Franke AA, Cooney RV. Exploring the feasibility and effects of a high-fruit and vegetable diet in healthy women. Cancer Epidem, Bio & Prev. 1999;8:919-924.
48. Bub A, Watzl B, Abrahamse L, et al. Moderate intervention with carotenoid-rich vegetable products reduces lipid peroxidation in men. J Nutr. 2000;130:2200-2206.
49. Record IR, Dreosti IE, McInerney. Changes in plasma antioxidant status following consumption of diets high or low in fruit and vegetables or following dietary supplementation with an antioxidant mixture. Brit J Nutr. 2001;85:459-464.
50. van den Berg R, van Vliet T, Broekmans WMR, et al. A vegetable/fruit concentrate with high antioxidant capacity has no effect on biomarkers of antioxidant status in male smokers. J Nutr. 2001;131:1714-1722.
51. Steinberg D, Lewis A. Oxidative modification of LDL and atherogenesis. Circulation. 1997;95:1062-1071.
52. Chopra M, O'Neill ME, Keogh N, Wortley G, Southon S, Thurnham DI. Influence of increased fruit and vegetable intake on plasma and lipoprotein carotenoids and LDL oxidation in smokers and nonsmokers. Clin Chem. 2000;46(11):1818-1829.
53. Southon S. Increased fruit and vegetable consumption with the EU: potential health benefits. Food Res Int. 2000;33:211-217.

References

54. Arendt BM, Boetzer AM, Lemoch H, et al. Plasma antioxidant capacity of HIV-seropositive and healthy subjects during long-term ingestion of fruit juices or a fruit-vegetable-concentrate containing antioxidant polyphenols. Eur J Clin Nutrition. 2001;55:786-792.
55. Conlin PR, Chow D, Miller ER, et al. The Effect of Dietary Patterns on Blood Pressure Control in Hypertensive Patients: Results from the Dietary Approaches to Stop Hypertension (DASH) Trial. Am J Hypertens. 2000;13:949-955.
56. Moore TJ, Conlin PR, Ard J, Svetkey LP. DASH (Dietary Approaches to Stop Hypertension) diet is effective treatment for stage 1 isolated systolic hypertension. Hypertension. 2001;38:155-158.
57. Moline J, Bukharovich IF, Wolff MS, Phillips R. Dietary flavonoids and hypertension: is there a link? Med Hypoth. 2000;55(4):306-309.
58. Joshipura KJ, Ascherio A, Manson JE, et al. Fruit and vegetable intake in relation to risk of ischemic stroke. JAMA. 1999;282:1233-1239.
59. Tabak C, Smit HA, Rasanen L, et al. Dietary factors and pulmonary function: a cross sectional study in middle aged men from three European countries. Thorax. 1999;54:1021-1026.
60. Smit HA, Grievink L, Tabak C. Dietary influences on chronic obstructive lung disease and asthma: A review of the epidemiological evidence. Proc Nutr Soc. 1999;58(2):309-319.
61. Tabak C, Arts IC, Smit HA, Heederik D, Kromhout D. Chronic obstructive pulmonary disease and intake of catechins, flavonols, and flavones. Am J Respir Crit Care Med. 2001;164:61-64.
62. Butland BK, Fehily AM, Elwood PC. Diet, lung function, and lung function decline in a cohort of 2512 middle aged men. Thorax. 2000;55:102-108.
63. Ford ES, Mokdad AH. Fruit and vegetable consumption and diabetes mellitus incidence among U.S. adults. Prev Med. 2001;32:33--39.
64. Meyer K, Kushi LH, Jacobs DR, Slavin J, Seller TA, Folsom AR. Carbohydrates, dietary fiber and incident type 2 diabetes in older women. Am J Clin Nutr. 2000;71:921-930.
65. Sargeant LA, Khaw KT, Bingham S, et al. Fruit and vegetable intake and population glycosylated haemoglobin levels: the EPIC-Norfolk study. Eur J Clin Nutrition. 2001;55:342-348.
66. McCrory MA, Fuss PJ, Saltzman E, Roberts SB. Dietary determinants of energy intake and weight regulation in healthy adults. J Nutr. 2000;130:276S-279S.
67. Rolls BJ. The role of energy density in the overconsumption of fat. J Nutr. 2000;130:268S-271S.
68. Roberts SB, Heyman MB. Dietary composition and obesity: Do we need to look beyond dietary fat? J Nutr. 2000;130:267S.
69. Bell EA, Rolls BJ. Energy density of foods affects energy intake across multiple levels of fat content in lean and obese women. Am J Clin Nutr. 2001;73:1010-1018.

References

70. Burton-Freeman B. Dietary fiber and energy regulation. J Nutr. 2000;130:272S-275S.
71. Van Horn L. Fiber, lipids, and coronary heart disease. Circulation. 1997;95:2701-2704.
72. Pereira MA, Ludwig DA. Dietary fiber and bodyweight regulation. Ped Clin North Am. 2001;48(4):969-979.
73. Osler M, Heitmann BL, Gerdes LU, Jorgensen LM, Schroll M. Dietary patterns and mortality in Danish men and women: A prospective observational study. Brit J Nutr. 2001;85:219-225.
74. Strandhagen E, Hansson P-O, Bosaeus I, Isaksson B, Eriksson H. High fruit intake may reduce mortality among middle-aged and elderly men. The study of men born in 1913. Eur J Clin Nutrition. 2000;54:337-341.
75. Muhlbauer RC. Effect of vegetables on bone metabolism. Nature.1999;401:343-344. American Cancer Society Inc. 2001. www.cancer/org. Surveillance Research, accessed 01/29/02.
76. Bushinsky, DA. Acid-base imbalance and the skeleton. European Journal of Nutrition. 2001; 40: 238-244.
77. Riond, Jean-Luc,. Animal nutrition and acid-base balance. European Journal of Nutrition. 2001; 40: 245-254.
78. Tucker, KL, Hannan, MT, Kiel, DP. The acid-base hypothesis: diet and bone in the Framingham Osteoporosis Study. European Journal of Nutrition. 2001; 40: 231-237.
79. Frassetto, L., Morris, RC, Sellmeyer, DE, Todd, K, Sebastian, A. Diet, evolution, and aging. The pathophysiological effects of the post-agricultural inversion of the potassium-to-sodium and base-to-chloride ratios in the human diet. European Journal of Nutrition. 2001; 40: 200-213.
80. Remer, T. Influence of nutrition on acid-base balance – metabolic aspects. European Journal of Nutrition. 2001; 40: 214-220.
81. Kiwull-Schone, H, Kalhoff, H, Manz, F, Diekmann, Kiwull, P. Minimal-invasive approach to study pulmonary, metabolic and renal responses to alimentary acid-base changes in conscious rabbits. European Journal of Nutrition. 2001; 40: 255-259
82. Kalhoff, H, Manz, F. Nutrition, acid-base status and growth in early childhood. European Journal of Nutrition. 2001; 40: 221-230.
83. Remer, T. Influence of diet on acid-base balance. Seminars in Dialysis. 2000: 13(4); 221-226
84. Lemann, J, Bushinksy, DA, Hamm, LL. Bone buffering of acid and base in humans. American Journal of Renal Physiology. 2003; 285: F811-F832.
85. Prynne, Cj, Ginty, F, Paul, AA, Bolton-Smith, C, Stear, SJ, Jones, SC, Prentice, A. Dietary acid-base balance and intake of bone-related nutrients in Cambridge teenagers. European Journal of Clinical Nutirtion . 2004; 58: 1462-1471.
86. Macdonald, Hm, New, SA, golden, MH, Campbell, MK, Reid, DM. Nutritional Associations with bone loss during the menopausal transition: evidence of a beneficial effect of calcium, alcohol, and fruit and vegetable

References

nutrients and of a detrimental effect of fatty acids. American Journal of Clinical Nutrition. 2004; 79:155-165.

Kidney Stones

1. Trinchieri, A, Zanetti, G, Curro, A, Lizzano, R. Effect of potential renal acid load of foods on calcium metabolism of renal calcium stone formers. European urology. 2001; 39: 33-36.
2. Simpson DP. Citrate excretion: a window on renal metabolism. Am J Physiol. 1983;244:F223-F234.
3. Nicar MJ, Skurla C, Sakhaee K, Pak CY. Low urinary citrate excretion in nephrolithiasis. Urology. 1983;21:8-14.
4. Pattaras JG, Moore RG. Citrate in the management of urolithiasis. J Endourol. 1999;13:687-692.
5. Menon M, Mahle CJ. Urinary citrate excretion in patients with renal calculi. J Urol. 1983;129:1158-1160.
6. Leumann E, Hoppe B, Neuhaus T. Management of primary hyperoxaluria: efficacy of oral citrate administration. Pediatr Nephrol. 1993;7:207-211.
7. Fegan J, Khan R, Poindexter J, Pak CY. Gastrointestinal citrate absorption in nephrolithiasis. J Urol. 1992;147:1212-1214.
8. Pak CY, Fuller C. Idiopathic hypocitraturic calcium-oxalate nephrolithiasis successfully treated with potassium citrate. Ann Intern Med. 1986;104:33-37.
9. Whalley NA, Meyers AM, Martins M, Margolius LP. Long-term effects of potassium citrate therapy on the formation of new stones in groups of recurrent stone formers with hypocitraturia. Br J Urol. 1996;78:10-14.
10. Lee YH, Huang WC, Tsai JY, Huang JK. The efficacy of potassium citrate based medical prophylaxis for preventing upper urinary tract calculi: a midterm followup study. J Urol. 1999;161:1453-1457.
11. Barcelo P, Wuhl O, Servitge E, Rousaud A, Pak CY. Randomized double-blind study of potassium citrate in idiopathic hypocitraturic calcium nephrolithiasis. J Urol. 1993;150:1761-1764.
12. Hamm LL, Hering-Smith KS. Pathophysiology of hypocitraturic nephrolithiasis. Endocrinol Metab Clin North Am. 2002;31:885-893, viii.
13. Preminger GM, Sakhaee K, Pak CY. Alkali action on the urinary crystallization of calcium salts: contrasting responses to sodium citrate and potassium citrate. J Urol. 1988;139:240-242.

References
Appendix A

U.S. Department of Agriculture, Agricultural Research Service. 2009. USDA National Nutrient Database for Standard Reference, Release 22. Nutrient Data Laboratory Home Page,

Index

A

acid, i, 6,-8, 10, 14-19, 20, 25, 26, 30-34, 44-50, 63,76
acidic, 3, 7, 8, 10, 15-17, 19, 21, 22, 25-28, 30, 38, 47, 51, 60, 63
acidity, 11, 14, 15-17, 21, 22, 25, 27, 28, 31, 32, 35, 38, 41, 46-48, 51, 57 63, 65, 70, 71, 76, 86, 163
adrenal gland, 21, 32, 341
agricultural revolution, 7
alcohol, 4, 25, 58, 64, 341
alkali ash residue, 48
alkaline, i, 7, 8, 14-19, 21, 25, 26, 45-47, 49-51, 57, 70-72
alkalinity, i, 15, 17, 19, 64, 65, 70, 76, 117
amino acid, 3, 19, 30, 32, 37, 40, 44, 60, 70
ammonia, 19
anabolism, 8
anterior pituitary gland, 34, 339
ash analysis, 49
athlete, i, 3, 26, 31, 32, 34, 40, 80, 116, 119, 344

B

basal metabolic rate (BMR), 7, 31, 39, 116, 120, 344
base i, ii, 16, 18, 31, 44-46, 49, 57
BCAA (branched chain amino acids), 31, 32, 65
bicarbonate, 7, 19, 35, 44, 45, 48, 49
bioavailability, 8, 44, 49
biomarker, 10, 57, 119, 121, 343
blood, 15, 16, 17, 18, 19, 21, 32-35, 39, 46, 122

blood glucose (blood sugar), 32, 34, 37, 38, 40, 58, 59, 62, 74
blood pressure, 116, 341 342
body composition, 3, 10, 33, 57, 71, 119
body mass index, 5, 119, 344
brain, 3, 9, 17, 30
buffer, 6, 7, 15, 17-21, 25, 26, 29, 44-46

C

calcium, 17, 20, 21, 25, 27, 28, 32, 4, 45, 47, 49
calorie, 3, 6, 7, 9, 25, 26, 31, 40, 44, 58, 62, 70, 73, 80, 116
carbohydrate, 7, 8, 9, 14, 25, 30, 32, 37, 58, 59, 63, 70, 71, 73, 76, 78 80
carbon dioxide, 19
cardiovascular, 6, 15, 45, 129
cardiovascular disease, 6, 45, 46, 74, 119, 120, 342, 344, 346
catabolism, 8
Chinese medicine, 44
chloride, 48, 49
chlorophyll, 65
cholesterol, 19, 37, 59
cortisol, 3, 14, 32, 33, 38, 40, 41, 341
creatine, 64
Cretans, 44

D

degenerative disease, 6, 40, 44, 45, 47
DHA, 74
diabetes, 5, 6, 7, 25, 33, 37, 38, 40, 46, 58, 59, 120, 346
diabetes insipidus, 38

Index

diabetes mellitus, 38
diet, i, ii, 4,-7, 8, 10, 11, 14, 17, 20, 25, 27, 33, 35, 38, 41, 44-47, 49, 51, 57, 59, 60, 62, 66, 69, 70, 73, 74, 163
dietary fat, 60, 61, 62
digestive enzyme, 15, 21
disease, i, 4, 5, 6, 7, 17, 28, 30, 35 40, 45-48, 60, 62, 63
diseases of civilization, 7
DNA, 28
dynamic warm up, 122

E

electrolytes, 19, 20, 26
endocrine, 35, 348
energy, 40, 44, 46, 58, 60, 61, 63, 66, 116, 163
enzyme, 9, 15, 17, 21, 32, 37, 60
EPA, 74
essential amino acid, 10, 32, 60, 70
essential fatty acid/EFA, 61, 62, 74
exercise, 3, 5, 16, 34, 40, 59, 63, 116-119

F

fasting, 25, 58, 59
fat loss, 4,14,25,26, 28, 33, 58, 59, 61, 76, 78, 116, 17,129,163
Fats That Heal, Fats That Kill , 61
Fibre, 7, 63
fish oil, 65, 74
food preparation, 71
fruit, 6, 17, 18, 25, 26, 44-46, 48, 50, 63, 66

G

Genetic, 7
GH deficiency, 35
GH-IGF-1 axis, 34, 35
glomerular filtration rate (GFR), 46
glucagon, 37
glucocorticoid, 32
gluconeogenesis, 30, 32
glucose, 30, 32, 34, 37
glutamine, 31, 32, 51, 64
glycemic index, 47, 59
glycogen 37, 59
glycogen synthesis 37, 59
grain, 14, 25,44, 45, 46,4 8, 63
growth hormone, 33, 34, 36, 40, 41, 339

H

health, 3,-6, 9, 10, 11, 14-16, 21, 26, 30, 33, 35,41,44,62,64,69,70, 116
heart disease, 5, 6, 30, 62, 341
homeostatic, 17
hormonal dysfunction, 14, 41, 57, 338
hormonal imbalance, 14
hormone, 10, 14, 17, 19,25,33,57,59
hunter-gatherers, 44
hydrochloric acid,8, 18, 45
hydrogen, 15, 19, 21, 61
hydrogen ion, 15, 19, 21
hydrogen molecule, 15, 61
hydrogenated, 61
hyperinsulinemia, 37
hyperplasia, 5, 35
hypertension, 5, 37, 46, 48, 119, 35
hypertrophy, 5, 35, 73
hypothyroidism, 39, 340

Index

I

immune, 30-32, 35, 60, 65
insulin, 14, 31, 33, 34, 37, 38, 40, 41, 58, 59, 61, 62, 76, 116, 339, 341, 342
insulin- growth factor (IGF-1), 8, 34, 35
insulin resistance, 37, 38, 41, 339, 342,
insulin sensitivity, 14, 31, 33, 38, 40, 58, 59, 76, 116
insulinemic index, 59, 61
interval training, 129
isoleucine, 32

K

ketoacidosis, 38
ketone, 3, 25, 38
kidney, 9, 17, 19, 21, 25, 27, 31-33, 35, 44-49, 60, 64
kidney stone, 7, 33, 40, 64

L

lactic acid, 8
Lance Armstrong, i, 16
latent acidosis, 18
lean body mass, 30, 120, 344
leucine, 32
libido, 33, 39, 340
liver, 21, 25, 30, 31, 32, 35, 37

M

magnesium (magnesium citrate), 7, 17, 2021, 25-27, 29, 46-49, 64
Manz, 49, 50

meal frequency, 9, 58
metabolic acidosis, 6, 16, 18, 35, 30, 31, 32, 33, 35, 38-40, 47, 48, 163,
metabolic syndrome, 59
metabolism, i, 8, 9, 15,-17, 19, 25, 26, 31, 32, 34, 38-40, 44, 47, 60, 64, 66,73, 116, 163, 339, 340, 341
Michael Phelps, 3, 80
mineral, 8, 17, 20, 21, 25, 26, 27, 28, 44, 46-49, 51, 63, 65, 71, 80
mineral content , 8, 28, 44, 71
mineral loss, 27, 71
monounsaturated fatty acid, 62
muscle, 3, 5,-7, 9, 16, 17, 20, 25-34, 36, 38-40, 49, 59, 60, 64, 65, 73, 116, 117, 120, 122,127, 129, 163, 344, 345
muscular, i, 26

N

nervous system, 30, 32, 122
net acid excretion, NAE, 49
nitrogen, 30
nutrient, 6, 7, 46, 51, 73
nutrition, i, 6, 9, 10, 34, 38, 44, 57-59, 69, 17
nutritional, 3
nutritional grading, 40
obesity, 4, 5, 6, 14, 31, 33, 58, 59

O

Okinawans, 45
olive oil, 62, 74
omega 3 fatty acid, 61, 62, 65
omega 6 fatty acid, 61, 62
omega 9 fatty acid, 62, 74

Index

organic acid, 49
organically bound minerals, 47
osteoporosis, 7, 27, 28, 46, 339, 341
oxygen dissociation curve, 16

P

pancreas, 21, 35, 37, 38
pepsin, 15
percent body fat, 119, 120, 345
pH, 7, 10, 15-19, 21, 25, 28, 38, 41, 44, 48, 57, 163
phosphorus, 45, 49
physical activity, 3, 4, 6, 9, 10, 63, 80, 163
polyunsaturated fatty acid, 61, 62
potassium, 7, 17, 20, 21, 25-27, 29, 46, 47, 48, 49
potential hydrogen, 15
PRAL, 10, 48, 49, 50, 51, 57, 63, 66
PRAL density, 51, 70, 76
prevention, i, 5, 30, 64
prostaglandin, 28
protein, 4, 7, 8, 9, 14, 15, 19, 25, 28, 32, 34, 37, 39, 44-50, 58, 59, 60, 61, 62, 63, 65, 70, 71, 72, 73, 74, 76, 78
protein synthesis, 9, 32, 34

R

recipes, 84
red blood cell, 16, 19
refined, 7, 14, 38, 46
Remer, 49, 50
resistance training, 116, 127, 129

S

saliva (testing), 10, 18, 21, 57, 163
salivary pH, 21, 163
salmon oil, 74
salt, 8, 35, 44-46, 48
saturated fatty acid, 7, 46, 62, 63, 73, .74
science, ii, 14,
scientist, 30
sodium, 20, 21, 26, 27, 29, 47, 48, 49
sodium chloride, 48
starvation, 3
stress, 3, 9, 21, 27, 30, 32, 34, 38, 39, 40, 63, 340, 341
stretch, 122
sulphur, 45, 49
supplement, 10, 17, 28, 31, 40, 51, 40, 51, 64, 65, 66
Surgeon Generals Report, 6
syndrome x (metabolic syndrome), 37, 38, 40, 59

T

table salt, 7, 48
Tanita ®, 119, 120
thermic effect of food, 60
Thomas Edison, i
thyroid gland, 39
thyroid hormone, 14, 33, 39, 40, 41, 59, 340
thyroid stimulating hormone (TSH), 39
thyroxine, 39
training, 80
triglyceride, 37
triiodothyronine, 39

Index

U

Udo Erasmus, 60
urinary pH, 21, 163
urine, 18, 19, 21, 31, 38, 49, 57
urine testing, 10

V

valine, 32
vegetable, 6, 17, 25, 26, 44-48, 50, 51, 63, 66, 71
vitamin , 8, 44, 46, 51, 53, 65, 71, 80
vitamin B, 66
vitamin C, 65
vitamin D, 28

W

waist hip ratio (WHR), 120
warm up, 122
water, 7, 15, 19, 20, 58, 64-66
weight, 3-6, 9, 14, 25, 27, 30, 33, 39, 40, 60, 65, 70, 73, 76, 119, 344, 345
weight gain, 4, 14, 33
weight loss, 3, 6, 80
weight training, 3, 73, 116-18

About the Author

Dr. Alwyn Wong has been involved in the fitness industry for over 15 years and brings with him a wealth of experience. He uses an integrated treatment approach, combining active release techniques (ART®), acupuncture, chiropractic, nutritional consulting, and program design to treat his patients, many of whom have included professional athletes from the NFL, NHL, NBA, MLB, and PGA, as well as Olympic and IFBB athletes.

Although his focus has shifted to more clinical work, he remains as passionate about fitness as he did in 1994. He has spent the last few years gaining international experience, not only treating athletes, but also teaching personal trainers and other fitness professionals. He is a sought after lecturer and guest speaker, and has traveled throughout North America sharing his knowledge.

He lives and practises in Toronto, Canada.

www.ingramcontent.com/pod-product-compliance
Lightning Source LLC
Chambersburg PA
CBHW031641170426
43195CB00035B/176